The Yale Guide to Ophthalmic Surgery

The Yale Guide to Ophthalmic Surgery

Senior Editor
C. Robert Bernardino, MD, FACS

Section Editors
Members of the Department
of Ophthalmology and Visual Sciences
at Yale School of Medicine

Lead Authors
Benjamin Erickson, MD and Yasha Modi, MD

Illustrated by
Benjamin Erickson, MD

Wolters Kluwer | Lippincott Williams & Wilkins
Health
Philadelphia · Baltimore · New York · London
Buenos Aires · Hong Kong · Sydney · Tokyo

Senior Executive Editor: Jonathan W. Pine, Jr.
Senior Product Manager: Emilie Moyer
Senior Manufacturing Manager: Benjamin Rivera
Marketing Manager: Lisa Lawrence
Design Coordinator: Teresa Mallon
Production Service: Absolute Service, Inc./Maryland Composition

**WW
18.2
Y17
2011**

Library of Congress Cataloging-in-Publication Data

Yale guide to ophthalmic surgery / senior editor, C. Robert Bernardino ; section editors, Members of the Department of Ophthalmology and Visual Sciences at Yale School of Medicine ; lead authors, Benjamin Erickson and Yasha Modi ; illustrated by Benjamin Erickson.
    p. ; cm.
  Guide to ophthalmic surgery
  Includes bibliographical references and index.
  ISBN 978-1-60913-705-2
  1. Eye diseases—Surgery—Outlines, syllabi, etc. 2. Ophthalmology—Outlines, syllabi, etc. I. Erickson, Benjamin. II. Modi, Yasha. III. Bernardino, C. Robert. IV. Yale University. Dept. of Ophthalmology and Visual Sciences. V. Title: Guide to ophthalmic surgery.
  [DNLM: 1. Eye Diseases—surgery—Outlines. 2. Ophthalmologic Surgical Procedures—Outlines. 3. Eye—physiopathology—Outlines. WW 18.2]
  RE80.Y35 2011
  617.7'1—dc22

                                         2010052103

CCS0311

Contributors

Senior Editor
C. Robert Bernardino, MD, FACS
Associate Professor
Department of Ophthalmology and Visual Sciences
Yale School of Medicine
Director of the Ophthalmic Plastics and Orbital
   Surgery Section
Yale Eye Center
Residency Program Director in Ophthalmology
Yale New Haven Hospital and Yale School
   of Medicine
New Haven, Connecticut

Lead Authors
Benjamin Erickson, MD
Class of 2010, Yale School of Medicine
Resident in Ophthalmology
Bascom Palmer Eye Institute
University of Miami Health System
Miami, Florida

Yasha Modi, MD
Class of 2010, Yale School of Medicine
Resident in Ophthalmology
Bascom Palmer Eye Institute
University of Miami Health System
Miami, Florida

Section Editors
Ron Adelman, MD, MPH, FACS
Associate Professor
Department of Ophthalmology and Visual Sciences
Yale School of Medicine
Retina Section
Yale Eye Center
New Haven, Connecticut

Susan Forster, MD
Associate Clinical Professor
Department of Ophthalmology and Visual Sciences
Director of Medical Studies
Department of Ophthalmology
Yale School of Medicine
Comprehensive Eye Service
Yale Eye Center

Paul A. Gaudio, MD
Assistant Clinical Professor
Department of Ophthalmology and Visual Sciences
Yale School of Medicine
Uveitis Section
Yale Eye Center
New Haven, Connecticut

John J. Huang, MD
Associate Professor
Department of Ophthalmology and Visual Sciences
Yale School of Medicine
Director, Uveitis and Retina Sections
Yale Eye Center
New Haven, Connecticut

James E. Kempton, MD
Director of Eye Care Services
Veteran's Affairs Connecticut Healthcare System
Assistant Professor of Ophthalmology
Yale University Associate Program Director
Yale New Haven Hospital
New Haven, Connecticut

Jimmy K. Lee, MD
Assistant Professor
Department of Ophthalmology and Visual Sciences
Yale School of Medicine
Director of Cornea and Refractive Surgery
Yale Eye Center
New Haven, Connecticut

Hylton R. Mayer, MD
Assistant Professor
Department of Ophthalmology and Visual Sciences
Yale School of Medicine
Glaucoma Section
Yale Eye Center
New Haven, Connecticut

Daniel J. Salchow, MD
Assistant Professor
Department of Ophthalmology and Visual Sciences
Director of Pediatric Ophthalmology and
   Strabismus Sections
Yale Eye Center
New Haven, Connecticut

M. Bruce Shields, MD
Marvin L. Sears, Professor and Chairman Emeritus
Department of Ophthalmology and Visual Science
Yale School of Medicine
Glaucoma Section
Yale Eye Center
New Haven, Connecticut

James C. Tsai, MD, MBA, FACS
Robert R. Young, Professor and Chairman
Department of Ophthalmology and Visual Science
Yale School of Medicine
Chief of Ophthalmology
Yale New Haven Hospitals
Director of the Glaucoma Section
Yale Eye Center
New Haven, Connecticut

Contents

Preface

MEDICAL STUDENTS, BEGINNING residents, and technicians all need to master the fundamentals of ophthalmic surgery. Because of the small operative field and rapid case turnover, however, it can be difficult to develop a comprehensive understanding of each case. On rotation, it is not always possible to obtain a full case schedule in advance of an operating day. Additionally, efficient use of upper level surgical texts can be difficult because they are written with the primary surgeon in mind and often assume understanding of unfamiliar terms and concepts.

Accordingly, we at Yale worked to produce an illustrated pocket guide that concisely outlines the surgical and laser procedures most likely to be encountered on rotation in each specialty field. The case narratives in our book follow a consistent format and can be read in 15 minutes or less, making it an ideal reference during a busy day in the operating room. The *Wills Eye Manual* provides trainees with a quick pocket reference for the ophthalmology clinic; we sought to produce a surgical equivalent that will enable trainees to better prepare for the operating room.

The guide outlines the surgical and laser procedures most likely to be observed in the following specialties: cornea, general and comprehensive ophthalmology, glaucoma, pediatrics, oculoplastics, retina, and trauma. The case narratives follow a common format for ease of use. After a brief procedure description, each narrative describes indications, medical and surgical alternatives, relevant anatomy and pathophysiology, preoperative assessment, anesthetic considerations, procedure steps, potential complications, postoperative care, and resources for further reading. More than 270 procedural line illustrations accompany the critical steps of each procedure to facilitate understanding. The appendix includes additional chapters relevant to surgical ophthalmology (i.e., local anesthesia), whereas the glossary defines terms that may be unfamiliar to students. A companion website provides the full text of the book and also features surgical videos, color images, and additional tables and checklists.

The perspective of the authors is also a unique asset to this resource. The primary authors are medical students entering ophthalmology residency, ensuring that the text is clear and accessible to trainees at all levels. This book makes no assumption of previous ophthalmologic knowledge and can be read as an introductory text. The editors, however, are experts within each specialty area, ensuring that the material remains comprehensive and accurate.

It is our hope that this guide will serve an important need by providing ophthalmology trainees and staff with a portable and simple introduction to ophthalmology procedures.

Senior Editor's Note

THE MOST SUCCESSFUL PHYSICIANS are those that practice lifelong learning, that is, to have an inquisitive mind, an insatiable thirst for knowledge, and the drive to feed that thirst. Learning can come from journal articles or major meetings, but certainly the best learning may not be so formalized. Learning from experience and observation is how many of us expand our knowledge. Those of us in academic medicine have an additional, treasured source: our medical students, residents, and fellows. For many of us, we learn from our students as much as we give to them. This is how this book came to fruition.

Benjamin Erickson and Yasha Modi were two typical medical students interested in ophthalmology. They were hardworking and inquisitive. They took advantage of their rotation by spending time both in the operating room and in clinics with the residents and staff. During this time, they noticed the great opportunity to participate and learn, but also realized the difficulty a novice learner may have in understanding medical and, in particular, surgical interventions. Ben and Yasha took the extra step, they wrote a simple guide for other medical students rotating in ophthalmology on surgery and the medical student's role. They then approached me, the residency program director, for advice on how to distribute this guide, and I saw the diamond in the rough. Thus, this book was born.

We would like to thank the Yale ophthalmology residents and fellows for their teaching and their insight into the educational needs of beginning trainees. Assembling this guide would not have been possible without the continuous assistance of the administrative assistants, ophthalmic technicians, and operating room staff of the Yale Eye Center and Yale New Haven Hospital.

C. Robert Bernardino, MD, FACS

Acknowledgements

AT THIS TIME, I WOULD LIKE to thank all the contributors for their hard work on this book. In particular, I would like to recognize Ben and Yasha, who not only had the initial idea, but through hard work, brought it to fruition. Hopefully, this text will allow more people to be involved in ophthalmic care by breaking the barrier of complex knowledge down. Finally, I want to thank my family: my wife Nana and my son Trevor, who both love and support me, giving me the energy and drive to pursue these worthwhile projects.

It is my hope, no matter what level of learner you are, that you will learn from this text and then share that knowledge with your friends, colleagues, and your patients.

CHAPTER 1

Introduction to Ophthalmic Surgery

C. Robert Bernardino

Ophthalmic surgery encompasses any surgical procedure performed around, on, or in the eye. This periocular region is fairly small defined by the bony orbit, soft tissues contained in the orbit, and the eyelids, which border its anterior-most portion. Within these confines, surgery ranges from basic eyelid reconstruction to the most refined and delicate retinal surgery; techniques have been developed that typically use magnification and specialized instrumentation to work around this small field. Basic knowledge of the anatomy, instrumentation, and surgical technique will go a long way for the medical student, technician, or resident early in his or her career to be an active participant during these complex procedures. Failure to be prepared for surgery relegates one's role to observer in the best scenario and liability in the worse case.

This book is designed to give an overview of the different surgical procedures performed by an ophthalmologist. The basic anatomy will be reviewed. Important pathologic scenarios will be described. The procedures will be delineated in a step-wise fashion. A high-yield review section is included with each surgical procedure, which includes surgical pearls. This guide should serve as the first resource in learning about ophthalmic surgical procedures, a review of principles prior to surgery, and a concise summary for postsurgical analysis and critique.

TARGET AUDIENCE

- Ophthalmic technician
- Medical student
- Ophthalmic surgical assistant or nurse
- Ophthalmology resident
- Practicing ophthalmologist

The Ophthalmic Technician

- The ophthalmic technician is often the first person a patient encounters when they visit an ophthalmologist. Therefore, they can be the face of an ophthalmic practice and can help mold how a patient views the practice and, in turn, its surgeons. When a patient is signed up for surgery, secondary questions about the surgery or filling out surgical forms are often left to the ophthalmic technician.

- Intimate knowledge of the surgical techniques used by the ophthalmic surgeon are important, so that when a question from a patient arises, the question can be answered appropriately. Patients are better equipped to handle surgery when they are properly educated; doubt in a patient's mind can lead to anxiety and fear of surgery. Hence, answering a patient's question about what to expect during surgery should not be responded with "don't worry, it will be a piece of cake." A more appropriate response would be to describe the surgery in simple terms and be specific when necessary. This is only possible when the ophthalmic technician has this knowledge at hand.

- This book is ideal in this situation—as an essential resource when first learning about an ophthalmic surgical technique or as a quick reference when a patient does ask a specific question.

The Medical Student

- Medical students are put in a difficult situation when it comes to ophthalmology. Most medical schools do not have an ophthalmology rotation, and therefore, the medical student must choose an elective in order to explore whether he or she is interested in ophthalmology. This is further hampered by the fact that most basic science curricula only include perhaps one lecture on ophthalmic anatomy and a few lectures on ophthalmic pathology. Therefore, the medical student may be ill equipped to determine whether they want to pursue ophthalmology as a career choice. This is further complicated by the early match for ophthalmology residency. If a medical student were interested in pursuing ophthalmology as a career, he or she has limited time to impress the ophthalmology faculty to obtain support for candidacy.

- Learning and assisting during ophthalmic surgery can be quite challenging. The operative field is quite small and the tissues are delicate. Surgeries are performed under a microscope, and learning basic orientation in the field is often difficult. Surgeries are often very quick and surgical steps can be subtle. Finally, any small misstep during surgery can lead to major consequences; therefore, surgeons may be gun shy to disrupt routine to teach and engage the medical student.

- Studying prior to assisting in surgery or reviewing after participating in a case will lead to better understanding of the surgical procedures. Standard textbooks or journal articles are quite complex and difficult for the novice ophthalmic learner. This book serves as an ideal first guide for ophthalmic surgery.

The Ophthalmic Surgical Assistant or Nurse

- Ophthalmic surgery can be very fast and very complex. The limiting factor in efficient surgery is often the interaction between the surgeon and the surgical assistant. The knowledgeable assistant can anticipate the surgeon's moves and can allow the surgeon to move rapidly through a procedure without looking outside of the microscopic field.

- Complicating this intricate dance between surgeon and surgical assistant is that most ophthalmic assistants are not dedicated strictly to ophthalmology. Often, their interaction with ophthalmology is through cross-training, or, in the worse-case scenario, are called in off hours for the occasional ophthalmology emergency.

- Review of procedures before or after a case will lead to better efficiency in the ophthalmic operating room (OR). Furthermore, for cross-training or for the occasional assistant, quick-glance review prior to a case will allow for safety particularly in the off hours emergency case, which is likely the most complex. As a reference for these uses, this book is ideal.

The Ophthalmology Resident

- Ophthalmic residency training is quite challenging. In a short span of 3 years, residents must become competent in the medical and surgical management of patients with eye disease. In many programs, surgical education is held off until later in the training, in some cases not until 3rd year. In other instances, limited exposure occurs in the 1st or 2nd year of ophthalmology training. With limited exposure, the resident needs to have command of the basic procedural knowledge in order to have a case "passed" to them. Also, in the hierarchical surgical training system, junior residents often evaluate and refer surgical candidates to their senior colleagues. Without intimate knowledge of these surgical procedures, counseling surgical patients is often difficult.

- Self-guided learning of ophthalmic surgical techniques is required for mastery. This includes understanding anatomy, pathology, instrumentation, procedural steps, and preoperative and postoperative patient management. However, this broad body of knowledge is typically not available in one text. This text will serve as that initial source.

The Practicing Ophthalmologist

- Whether practicing comprehensive ophthalmology or subspecialty care, all ophthalmologists require knowledge of all of the basic concepts of ophthalmology in surgical care. This is vital when caring for patients directly or referring patients for specific subspecialty care. Furthermore, all ophthalmologists are educators and administrators of their practices, and therefore, need to teach their staff about specific nuances of surgical ophthalmologic care in order to deliver top care. Occasionally, an ophthalmologist will also have to team up with a subspecialty colleague to offer combined surgery; knowledge of your colleagues' techniques will allow for better surgical planning and, ultimately, efficiency in the OR. Finally, all ophthalmologists now need to maintain certification with the medical board, and this knowledge often includes broad-based surgical ophthalmic care.

- Review of concepts and techniques, before and after surgical procedures, either when teaching staff or reviewing for the maintenance of certification exam is ideal. A one-stop source of this knowledge is ideal, and this book is designed to fill this need.

CHAPTER 2

The Ophthalmology Operating Room

C. Robert Bernardino

Most ophthalmic surgeries incorporate an operating microscope. Exceptions include oculoplastic and most strabismus procedures, which are generally performed with the aid of loupe magnifiers. The operating microscope permits a detailed, stereoscopic view of the surgical field, but is inconvenient for cases that require the surgeon to switch rapidly between different planes of focus.

Scrubbed members include the primary surgeon (attending or senior resident), the assistant (typically a resident), and the scrub technician who hands the primary surgeon the necessary instruments. Outside of the surgical field, there is a circulating technician who manages the operating room (OR) and all logistical problems that may arise. Also, most surgeries are performed in the presence of an anesthesiologist or certified registered nurse anesthetist (CRNA). Any additional members (such as medical students) generally observe the surgery via a third viewing ocular or a projected monitor.

THE OPERATING MICROSCOPE

The following are several key components with which to become familiar:

- Oculars: There are generally two to three viewing pieces depending on the microscope. If given the chance to observe under the microscope, you should set the pupillary distance (PD) to a level that provides stereoscopic vision. Ideally, you will adjust your PD prior to scrubbing. Once you are scrubbed, however, you may adjust the PD after placement of a sterile knob or use of sterile baggies.
- Magnification system: The greater the magnification, the smaller the field of view and the narrower the depth of focus. Under high

magnification, the field can be as small as 150 mm². Accordingly, it is important to retain a frame of reference so as not to lose track of the operative location. This can be accomplished by periodically looking directly at the surgical field rather than through the oculars.

- Inverter: Retina cases (e.g., vitrectomy) generally involve use of an additional lens that is placed on the cornea to afford the surgeon a detailed view of the posterior segment of the eye. The optical properties of these lenses result in inversion of the microscope image (e.g., an instrument inserted at the 12 o'clock position will appear to be coming from 6 o'clock). An "inverter" switch on the microscope can be used to "re-flip" the image so that it corresponds with the anatomic view.
- Laser filters: For your protection, it is important to confirm your scope head has a filter in place prior to the use of any surgical lasers. Filters generally do not degrade the quality of the surgeon's view, but they can change the red reflex and the hue of the surgical field.
- Foot pedal: Controls the image focus, the magnification, and the optical axis of the microscope. On some foot pedals, the operating microscope light intensity and room lights can be adjusted.

SOME PRINCIPLES OF OCULAR MICROSURGERY:

- It is critical to observe a sterile procedure. Ophthalmology ORs are often crowded with numerous pieces of equipment. Be aware of your surroundings. Be especially careful when moving backward that your backside does not bump into any sterile field. If you suspect you have touched something nonsterile or broken the sterile field, swallow your pride and request a new glove or quietly notify the attending surgeon. If you feel you have identified another member of the team who has breached the sterile field, quietly notify that person and potentially the attending or scrub nurse. Safety first.

- Generally, ophthalmic surgeries are conducted while seated. The primary surgeon and the assistant sit 90 degrees to one another on the side of the operated eye. The scrub technician's Mayo stand, which holds the most commonly used instruments, is positioned over the thorax/abdomen. Students or observers, if scrubbed, may observe through a third ocular positioned on the side of the nonoperative eye. If they are not scrubbed, however, a viewing monitor may be placed in the room outside of the immediate surgical area.

- It can be tiring to sit at the operating scope if you are not positioned comfortably. You should be able to use the oculars while sitting erect with a slight forward lean. Your feet should be flat on the ground and your knees bent at 90 degrees. If hunched or stretching, it is often possible to adjust the surgical stool height without breaking scrub by using a foot pedal. Most oculars also have a hinge that allows them to pivot vertically. Avoid repositioning yourself or the microscope while the primary surgeon is actively operating, as small bumps against the bed, microscope, or primary surgeon can create large problems.

- Additional foot pedals: For many procedures, such as vitrectomy, laser application, cautery, irrigation-aspiration, and phacoemulsification, an additional foot pedal is used to control the instrument settings. Most commonly, the dominant foot (right foot) is used to control these instruments, while the other foot (left foot) is used to adjust the microscope settings.

- Hand–eye coordination: The surgeon and assistant operate while looking through the oculars, which are not in line with the surgical field. Learning to perform delicate maneuvers without looking directly at one's hands can be challenging. If scrubbed, a student may be asked to periodically wet the cornea with balanced saline solution (BSS) delivered through a cannula. This seemingly simple task provides an introduction to the challenges of operating with a microscope. When first assisting under an operating microscope, it is recommended to approach the eye with instruments or materials without using the microscope. Once the materials are in a safe position and your hand is resting on the patient's face or the wrist rest, look through the ocular to complete your approach to your final destination within the surgical field. Experienced surgeons typically do not need to watch their hands approach the surgical field, and they will maintain their view through the microscope oculars while receiving and handing off instruments.

- Hand stabilization: When performing microsurgery, it is almost always necessary to have your hands stabilized against some fixed object. A wrist rest or forearm rest is often used, or the surgeon can rest his or her hands on the brow and/or cheek of the patient for stabilization. Depending on the surgical maneuver, the surgeon will usually rest either his or her wrist or metacarpal pad of the thumb or fifth finger against a fixed object.

- Good surgical technique should result in natural, stable, and controlled hand movements. If you are struggling to maintain controlled movements or, if the surgical maneuver requires it, you may need to reposition your chair, microscope, or wrists. Your elbows should stay tight against your body for most surgical maneuvers. Occasionally, it is useful to use your nondominant hand to help stabilize your dominant hand, such as during the capsulorrhexis. While most surgeons have a dominant hand that they prefer for complex maneuvers, ideally, a surgeon should be comfortable using either hand for any technique. Even if you are not truly ambidextrous, you should prepare to use both hands in coordination. The nondominant hand plays an important role facilitating many surgical maneuvers, such as during suturing. Additionally, a nondominant hand that is not actively performing a maneuver should not drift away or push into the eye inadvertently.

- As an assistant, it is important to be familiar with the surgical steps so that you may proactively assist with the surgery. Ask the primary surgeon's permission regarding how much assistance they would like from you during the procedure. For example, ask for scissors or a small blade while the primary surgeon is suturing. Use BSS to clear away heme or when wet-field cautery is used. Generally, it is a good idea to avoid reaching over the primary surgeon's hands.

- Always be aware of the location and movement of sharps (especially when you are assisting). In general, it is a good idea to move slowly and predictably, particularly when dealing with sharps. When receiving or handing off instruments or sharps, grasp the instrument firmly and pause briefly to confirm the exchange with the scrub tech. When handing off suture needles, it is ideal to capture the suture with the instrument rather than the needle itself. This allows the needle to dangle loosely, and will decrease the possibility of it inadvertently sticking your colleagues. Clearly communicate the position of sharps if you place them on the instrument stand ("needle back").

OPHTHALMIC SURGERY ETIQUETTE

- Treat all members of the surgical team with respect. Maintaining a calm voice, even during stressful moments, will keep your patient and surgical staff at ease and will improve your surgical team's confidence in you.

- Be aware that most ophthalmology patients are awake during surgery. Avoid inappropriate or loud conversation. Avoid talking with patients who are actively undergoing surgery, as they will move excessively while talking with you.

- Avoid talking to the primary surgeon, particularly while they are engaged in complex maneuvers (unless they initiate the conversation).

- Do not say anything that may be interpreted by the patient that there is a problem, such as "oops" or "did you mean to do that." Refer to blood as "RBCs" or "heme."

Further Reading

Text

Eisner G. *Eye Surgery.* 2nd ed. New York, NY: Springer-Verlag; 1990.

Primary Source

Maloney WF. Advances in small incision cataract surgery. *Focal Points.* 2000;18(1).

CHAPTER 3

Cornea

Jimmy K. Lee and Paul A. Gaudio

3.1 KERATOPLASTY

Keratoplasty is full-thickness (penetrating) or partial-thickness (lamellar) removal of a damaged central cornea, followed by replacement with donor tissue of equivalent dimensions.

The cornea is immunologically privileged, and transplant generally does not require systemic immunosuppression.

INDICATIONS

A keratoplasty graft may be used to strengthen a weak cornea, restore visual acuity, halt disease progression, and/or improve cosmesis.

Penetrating Keratoplasty (PKP) (FIG. 3.1.1A)

PKP is performed for the following reasons:

- Defects that affect the full stromal thickness and/or endothelial layer

- Late stage or acute keratoconus

- Accidental penetration of the anterior chamber during a lamellar procedure

- Emergency treatment of a perforated corneal ulcer

Advantages

- Surgeons generally have the most experience with this procedure, so outcomes tend to be reliable. Historically, it offers the best visual prognosis.

Disadvantages

- Because the entire central cornea is replaced, this procedure often produces significant post-operative astigmatism and ocular surface changes. Correction may require the use of a hard contact lens.

- It renders the cornea vulnerable to comparatively minor trauma, since strength is significantly reduced even after wound healing.

- In contrast to anterior lamellar procedures, the graft requires careful preoperative screening to ensure adequate donor endothelial cell density. Insufficient cell density leads to graft edema and opacity.

- Since PKP grafts include the highly cellular endothelial layer, the risk of rejection is greater. The corneal stroma consists of laminar collagen and diffuse keratocytes, which are less likely to trigger a host immune reaction.

- There is an increased risk of suprachoroidal hemorrhage and endophthalmitis due to anterior chamber entry.

Anterior Lamellar Keratoplasty (ALK) (FIG. 3.1.1B)

- ALK is superficial stromal opacity or scarring with an intact Descemet's membrane and healthy endothelium.

Advantages

- The plane of dissection is in the superficial corneal stroma, so the risk of inadvertent anterior chamber penetration is lower than with deep lamellar procedures.

- Donor tissue is easier to obtain and store because the graft does not require viable endothelial cells. Consequently, the risk of rejection is also lower.

- Rehabilitation tends to be quicker than for penetrating procedures, with reduced steroid requirements.

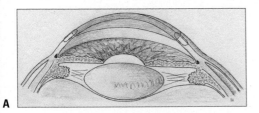
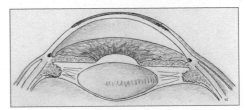
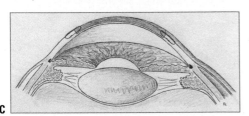
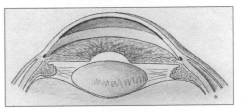

FIGURE 3.1.1 ♦ **(A)** *Penetrating keratoplasty (PKP):* Replacement of the full central corneal thickness with a sutured donor graft. **(B)** *Anterior lamellar keratoplasty (ALK):* Replacement of the corneal epithelium and superficial stroma with a sutured partial-thickness graft. **(C)** *Deep anterior lamellar keratoplasty (DALK):* Replacement of the corneal epithelium and full stromal thickness with a sutured donor graft. The plane of dissection for the host corneal bed is at the interface between the posterior stroma and Descemet's membrane. **(D)** *Posterior lamellar keratoplasty (e.g., DSEK):* Replacement of the corneal endothelium and Descemet's membrane and with a donor graft.

- This procedure is better tolerated in inflamed eyes since the anterior chamber is not entered.

Disadvantages

- Lamellar dissection is more difficult than en bloc removal of the central cornea for PKP.
- Uneven dissection of the donor or recipient cornea can adversely impact postoperative visual acuity.
- Opacity or vascularization may develop at the host–donor interface.

Deep Anterior Lamellar Keratoplasty (DALK) (FIG. 3.1.1C)

- DALK is deeper stromal opacities or scarring with an intact Descemet's membrane and healthy endothelium.

Advantages

- The plane of dissection is along Descemet's membrane rather than within the stroma, producing a smoother recipient corneal bed. This theoretically benefits postoperative visual acuity.

Disadvantages

- Deeper dissection increases the risk of accidental anterior chamber perforation. This requires conversion to PKP with its associated risks.

Posterior Lamellar Keratoplasty (FIG. 3.1.1D)

- The preferred treatment for corneal opacity due to endothelial defects that are not associated with independent stromal damage (e.g., bullous keratopathy, Fuchs endothelial dystrophy).

Advantages

- Transplant can be completed through a small limbal or scleral incision. This helps maintain the anterior corneal curvature, limiting postoperative refractive changes and astigmatism.
- Because refractive changes are more predictable, it is possible to perform simultaneous cataract extraction with intraocular lens (IOL) placement.
- Grafts generally adhere to the recipient corneal bed without the need for sutures. Some techniques also permit use of self-sealing incisions.
- Wound healing is generally much faster and less complicated than with PKP. It is therefore safer to suppress endothelial rejection with steroids.
- There is less vulnerability to postoperative trauma, since the required incisions are much smaller.

Disadvantages

- This is the most technically challenging approach because of the need to excise host cornea and manipulate donor tissue through a small incision.

- As with PKP, these procedures require donor tissue with a high endothelial cell density. The rejection risk is therefore greater than for anterior lamellar procedures.
- Despite the use of smaller incisions, there is still a risk of endophthalmitis due to anterior chamber entry.
- Multiple techniques have been developed over the past decade:
  - Deep lamellar endothelial keratoplasty (DLEK): A curved blade is used to perform lamellar dissection at 80% to 90% of the stromal depth. Deep stroma, Descemet's membrane, and the endothelium are then removed and replaced with donor tissue.
  - Descemet's stripping endothelial keratoplasty (DSEK): Descemet's membrane and endothelium are peeled away without the need for stromal dissection. The graft includes deep stroma, Descemet's membrane, and the endothelium.
  - Descemet's stripping automated endothelial keratoplasty (DSAEK): Identical to DSEK, except that the donor cornea is dissected with a microkeratome rather than by hand.
  - Descemet's membrane endothelial keratoplasty (DMEK): Similar to DSEK, but the donor cornea is prepared to include only Descemet's membrane and endothelium. This procedure most closely replicates the preoperative corneal thickness, resulting in the smallest and most predictable refractive change.

ALTERNATIVES

Medical Therapy

Timely intervention may eliminate the need for surgery in some instances (e.g., prompt antibiotic therapy for bacterial keratitis can prevent ulceration and perforation).

- Keratoconus: Hard contact lenses are helpful in early stages, but do not modify disease progression.
- Fuchs endothelial dystrophy: In early stages, topical hyperosmolar solutions can be applied to dehydrate the cornea, temporarily reducing edema and opacity.

Laser/Surgery

- Phototherapeutic keratectomy: Corneal scars can be ablated with an excimer laser if they are confined to the anterior stroma. Up to 20% of the stromal thickness can be removed with this technique.
- Keratoprosthesis: Opaque central cornea is replaced with a clear synthetic implant. This procedure is considered in cases where traditional keratoplasty is expected to fail (e.g., history of recurrent graft rejection or severe ocular surface inflammation).

RELEVANT PHYSIOLOGY/ANATOMY

Cornea Overview

- Clear refractive media: $\sim$ 43 diopters (provides $\geq$ two-thirds of total refraction).
- Average central thickness: 560 microns (increases with hydration).
- Nourishment: Provided by the limbal capillaries laterally, tear film anteriorly, and aqueous humor posteriorly.
- Sensation: Transmitted by the ophthalmic division of the trigeminal nerve. The corneal reflex is conducted by CN V_1 afferent fibers and CN VII efferent fibers.

Corneal Anatomy (FIG. 3.1.2)
Five distinct layers
Epithelium:

- Nonkeratinized stratified squamous epithelium with a thin basement membrane.
- Protects the inner layers from pathogens and the corneal nerve endings from irritation (epithelial defects cause pain and foreign body sensation because the nerve endings are exposed).
- Regenerates rapidly from stem cells located at the corneal limbus.

Bowman's Layer:

- A thin layer of highly organized anterior stroma that is more durable than the overlying epithelium.
- Injury can lead to corneal scarring because it has a limited regenerative capacity.

Stroma:

- Consists of hydrated laminar collagen produced by keratocytes (corneal fibroblasts). Water content is maintained at approximately 70% by the

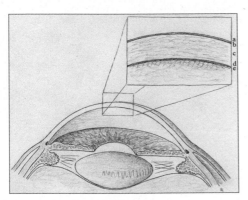

FIGURE 3.1.2 ◆ *Corneal anatomy:* The cornea is composed of five distinct layers: nonkeratinized epithelium (a), Bowman's membrane (b), laminar collagen stroma (c), Descemet's membrane (d), and endothelium (e).

endothelial pump mechanism, which preserves optic clarity. Greater hydration leads to corneal opacity.

- Avascular tissue has slow metabolism and limited cell content. Therefore, this layer is immunologically privileged but easily damaged by infection.
- Chemical injury or prolonged inflammation can induce vascularization, which increases the risk of transplant rejection.

Descemet's Membrane:

- A thick, durable basement membrane generated by the adjacent endothelial cells.
- As the strongest layer of the cornea, it plays an important role in defining the shape of the anterior chamber.

Corneal Endothelium:

- Regulates stromal hydration with an adenosine triphosphate (ATP)-driven pump-leak system that is critical to maintaining corneal transparency.
- Cell density decreases with age and anterior chamber interventions such as phacoemulsification.
- The normal adult cell count is approximately 2,500 cells/mm^2. Below 300 cells/mm^2, edema is inevitable due to inadequate pumping.
- Defects in this layer are filled by enlargement and migration since these hexagonal cells cannot

divide. Loss of cell symmetry and significant variation in cell size are signs of an unhealthy endothelium.

Relevant Disease Processes

Keratoconus

- Progressive thinning of the cornea causes conical protrusion with severe, irregular astigmatism.
- It can occur sporadically, but there are also known familial and syndromic associations (e.g., Marfan syndrome, Down syndrome, and Ehlers-Danlos syndrome).
- Acute keratoconus results in sudden corneal destabilization and edema due to tears in Descemet's membrane.

Corneal Dystrophies

- Hereditary metabolic diseases that can affect any layer of the cornea and can lead to bilateral opacity.
- Fuchs endothelial dystrophy is the most common.

Bullous Keratopathy

- Loss of functioning endothelial cells leads to stromal edema and opacity. The overlying epithelium becomes less adherent and develops fluid-filled cysts in the basal layers.
- May be caused by trauma, intraocular inflammation, endothelial dystrophy, or anterior segment surgery.

Corneal Ulcer

- Can be bacterial (most common), viral, fungal, or parasitic.
- May develop within hours of inoculation depending on the pathogen virulence and host immune status.
- Progression: Epithelial lesion, stromal invasion, corneal ulcer, descemetocele (stromal melt exposes Descemet's membrane), corneal perforation with aqueous leakage, and endophthalmitis.

PREOPERATIVE SCREENING

Evaluate the patient's visual potential and motivation to comply with lengthy postoperative rehabilitation.

Assess the tear film and lid function since abnormalities can cause ocular surface defects that will delay wound healing.

Slit lamp exam: Check for corneal opacities, edema, and vascularization, as well as for evidence of anterior chamber inflammation (e.g., cell and flare, hypopyon, and synechiae). Accurate assessment of the depth, thickness, and origin of corneal defects is critical to selecting an appropriate procedure.

Specular microscopy: Quantify endothelial cell density using a magnified image to count the several cells within 1 mm². In addition to central corneal thickness, coefficients for cell symmetry and size variation can be calculated.

Keratometry/video keratography: Measure and document preoperative astigmatism to provide a reference point, since keratoplasty may significantly alter the corneal curvature.

Donor Screening: The eye bank will check for HIV and hepatitis as well as for history of ocular inflammation, malignancy, anterior chamber disease, and prior surgery. Though not routine, human leukocyte antigen (HLA) cross-matching may improve outcomes in patients at high risk of rejection (e.g., prior graft rejection).

ANESTHESIA

Retrobulbar or peribulbar anesthesia is sufficient for most patients undergoing keratoplasty.

Topical anesthesia can be used for some posterior lamellar procedures, but does not provide globe akinesia.

General anesthesia may be necessary for pediatric and uncooperative patients, as well as for obese patients undergoing PKP (the risk of suprachoroidal hemorrhage increases with high intrathoracic pressures, so the patient should be as relaxed as possible).

PROCEDURE

 Penetrating and Anterior Lamellar Keratoplasty: (SEE TABLES 3.1.1 Rapid Review of Steps and 3.1.2 Surgical Pearls, and WEB TABLES 3.1.1 to 3.1.4 for equipment and medication lists).

1. *Preoperative Medication:* In preparation for PKP, the globe is decompressed pharmacologically (with IV mannitol) or mechanically (with a Honan balloon, FIG. 3.1.3) to reduce the risk of suprachoroidal hemorrhage and intraocular content

TABLE 3.1.1 Rapid Review of Steps for Keratoplasty
(1) Decompression (pharmacologic vs. mechanical with Honan balloon)
(2) Radial corneal marking
(3) Partial thickness trephination
(4) Lamellar dissection for ALK, DALK vs. removal of central cornea for PKP
(5) Donor eye prep with trephine + lamellar dissection for ALK, DALK
(6) Suturing of graft (+/− intraoperative keratometry)

prolapse. Miotics are often used to constrict the pupil in phakic patients, protecting the native lens from intraoperative trauma. These measures are not necessary in anterior lamellar procedures, since the anterior chamber is not entered.

2. *Globe Stabilization:* The globe can be stabilized with traction sutures placed near the limbus or beneath the rectus muscles (FIG. 3.1.4), or with a Flieringa scleral fixation ring.

3. *Trephination:* Castroviejo calipers are used to locate the center of the cornea and to mark the desired radius of excision (FIG. 3.1.5). Radial lines are then stained onto the corneal epithelium, using a radial keratotomy marker (FIG. 3.1.6A,B). This aids in centering the graft and in optimizing suture locations. A partial-thickness circular incision is then made in the cornea with a vacuum

TABLE 3.1.2 Surgical Pearls
Preoperative:
• Check donor cornea. To reduce risk of suprachoroidal hemorrhage, make sure blood pressure is under control. If retrobulbar anesthesia is given, check for akinesia and anesthesia. Reduce posterior pressure with Honan balloon.
Intraoperative:
• Suture the first four cardinal sutures as soon as possible. Inflate the anterior chamber with viscoelastic device. Complete suturing of donor cornea with interrupted or running sutures.
Postoperative:
• Warn patients against coughing, straining, heavy lifting. Review symptoms of early primary graft rejection (decreased vision, pain, photophobia).

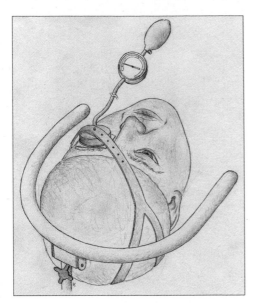

FIGURE 3.1.3 ◆ *Decompression:* A Honan balloon compresses the vitreous, lowering intraocular pressure, and decreasing the risk of suprachoroidal hemorrhage and ocular content extrusion during PKP.

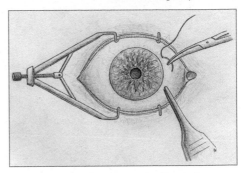

FIGURE 3.1.4 ◆ *Traction sutures:* Retrobulbar anesthesia paralyzes the extraocular muscles, but the globe can be further stabilized prior to surgery by placing limbal traction sutures.

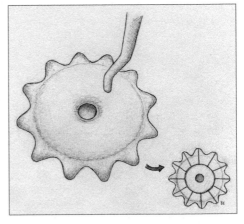

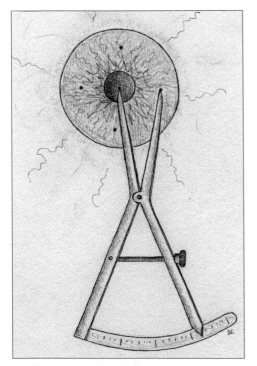

FIGURE 3.1.5 ◆ *Corneal measurement:* Castroviejo calipers are used to locate the center of the cornea and to mark the desired radius of host corneal excision.

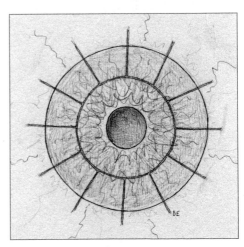

FIGURE 3.1.6 ◆ *Keratotomy marking:* Radial lines are stained onto the corneal epithelium with vital dye, using a radial keratotomy marker. These aid in centering the graft and in placing the anchoring sutures at appropriate intervals.

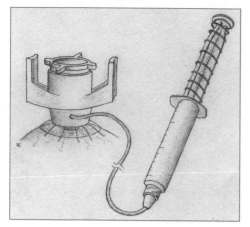

FIGURE 3.1.7 ◆ *Vacuum trephine placement:* A trephine is carefully centered on the cornea while the spring-loaded plunger is depressed. When it is released (shown above), vacuum pressure firmly anchors the trephine to the corneal surface.

trephine (FIG. 3.1.7). It should be large enough in diameter to remove the defect of interest and avoid the visual axis, while maintaining sufficient distance from the limbal vessels, which carry inflammatory cells that mediate graft rejection. Incision depth depends on the several trephine revolutions (one-fourth turn = 60 microns) (FIG. 3.1.8). In lamellar procedures, lateral dissection with a blade, microkeratome, or laser permits

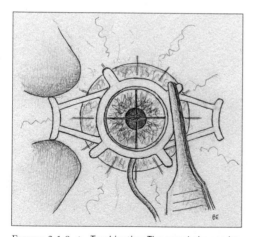

FIGURE 3.1.8 ◆ *Trephination:* The crosshairs used to center the trephine on the cornea can be seen from above. The trephine knob is carefully rotated with forceps the several turns necessary to produce an incision of the desired depth (one-fourth turn = 60 microns).

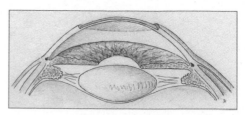

FIGURE 3.1.9 ◆ *Lamellar dissection:* In lamellar procedures, lateral dissection with a blade, microkeratome, or laser permits removal of epithelium and stroma with exposure of the underlying "recipient bed."

removal of epithelium and stroma with exposure of the underlying "recipient bed" (FIG. 3.1.9). In penetrating procedures, the circular incision is completed in a controlled fashion with a fine scalpel and scissors (FIG. 3.1.10A,B).

4. *Donor Eye Preparation:* For lamellar keratoplasty, trephination and lateral dissection can be used to harvest a corneal graft of the desired diameter and thickness from the donor eye. Alternatively, microkeratome-prepared cornea can be obtained in various thicknesses. It theoretically improves visual potential by providing a smoother donor–host interface than free-hand dissection. For PKP, a full-thickness graft of the appropriate diameter is harvested from the donor cornea with a trephine, taking care to avoid damage to the endothelial surface (FIG. 3.1.11).

5. *Graft implantation:* For lamellar procedures, the graft is placed onto the recipient bed and secured with radial 10-0 sutures through 90% of the host corneal thickness. For PKP, four "cardinal" sutures are initially placed at the 12, 3, 6, and 9 o'clock positions after injection of viscoelastic to support the anterior chamber (FIG. 3.1.12). Closure is then completed with running or interrupted sutures after viscoelastic aspiration (FIG. 3.1.13). A keratometer can be used intraoperatively to guide suture tensioning and to minimize postoperative astigmatism. After closure is complete, the wound is tested for leaks by infusing balanced salt solution (BSS) through a paracentesis tract in the peripheral cornea.

 Posterior Lamellar Keratoplasty: DSEK/ DSAEK/DMEK: (SEE TABLES 3.1.3 Rapid Review of Steps and 3.1.4 Surgical Pearls, and WEB TABLES 3.1.5, 3.1.6, and 3.1.7 for equipment and medication lists).

1. *Preoperative Medication:* As with PKP, the globe is decompressed.

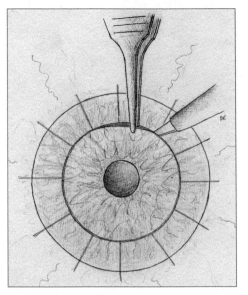

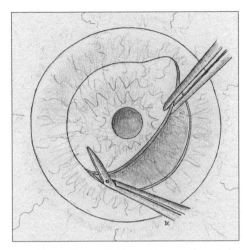

FIGURE 3.1.10 ✦ *Penetrating keratoplasty:* In penetrating procedures, a fine scalpel is used to enter the anterior chamber in a controlled fashion. Scissors may then be used to complete the removal of host cornea.

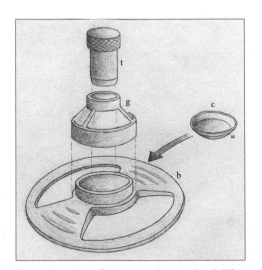

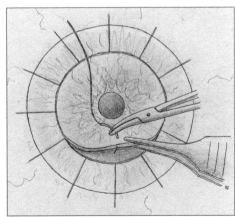

FIGURE 3.1.11 ✦ *Donor corneal preparation:* A different trephine is used to remove an appropriately sized donor graft from the banked cornea (c). The cylindrical blade (t) is pressed through the guide (g) to cut the donor tissue, which is cupped in the trephine base (b).

FIGURE 3.1.12 ✦ *Suturing:* The graft is secured with radial 10-0 sutures through 90% of the corneal thickness. For penetrating procedures (pictured), 4 cardinal sutures are initially placed at 12, 3, 6, and 9 o'clock. The radial keratotomy mark facilitates suture placement at appropriate intervals.

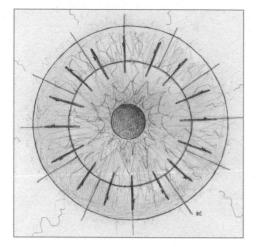

FIGURE 3.1.13 ◆ *Sutures in situ:* Use of 16 interrupted corneal sutures is the gold standard for penetrating keratoplasty. After the sutures are placed, the knots are rotated and buried within the cornea so as not to irritate the palpebral conjunctiva during lid closure. Various running suture patterns may also be used.

2. *Corneal Marking:* Castroviejo calipers are used to locate the center of the cornea and to mark the desired radius of Descemet's membrane stripping. A circular outline is then stained onto the corneal epithelium (FIG. 3.1.14).

3. *Scleral/Limbal Tunnel:* A flap of temporal conjunctiva adjacent to the limbus is elevated with sharp dissection. Specialized blades are then used to create a tunnel through the underlying sclera and into the peripheral anterior chamber (FIG. 3.1.15). This tunnel must be wide enough to accommodate the folded donor graft. Corneal curvature will be reduced in the meridian of this

TABLE 3.1.3 Rapid Review of Steps for DSEK/DMEK
(1) Corneal epithelial marking to delineate area of Descemet's stripping
(2) Creation of limbal, scleral, or clear corneal tunnel
(3) Descemet's membrane stripping and removal
(4) Recipient corneal bed preparation
(5) Graft preparation and insertion
(6) Graft fixation (air injected for tamponade)
(7) Manipulation free period
(8) BSS injection (leaving residual air bubble)
(9) Tunnel closure (limbal and scleral wounds require sutures)

TABLE 3.1.4 Surgical Pearls
Preoperative:
• For combined cataract extraction/IOL implant/ DSAEK cases, select a lens power that would result in −1.5 diopter (since the corneal graft induces on average +1.5 diopter hyperopic shift. Presoaking donor cornea in balance salt solution chelates the detergent from donor cornea storage media and reduces the risk of graft slippage or dislocation.
Intraoperative:
• A long wound (corneal or scleral) is critical to maintain anterior chamber stability during graft insertion. Peripheral stromal roughening creates a "Velcro-like" interface, which facilitates adherence of the graft.
Postoperative:
• Instruct the patient to lie flat (face parallel to the floor), explaining how the air bubble tamponades the donor cornea best in that position. Allow the patient to sit/stand for 10–15 minutes every hour if lying flat is uncomfortable. Discourage eye rubbing, straining, heavy lifting.

incision, producing astigmatism. The degree of flattening is directly related to incision length, and inversely related to distance from the central cornea. Since the required incision is longer than those used for cataract phacoemulsification, it is generally placed further from the central cornea. If transplant is combined with cataract surgery, however, some surgeons will perform both procedures through a limbal or clear corneal incision.

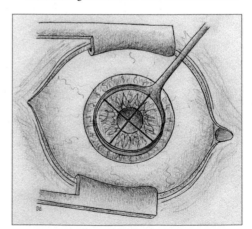

FIGURE 3.1.14 ◆ *DSEK/DMEK corneal marking:* A circular outline is marked on the corneal epithelium to delineate the desired area of Descemet's membrane stripping.

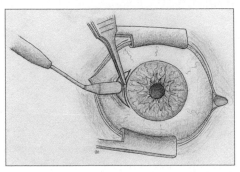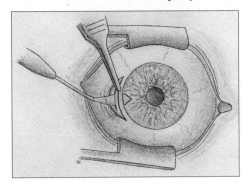

FIGURE 3.1.15 ◆ *Scleral tunnel:* After a flap of temporal conjunctiva is elevated with sharp dissection, specialized blades are used to make a tunnel through the sclera and into the peripheral anterior chamber. A scleral tunnel produces the least postoperative astigmatism, but a limbal or clear corneal tunnel is occasionally substituted if the patient is undergoing simultaneous cataract extraction.

4. *Host Tissue Removal:* The anterior chamber is filled with viscoelastic to maintain its curvature during scoring of Descemet's membrane. A reverse Sinskey hook is then inserted through a paracentesis wound. The tip of the hook is used to penetrate Descemet's membrane and it is swept in a circular motion using the epithelial marking as a guide (FIG. 3.1.16). The posterior layers of the central cornea, including Descemet's membrane and endothelium, are then bluntly dissected away from the anterior cornea and removed from the anterior chamber with Utrata forceps (FIG. 3.1.17). This creates a smooth recipient bed for donor tissue implantation.

5. *Recipient Bed Preparation:* Since the incidence of postoperative graft dislocation is relatively high, some surgeons attempt to increase donor tissue adhesion by roughening the peripheral recipient

bed with a scraping tool. An irrigation-aspiration unit is then used to remove the viscoelastic and remnants of Descemet's membrane.

6. *Graft Preparation and Insertion:* The donor cornea is dissected into anterior and posterior layers, either by hand or with a microkeratome. Many eye banks now offer predissected cornea. After lamellar dissection, a trephine is used to harvest a circular graft of appropriate diameter. Grafts for DSEK and DEAEK include deep stroma, Descemet's membrane, and endothelium, while those for DMEK omit the deep stroma. After the endothelial surface of the graft is coated with viscoelastic for protection, it is folded in half and inserted through the scleral tunnel with

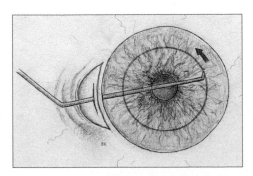

FIGURE 3.1.16 ◆ *Descemet's membrane penetration:* A reverse Sinskey hook is inserted into the anterior chamber through the tunnel. The tip of the hook is used to penetrate Descemet's membrane. It is then swept in a circular motion using the epithelial marking as a guide.

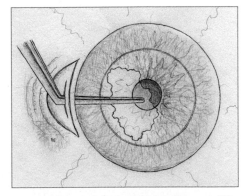

FIGURE 3.1.17 ◆ *Descemet's/endothelial removal:* The posterior layers of the central cornea, including Descemet's membrane and endothelium, are then bluntly dissected from the anterior cornea and removed from the anterior chamber with forceps. This creates a smooth recipient bed for donor tissue implantation.

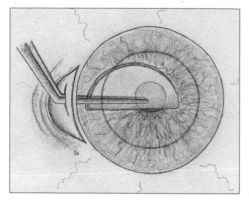

FIGURE 3.1.18 ✦ *Graft insertion:* The endothelial surface of the graft is coated with viscoelastic for protection. It is then folded in half to permit insertion into the anterior chamber with forceps.

forceps (FIG. 3.1.18). Some surgeons have begun to insert the folded graft using an intraocular lens injection system, which can be used in conjunction with a smaller clear corneal incision.

7. *Fixation of Donor Graft:* The graft is then unfolded by reinflating the anterior chamber with BSS on a cannula and centered using gentle manipulation. Air is injected posterior to the graft, filling the entire anterior chamber and tamponading the donor tissue firmly against the recipient stromal surface. Some surgeons massage the cornea with a laser-assisted in situ keratomileusis (LASIK) flap roller to squeeze residual fluid from the host–donor interface. Careful removal of all interface fluid decreases the incidence of postoperative displacement. The presence of air in the anterior chamber can produce pupillary block and precipitate acute angle closure (FIG. 3.1.19). This is prevented with routine peripheral iridectomy (FIG. 3.1.20) or pharmacologic pupillary dilation.

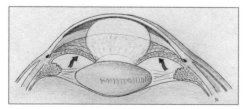

FIGURE 3.1.19 ✦ *Tamponade:* An air bubble is injected to tamponade the graft against the recipient corneal bed. The presence of air in the anterior chamber, however, can produce pupillary block and precipitate acute angle closure.

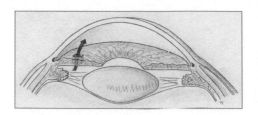

FIGURE 3.1.20 ✦ *Iridotomy:* It is therefore essential to prevent pupillary block by performing a peripheral iridotomy (shown) or by dilating the pupil with anticholinergic medication.

8. *Closure:* After a 10-minute manipulation-free period, BSS in injected, leaving a residual air bubble that occupies 30% of the anterior chamber volume. The temporal tunnel is often closed with dissolvable 9-0 Vicryl sutures, though corneal and limbal incisions may be self-sealing. The conjunctival flap is then reapproximated and closed with Vicryl sutures.

COMPLICATIONS

Intraoperative

- Suprachoroidal hemorrhage: Accumulation of blood between the choroid and sclera. The risk increases with high thoracic or IOP (PKP).
- Prolapse of intraocular contents: Expulsion of intraocular tissue through the corneal incision. The risk increases with high IOP (PKP).
- Anterior chamber perforation: Necessitates conversion to PKP (anterior lamellar procedures).

Postoperative

- Astigmatism: The single most common factor limiting postoperative visual acuity, assuming a healthy posterior segment. In management, corrective suture removal or adjustment must be balanced against adequate corneal wound healing (PKP, anterior lamellar).
- Wound leakage: Causes anterior chamber shallowing, hypotony, and increased risk of infection. Detected with the Seidel test: Leaking aqueous will dilute fluorescein placed over the surgical wound (PKP, rarely posterior lamellar).
- Graft dislocation: The most common complication of posterior lamellar procedures. Detached grafts can be repositioned and anchored by reinjecting air into the anterior chamber.

- Persistent epithelial defects: May result from an uneven interface between the host and donor corneal surfaces. This complication is especially common in eyes with prior surface defects (PKP, anterior lamellar).
- Loose sutures: Can serve as a nidus for corneal vascularization and/or infections such as suture abscess (PKP, anterior lamellar).
- Corneal ulcers: May form in the setting of persistent epithelial defects or suture abscess. They can also present due to recurrence of preoperative corneal infection.
- IOP elevation: In PKP, this is most often due to occlusion of the trabecular meshwork with inflammatory cells, hyphema, or residual viscoelastic material. In posterior lamellar procedures, injection of air into the anterior chamber can precipitate angle closure.
- Primary graft failure: The cornea remains opaque after transplantation due to inadequate pumping by the endothelial layer. In general, wait 2 to 4 weeks to see if the graft will ultimately clear before reintervention (PKP, posterior lamellar).
- Endophthalmitis: The risk of intraocular infection increases with anterior chamber entry (PKP, posterior lamellar).
- Interface irregularity: Optical distortion at the host–donor interface in anterior lamellar procedures. The risk is greater with free-hand stromal dissection.
- Interface opacity and/or vascularization: Occasionally seen with anterior lamellar procedures.
- Graft rejection: Mostly seen with PKP and posterior lamellar procedures due to greater graft cellularity. Treated with corticosteroids, it occurs in three forms.
  - Epithelial rejection: Lymphocytes from the limbal vasculature destroy peripheral cells; visible as punctate fluorescein staining on the slit lamp exam. This form of rejection is self-limited, since the donor epithelium is ultimately replaced with host tissue.
  - Subepithelial infiltrates: Signs of stromal rejection include discrete areas of opacity that may leave scars following resolution.
  - Endothelial rejection: This can lead to rapid corneal opacity due to pump mechanism failure. Anterior chamber inflammation and/or keratic precipitates may be visible on the slit lamp exam. A leading rejection line (Khodadoust line) is often apparent on the posterior corneal surface.

POSTOPERATIVE CARE

Instruct patients who have undergone posterior lamellar procedures utilizing an air bubble to lie face up in the recovery room (maintains graft position). They must also be cautioned to avoid rubbing their eyes.

On the first postoperative day, assess pain, intraocular pressure, visual acuity, and graft position. Perform slit lamp and fundus exams.

With PKP, apply topical corticosteroids for 1 month, then taper based on appearance of the graft. Eyes with high rejection risk may require a very long steroid taper and/or an indefinite basal dose. With lamellar procedures, steroids are generally necessary for shorter periods.

Administer antibiotics until the epithelial defects heal.

Eye protection is essential, especially following PKP. Counsel the patient to wear glasses or an eye shield at all times during the postoperative period. The patient must also avoid the Valsalva maneuver or heavy lifting.

Monitor graft edema with serial ultrasound pachymetry (central corneal thickness increases with hydration).

After several weeks of healing, manage astigmatism by adjusting running sutures or removing select interrupted sutures in clinic. The timing of final suture removal is highly variable and must be individualized.

Further Reading

Text

Lang GK. Cornea. In: Lang GK, ed. *Ophthalmology–A Pocket Textbook Atlas* 2nd ed. New York, NY: Georg Thieme Verlag; 2007:chap 5.

Marten L, Wang MX, Karp CL, et al. Corneal surgery. In: Yanoff M, Duker J, eds. *Ophthalmology*. 3rd ed. Philadelphia, PA: Mosby; 2009:351–360.

Panda A, Vanathi M, Kumar A, et al. Corneal graft rejection. *Surv Ophthalmol.* 2007;52(4):375–396.

Price MO, Price FW. Descemet's stripping endothelial keratoplasty. *Curr Opin Ophthalmol.* 2007;18(4): 290–294.

Tan DT, Mehta JS. Future directions in lamellar corneal transplantation. *Cornea.* 2007;26(9 Suppl 1):S21–28.

Primary Sources

Bahar I, Kaiserman I, McAllum P, et al. Comparison of posterior lamellar keratoplasty techniques to penetrating keratoplasty. *Ophthalmology.* 2008;115(9):1525–1533.

Ham L, Dapena I, van Luijk C, et al. Descemet membrane endothelial keratoplasty (DMEK) for Fuchs endothelial dystrophy: Review of the first 50 consecutive cases. *Eye.* 2009;23(10): 1990–1998.

Price FW Jr, Price MO. Descemet's stripping with endothelial keratoplasty in 200 eyes: Early challenges and techniques to enhance donor adherence. *J Cataract Refract Surg.* 2006;32(3):411–418.

3.2   KERATOPROSTHESIS (KPro)

A clear synthetic prosthesis, secured to a ring of donor tissue, is used to replace severely opacified host cornea.

The Boston Type 1 prosthesis, originally known as the Dohlman-Doane device, is the most commonly used KPro and has been FDA approved since 1992 (FIG. 3.2.1). The Alpha Cor prosthesis is a common alternative.

The Boston Type 2 prosthesis is similar to the Type 1, but the optic extends in order to penetrate a skin flap or mucosal graft covering an eye with end-stage surface damage (FIG. 3.2.2).

INDICATIONS

KPro use is reserved for cases of severe corneal opacity, where traditional penetrating keratoplasty (PKP) is expected to fail. Examples include:

- History of recurrent graft rejection;
- Severe chemical burns, keratoconjunctivitis sicca, or corneal vascularization; and
- Severe surface inflammation (e.g., ocular cicatricial pemphigoid or Stevens-Johnson syndrome).

ALTERNATIVES

Medical Therapy

- Medical management alone cannot reverse severe corneal opacity.
- Lubricants and soft contact lenses may be used to prevent further damage due to dry eye conditions.

Surgery

- Keratoplasty: The preferred treatment for corneal opacity that obstructs the visual axis. Full-thickness or lamellar techniques are selected depending on which layers of the cornea are affected (see Chapter 3.1 Keratoplasty).
- Limbal stem cell transplant: Stem cells located at the limbus are responsible for regenerating the corneal epithelium. In some cases, successful transplant from the fellow eye may restore a healthy ocular surface.

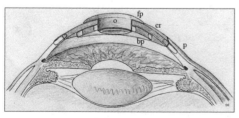

FIGURE 3.2.1 ✦ *Boston Keratoprosthesis:* Type 1 prosthesis is the most commonly used KPro both in the US and worldwide. It is depicted here in relation to anterior segment structures. Light is transmitted through a clear central optic (o) made of polymethylmethacrylate (PMMA). Front (fp) and back plates (bp) secure it to a rim of donor corneal tissue (cr), which is sutured to the peripheral host cornea (p).

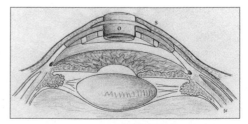

FIGURE 3.2.2 ✦ *Boston Keratoprosthesis:* Type 2 prosthesis is similar in design to the Type 1, but the optic (o) extends further to penetrate a skin flap (s) that has been used to cover an eye with very severe surface damage.

- Amniotic membrane transplant: Covering the cornea with banked allograft during episodes of acute inflammation may help to reduce ocular surface damage.

- Adjuncts to KPro implantation: If corneal opacity is due to a severe inflammatory condition, it may be advisable to simultaneously place a glaucoma drainage implant and/or remove opacified lens and vitreous as well as fibrotic iris tissue.

The back plate, which lies in the anterior chamber, has holes at regular intervals that permit the passage of aqueous to nourish the donor cornea.

Loosening of the plates is prevented with a titanium lock ring.

Host corneal preparation is identical to penetrating keratoplasty (see Chapter 3.1 Keratoplasty).

The donor cornea endothelial cell count is not as critical, because this tissue does not need to serve an optical function.

BOSTON TYPE 1 KPro OVERVIEW

Boston type 1 KPro is made of inert polymethylmethacrylate (PMMA).

It consists of front and back plates connected by a clear 3 to 3.5 mm diameter optic "stem" that permits transmission of images to the retina (Fig. 3.2.3A,B).

The front and back plates secure a full-thickness ring of donor cornea around the optic stem. This collar of tissue can then be sutured to the remaining host cornea.

The front plate has a tapered contour to permit smooth eyelid passage at the interface with peripheral cornea.

RELEVANT ANATOMY/PATHOPHYSIOLOGY

Cornea Overview

- Clear refractive media: $\sim$ 243 diopters (provides $\geq$ two-thirds of total refraction).

- Average central thickness: 560 microns (increases with hydration).

- Nourishment: Provided by the limbal capillaries laterally, tear film anteriorly, and aqueous humor posteriorly.

- Sensation: Transmitted by the ophthalmic division of the trigeminal nerve. The corneal reflex is conducted by CN V_1 afferent fibers and CN VII efferent fibers.

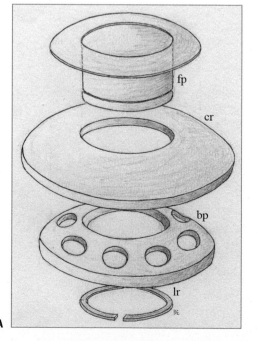

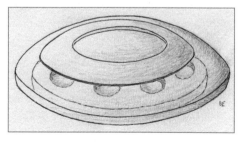

FIGURE 3.2.3 ◆ *Boston Type I components* **(A)** The front plate is attached to the optic stem, which fits into the back plate and is secured by a titanium lock ring. Assembled prosthesis **(B)** A ring of donor corneal tissue surrounds the optic stem, and is held in place by the front and back plates.

A

Corneal Anatomy (FIG. 3.2.4)
Five Distinct Layers
Epithelium:

- Nonkeratinized stratified squamous epithelium with a thin basement membrane.

- Protects the inner layers from pathogens and the corneal nerve endings from irritation (epithelial defects cause pain and foreign body sensation because the nerve endings are exposed).

- Regenerates rapidly from stem cells located at the corneal limbus.

Bowman's Layer:

- A thin layer of highly organized anterior stroma that is more durable than the overlying epithelium.

- Injury can lead to corneal scarring because it has a limited regenerative capacity.

Stroma:

- Consists of hydrated laminar collagen formed by keratocytes (corneal fibroblasts). Water content is maintained at approximately 70% by the endothelial pump mechanism, which preserves optic clarity. Greater hydration leads to corneal opacity.

- Avascular tissue with slow metabolism and limited cell content. This layer is therefore immunologically privileged but easily damaged by infection.

- Chemical injury or prolonged inflammation can induce vascularization, which increases the risk of transplant rejection.

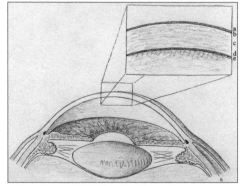

FIGURE 3.2.4 ◆ *Corneal Anatomy:* The cornea is composed of five distinct layers: epithelium (a), Bowman's membrane (b), stroma (c), Descemet's membrane (d), and endothelium (e).

Descemet's Membrane:

- A thick, durable basement membrane generated by the adjacent endothelial cells.

- As the strongest layer of the cornea, it plays an important role in defining the shape of the anterior chamber.

Corneal Endothelium:

- Regulates stromal hydration with an adenosine triphosphate (ATP)-driven pump-leak system that is critical to maintaining corneal transparency.

- Cell density decreases with age and anterior chamber interventions such as phacoemulsification.

- The normal adult cell count is approximately 2,500 cells/mm^2. Below 300 cells/mm^2, edema is inevitable due to inadequate pumping.

- Defects in this layer are filled by enlargement and migration since these hexagonal cells cannot divide. Loss of cell symmetry and significant variation in cell size are signs of an unhealthy endothelium.

Relevant Disease Processes
Burns and Chemical Injury

- These exposures can damage the conjunctival goblet cells and limbal stem cells, which are critical to maintaining a healthy ocular surface.

- Goblet cells produce mucin, which helps to maintain a smooth, moist conjunctival surface. The limbal stem cells are critical to the closure of defects in the corneal epithelium.

- Acids denature the proteins in ocular tissue, creating a barrier to further penetration. Alkali chemicals are therefore generally more dangerous.

Ocular Cicatricial Pemphigoid (OCP)

- An autoimmune disease affecting the skin and mucous membranes.

- The primary ocular manifestation is fibrosis and scarring of the conjunctiva.

- This secondarily reduces mucin and tear production. Coupled with the onset of trichiasis and other lid and lash defects, this may lead to corneal scarring and vascularization.

Stevens-Johnson Syndrome

- A hypersensitivity reaction affecting the skin and mucous membranes.

- Triggered by exposure to various drugs and pathogens.
- Produces conjunctival and corneal pathology similar to OCP.

PREOPERATIVE SCREENING

Assess lid function and integrity of the tear film.

- Slit lamp exam: Assess for ocular surface abnormalities, corneal opacities, edema, and vascularization, as well as for anterior chamber inflammation (cell and flare, hypopyon, and synechiae).
- Donor Screening: The eye bank will check for HIV and hepatitis as well as for history of ocular inflammation, malignancy, anterior chamber disease, and prior surgery.

ANESTHESIA

Performed under general anesthesia or monitored anesthesia care with retrobulbar block.

PROCEDURE

See Tables 3.2.1 Rapid Review of Steps and 3.2.2 Surgical Pearls, and Web Tables 3.2.1, 3.2.2, and 3.2.3 for equipment and medication lists.

1. *Preoperative Medication:* Dilating drops are administered if pars plana vitrectomy is also planned in conjunction with a temporary keratoprosthesis (see Chapter 8.2 Pars Plana Vitrectomy). The globe

---

TABLE 3.2.1 Rapid Review of Steps for Keratoprosthesis

(1) If retrobulbar anesthesia given, decompression of globe (pharmacologic vs. mechanical with Honan balloon)
(2) Radial corneal marking
(3) Partial thickness trephination of cornea
(4) Removal of central cornea
(5) Prep of donor eye with trephines to create corneal ring
(6) Insertion of keratoprosthesis into donor ring
(7) Suturing of donor ring/prosthesis to host corneal rim

TABLE 3.2.2 Surgical Pearls

Preoperative:
- Determine whether concurrent vitrectomy or glaucoma drainage implant surgery is also necessary. Be sure to get axial length if aphakic KPro is ordered.

Intraoperative:
- Do not assemble the KPro device until retina service finishes working on the retina for combined cases. If the retina is detached, refilling with silicone oil may be necessary.

Postoperative:
- The patient will be on antibiotics, steroids for the rest of the life. A large diameter contact lens is also required to protect the tarsal conjunctiva from the plastic KPro material.

---

is then decompressed pharmacologically (with IV mannitol) or mechanically (with a Honan balloon, Fig. 3.2.5) to reduce the risk of suprachoroidal hemorrhage and ocular content prolapse.

2. *Globe Stabilization:* The globe can be stabilized with traction sutures placed near the limbus or beneath the rectus muscles (Fig. 3.2.6), or with a Flieringa scleral fixation ring.

3. *Trephination:* Castroviejo calipers are used to locate the center of the cornea and to mark the

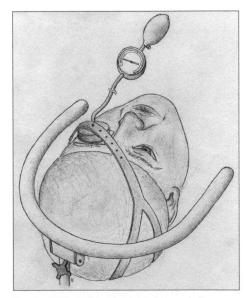

Figure 3.2.5 ◆ *Decompression:* A Honan balloon compresses the vitreous, lowering intraocular pressure and decreasing the risk of suprachoroidal hemorrhage and ocular content extrusion when the cornea is penetrated.

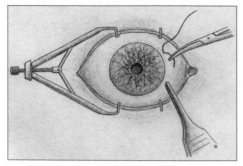

FIGURE 3.2.6 ◆ *Traction sutures:* Retrobulbar anesthesia paralyzes the extraocular muscles, but the globe can be further stabilized by placement of limbal traction sutures.

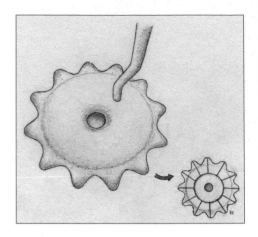

desired radius of host corneal excision (FIG. 3.2.7). Radial lines are then stained onto the corneal epithelium using a radial keratotomy marker (FIG. 3.2.8A,B). This aids in centering the prosthesis and in optimizing suture locations. A partial-thickness circular incision is then made in the cornea with a vacuum trephine (FIG. 3.2.9). Incision depth depends on

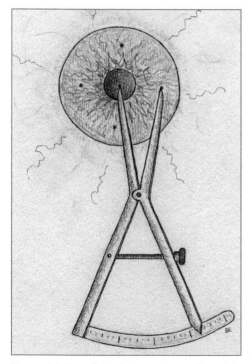

FIGURE 3.2.7 ◆ *Corneal measurements:* Castroviejo calipers are used to locate the center of the cornea and to mark the desired radius of corneal excision.

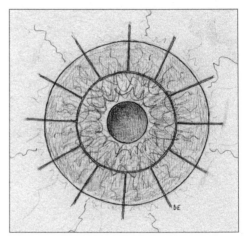

FIGURE 3.2.8 ◆ *Keratotomy marking:* Radial lines are stained onto the corneal epithelium with vital dye, using a radial keratotomy marker. These aid in centering the graft and in placing the anchoring sutures at appropriate intervals.

the several trephine revolutions (one-fourth turn = 60 microns) (FIG. 3.2.10). This incision is then completed in a controlled fashion with a fine scalpel and scissors (FIG. 3.2.11A,B).

4. *Donor Eye Preparation:* A full-thickness graft of the appropriate diameter is harvested from the donor cornea with another trephine (FIG. 3.2.12). A smaller diameter trephine is then used to remove a 3- to 3.5-mm core of tissue from the center of the graft. This creates a ring of donor cornea, which will fit snugly around the prosthesis optic.

5. *Prosthesis Assembly:* The optic is placed through the donor cornea ring, taking care to match the front plate with the anterior surface of the graft.

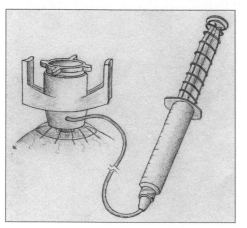

FIGURE 3.2.9 ✦ *Vacuum trephine placement:* A trephine is carefully centered on the cornea while the spring-loaded plunger is depressed. When the plunger is released (shown), vacuum pressure firmly anchors the trephine to the corneal surface.

The back plate is then placed over the optic stem and secured with a titanium lock ring.

6. *Donor implantation:* The exposed rim of donor tissue is anchored to the peripheral host cornea with partial thickness 10-0 sutures (FIG. 3.2.13). As with PKP, the gold standard is 16 evenly spaced, interrupted sutures. The wound is then tested for leakage by infusing balanced salt solution through a paracentesis tract in the peripheral cornea.

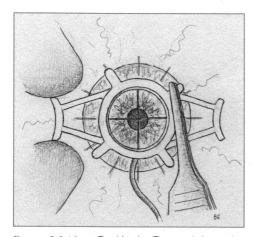

FIGURE 3.2.10 ✦ *Trephination:* The crosshairs used to center the trephine on the cornea are seen from above. The trephine knob is carefully rotated with forceps, the several turns necessary to produce an incision of the desired depth (one-fourth turn = 60 microns).

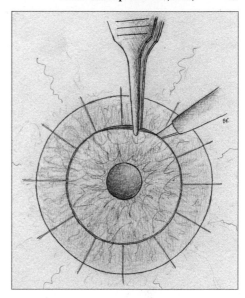

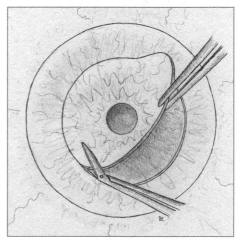

FIGURE 3.2.11 ✦ *Penetrating Keratoplasty:* A fine scalpel is used to enter the anterior chamber in a controlled fashion. Once the chamber is entered, special scissors may be used to finish removing the host cornea.

7. *Prosthesis Coverage:* It is very important to prevent drying of the ocular surface because this increases the risk of corneal breakdown or necrosis at the interface between the donor tissue and prosthesis. Recently, it has become common to protect this interface using a large-diameter soft contact lens. A colored lens that matches the contralateral iris may be selected for optimal cosmetic effect.

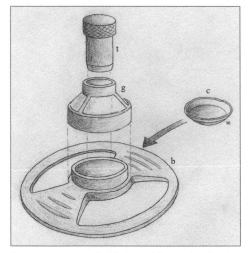

FIGURE 3.2.12 ◆ *Donor Corneal Preparation:* Another trephine is used to remove an appropriately sized donor graft from the banked cornea (c). The cylindrical blade (t) is pressed through the guide (g) to cut the donor tissue, which is cupped in the trephine base (b).

COMPLICATIONS

Intraoperative

- Suprachoroidal hemorrhage: Accumulation of blood between the choroid and sclera. The risk increases with high thoracic or intraocular pressure.

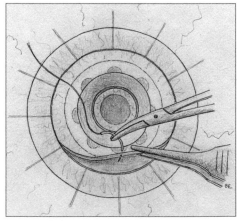

FIGURE 3.2.13 ◆ *Suturing:* Once the prosthesis and graft have been assembled, the exposed rim of donor tissue is then secured to the peripheral host cornea with partial thickness 10-0 sutures.

- Prolapse of intraocular contents: Expulsion of intraocular tissue through the corneal incision
- The risk increases with high IOP.

Postoperative

- Donor tissue melting/necrosis: Breakdown of donor tissue abutting the prosthesis can lead to aqueous leakage and infection.
- Corneal wound leakage: Leakage at the interface between host and donor cornea can lead to anterior chamber shallowing, hypotony, and increased risk of infection. It is detected with the Seidel test: Leaking aqueous will dilute fluorescein that is placed over the surgical wound.
- Retroprosthetic membrane: Postoperative uveitis can result in the formation of an avascular membrane that obstructs the KPro optic. Generally, this membrane can be removed with a neodymium-doped yttrium aluminum garnet (Nd:YAG) laser. Surgery is only occasionally required.
- Glaucoma: It is usually multifactorial in etiology. Pressure monitoring is difficult since the Goldmann applanation tonometer will not work with a KPro in place. Pressures must, therefore, be approximated with manual palpation of the eye and serial optic disc photos.
- Endophthalmitis: This may be sterile (a reaction to antigens released during tissue necrosis) or infectious (caused by inoculation of bacteria or fungi).
- Retinal detachment: Detachment is due to traction from inflammatory membranes caused by postoperative uveitis.

POSTOPERATIVE CARE

Monitor frequently for complications beginning on postoperative day one.

Administer oral antibiotics and injected steroids to control postoperative uveitis.

Instruct the patient to continuously wear a soft contact lens over the prosthesis. Applying prophylactic antibiotic drops decreases the risk of infection.

Further Reading

Text

Aquavella JV, Qian Y, McCormick GJ, et al. Keratoprosthesis: the Dohlman-Doane device. *Am J Ophthalmol.* 2005;140(6):1032–1038.

Ilhan-Sarac O, Akpek EK. Current concepts and techniques in keratoprosthesis. *Curr Opin Ophthalmol.* 2005;16(4): 246–250.

Lang G. Cornea. *Ophthalmology—A Pocket Textbook Atlas.* 2nd ed. New York, NY: Georg Thieme Verlag; 2007:chap 5.

Liu C, Hille K, Tan D, et al. Keratoprosthesis surgery. *Dev Ophthalmol.* 2008;41:171–186.

Massachusetts Eye & Ear Infirmary. *Artificial Cornea— The Boston Keratoprosthesis.* www.masseyeandear.org/specialties/ophthalmology/cornea-and-refractive-surgery/keratoprosthesis/

Primary Sources

Aldave AJ, Kamal KM, Vo RC, et al. The Boston type I keratoprosthesis: improving outcomes and expanding indications. *Ophthalmology.* 2009;116(4):640–651.

Harissi-Dagher M, Beyer J, Dohlman CH. The role of soft contact lenses as an adjunct to the Boston keratoprosthesis. *Int Ophthalmol Clin.* 2008;48(2):43–51.

Zerbe BL, Belin MW, Ciolino JB. Boston Type 1 Keratoprosthesis Study Group. Results from the multicenter Boston Type 1 Keratoprosthesis Study. *Ophthalmology.* 2006; 113(10):1779.e1–7.

3.3   KERATOREFRACTIVE SURGERY

Surgical correction of refractive error such as myopia, hyperopia, astigmatism, and presbyopia

The refractive error is corrected by modifying the radius of curvature of the anterior surface of the cornea.

INDICATIONS

Elective procedure for patients with refractive error stable for at least 1 year desiring independence from glasses or contact lenses.

CONTRAINDICATIONS

Systemic

- Autoimmune, collagen vascular, and thyroid disease
- Diabetes
- With pregnancy/nursing: induces variability in refractive error as well as changes in the tear layer
- History of abnormal wound healing: increased postoperative complications (e.g., corneal haze)
- Medications (e.g., amiodarone, retinal deposits; isotretinoin, increased risk of corneal scarring)

Ophthalmic

- Disorders that affect tear layer (e.g., dry eye, keratoconjunctivitis sicca)

- Disorders that interfere with wound healing (e.g., neurotrophic corneas, previous radial keratotomy)
- Glaucoma: Corticosteroids required after surgery can exacerbate glaucoma. Note: After corneal ablation, the central corneal thickness is decreased leading to an apparent reduction in intraocular pressure (IOP). Pachymetry is required to accurately assess central corneal thickness and adjust for measured IOP.
- Corneal aberrations (e.g., keratoconus, irregular astigmatism, pellucid marginal degeneration). Note: With new wavefront technology, milder forms of irregular astigmatism can be addressed with customized excimer ablation.
- Infectious ocular conditions (e.g., herpes keratitis)

NOTE: *Many of the above conditions are relative vs. absolute contraindications based largely on the severity of the condition.*

ALTERNATIVES

Glasses/Spectacles

- Minus lenses correct myopia and plus lenses correct hyperopia. Both of these lenses are spherical in shape.
- Astigmatism is treated with placement of cylindrical lens.

- Concurrent myopia/hyperopia with astigmatism can be treated with placement of a spherocylindrical lens.

Contact Lenses

- Contact lenses correct refractive error by altering the functional curvature of the anterior cornea.

- Hard contact lenses can modify certain forms of astigmatism by molding the anterior cornea into a spherical shape (for use in early keratoconus). The most commonly used polymers are referred to as rigid gas permeables (RGP) allowing for adequate oxygen permeability and nutrition to the anterior cornea.

- Soft contact lenses: Base curves are determined by keratometry as it matches the patient's corneal shape. The front curvature of the lens is determined by refractive error. Silicone hydrogels are the most commonly used materials, providing significant oxygen diffusion to the anterior cornea. Based largely on oxygen permeability, soft contact lenses are marketed as:
  - Daily wear (DW): to be removed prior to sleeping
  - Extended wear (EW): can be worn overnight for up to 6 days
  - Continuous wear (CW): can be worn for 1 month without removal. These lenses have 5–6 times greater oxygen permeability than conventional soft contact lenses. Adverse effects of long-term wear include:
    - Corneal infections/ulcers: due to poor lens hygiene, tear film abnormalities, bacterial stagnation
    - Allergic or giant papillary conjunctivitis due to continuous wear with a poorly fitting contact lens
    - Toric soft contact lenses can also modify astigmatism by placing a cylindrical correction in the contact lens. Orientation of the lens is therefore critical.

Alternative Refractive Surgeries

- Intraocular lens exchange: Removing a non-cataractous lens by phacoemulsification with placement of an accommodating or multifocal lens to correct the refractive error. This procedure is almost identical to that of cataract surgery.

- Implantable contact lens (ICL): Placement of a contact lens posterior to the iris and anterior to the natural lens.

RELEVANT PHYSIOLOGY/ANATOMY

Corneal Anatomy (FIG. 3.3.1)
Refractive Error Overview

- Emmetropia: Absence of refractive error

- Ametropia: Presence of refractive error

- Diopter (D): Measurement of refractive power of the lens. It is the reciprocal of the focal length of a lens (D = 1/f).

- Accommodation: Change in the refractive power of the lens to bring near objects into focus. Ciliary muscle contracts leading to increased curvature of the lens (likely via relaxation of the zonules/lens capsule) adding plus diopters to the lens. A 25 year old has ~ 10 (diopter) D of accommodation while a 50 year old has ~ 2 D of accommodation (presbyopia).

- Presbyopia: Loss of accommodation with aging. Previously emmetropic patients in their mid-to-late 40s will have difficulty reading or seeing close objects clearly. This loss of accommodation persists through the mid-50s before stabilizing. A plus lens is used to correct presbyopia because the lens does not increase the radius of curvature with relaxation of the zonules.

- Myopia ("nearsighted"): Distant images focus/converge anterior to the retina in an unaccommodated eye. Distance vision is out of focus and requires a minus lens for adequate correction. The *far point* is the point at which a distant object is focused most clearly on the retina. The reciprocal of the far point is roughly the diopter correction necessary to achieve

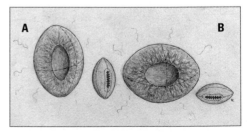

FIGURE 3.3.1 ◆ *"Against the Rule"* astigmatism **(A)** The horizontal meridian is the steepest, like a football standing on its point. This is more common in adults. *"With the Rule"* astigmatism **(B)** The vertical meridian is the steepest, like a football lying on its side. This is more common in children.

emmetropia (e.g., far point of 0.2 m = approximately a 5 D minus lens.)

a. Axial myopia: Eye is longer than average (for each millimeter of increased axial length, the patient becomes 3 D more myopic).

b. Refractive/curvature myopia: Refractive elements (e.g., corneal tear film or lens curvature) induce "overrefraction."

- Hyperopia ("farsightedness"): Images focus/converge posterior to the retina in an unaccommodated eye. Without accommodation, near vision is out of focus and requires a plus lens for adequate correction.

a. Axial hyperopia: Eye is shorter than average (e.g., congenital).

b. Refractive/curvature hyperopia: Refractive elements induce "underrefraction" (e.g., aphakia).

c. Latent hyperopia: The degree of total hyperopia corrected by accommodation; prepresbyopic patients can counteract a few diopters of hyperopia by accommodation. The extent of latent hyperopia is revealed by refraction with a cycloplegic (eliminates accommodation).

d. Manifest hyperopia: Hyperopia that cannot be corrected by accommodation. If congenital, this can be a cause of deprivation amblyopia.

e. Pediatric hyperopes: There is a connection between accommodation and convergence of the eyes. Therefore, severe hyperopes requiring significant accommodation to focus images might present with esotropia (potentially progressing to amblyopia).

- Astigmatism: Irregular corneal or lens shape that leads to different degrees of refraction and multiple focal points (thus distorting images).

a. Regular astigmatism: The cornea or lens is shaped like a football with two regular (constant power), but different radii (one shorter than the other) that are 908 apart. This leads to two different focal points in two different planes (meridians).

  ○ "With the Rule" astigmatism: The vertical meridian is the steepest (a football lying on its side). Technically, the principle meridians must be at right angles and the steeper axis is within 208 of the vertical meridian. This is more common in children.

  ○ "Against the Rule" astigmatism: The horizontal meridian is the steepest (a football standing on its point). Technically, the principle meridians must be at right angles and the steeper

axis is within 20 degrees of the horizontal meridian. This is more common in adults.

  ○ Oblique astigmatism: Principle meridians are outside 20 degrees of the horizontal or vertical meridian (obliquely placed football).

b. Irregular astigmatism: Irregularly shaped cornea in which the principal meridians are not perpendicular and have variable power. When discussing keratorefractive procedures, irregular corneal astigmatism is sometimes referred to as "higher order aberrations."

- Anisometropia: Difference in refractive error between the two eyes. In children, this can lead to monocular amblyopia because the eyes cannot accommodate differentially. That is, because the left and right images cannot be focused simultaneously, the child suppresses the nondominant image.

Classification

The history of keratorefractive surgery is extensive. However, the most procedures developed over time are rarely performed today. The most current keratorefractive surgeries involve central corneal manipulation with laser ablation superficially (Bowman's membrane) or deeper (stroma). These include photorefractive keratectomy (PRK) and laser-assisted in situ keratomileusis (LASIK), respectively. As technology improves, there has also been an increase in the several laser epithelial keratomileusis (LASEK) and laser-assisted subepithelial keratomileusis (EPI-LASEK) procedures as well.

- Photorefractive keratectomy (PRK): Surface reshaping using excimer laser on Bowman's membrane.
  - Epithelium is removed with alcohol.
  - An excimer laser ablates corneal thickness centrally to treat myopia (relative flattening of the corneal surface) or peripherally to treat hyperopia (relatively steepening the corneal surface).
  - The epithelium regenerates over time. Of the procedures listed here, this one carries the highest risk of postoperative corneal haze (see below).
  - This is a painful procedure as the epithelium is chemically removed. The patient wears a soft contact lens bandage while the corneal epithelium heals.

- Laser-assisted in situ keratomileusis (LASIK): A hinged lamellar keratectomy is created using an automated microkeratome knife or laser (creation of a 100–180 micron flap).

- Excimer laser ablation is applied to the corneal stroma followed by sutureless replacement of the flap.
- This procedure has the fastest recovery time with the lowest risk of postoperative corneal haze.
- This procedure is generally not painful but has increased risk of flap complications (see below). No soft contact lens is necessary.
- Contraindication: patients with thin corneas; after stromal ablation, 250 microns of tissue must remain.

- Laser subepithelial keratomileusis (LASEK): Removal of a thin epithelial sheet with a microkeratome blade (creating a 50 micron flap).
  - This procedure involves alcohol application to dislodge the epithelium after the initial cut by the microkeratome.
  - The excimer laser ablation occurs on Bowman's membrane.
  - This is an ideal procedure for thin corneas (which is a contraindication for LASIK).
  - Advantages over LASIK: No flap complications as this flap only involves the epithelium (can regenerate if damaged).
  - Advantages over PRK include a partially preserved epithelium. This procedure is still painful, however, as part of the epithelium is abraded (alcohol usage). This procedure also requires a soft contact lens bandage while the epithelium heals.
  - This procedure has a longer recovery time than LASIK.

- EPI-LASIK: Similar to LASEK. An epi-keratome is used to remove the epithelium (making a very thin corneal flap) followed by subsequent ablation on Bowman's membrane.
  - This specialized blade does not warrant subsequent alcohol usage to separate epithelium from Bowman's membrane (less epithelial damage the LASEK).
  - Like LASEK, this procedure is ideal for thin corneas.
  - Advantages over LASIK: No flap complications as this flap only involves the epithelium (can regenerate if damaged).
  - Painful procedure necessitating a soft contact lens bandage during the period of epithelial regeneration.

- Longer recovery time compared to LASIK, comparable to LASEK, but shorter than PRK.

PRINCIPLES OF EXCIMER LASER ABLATION

Excimer ("Excited Dimer") Laser: An 193-nm laser (ultraviolet spectrum) that ablates tissue (rather than creating burns or cuts). The laser is produced by a combination of an inert gas (argon, krypton, or xenon) with a reactive gas (fluorine or chlorine). It is used for both PRK and LASIK.

With the ArF laser, each pulse removes approximately 25 microns of tissue without damaging surrounding tissue.

- Myopic ablations: Requires more ablation in the center of the cornea.
- Hyperopic ablations: Requires more tissue removal in the periphery.
- Astigmatic ablations: Requires greater ablation in the steeper meridian.

The larger the optical zone size, the greater the depth of ablation required to achieve the same refractive correction. (Optical zone size must be greater than the scotopic pupil size in order to avoid glare/light insensitivity.)

Tracking systems: Despite perfect patient fixation, the eye still has saccadic movements. This system allows the laser to track these fine movements allowing for more accurate ablation profiles. The result of this innovation has led to "Wavefront-guided LASIK" or "custom LASIK," which minimizes "higher-order corneal aberrations" (irregular astigmatism) induced by traditional excimer lasers without a tracking device.

The laser is sensitive to humidity, temperature, and air impurities. A room that maintains exact levels of humidity/temperature and contains an air purification system is necessary to house the laser.

PREOPERATIVE SCREENING (FOR PRK AND LASIK)

Soft contact lenses must be removed 1–2 weeks before preoperative exam; hard contact lenses must be removed 3 weeks before preoperative exam. This allows for normalization of any corneal changes induced by the contact lens.

- Corneal topography: Use of keratometry/videokeratography to determine corneal shape (e.g., extent of astigmatism) and power/ refractive error of the central cornea (e.g., myopia/hyperopia).

- Pachymetry: Measures central corneal thickness. Measures central corneal thickness to determine how much stroma can safely be ablated (after ablation, a minimum of 250 microns of residual cornea is recommended).

- Determination of ocular dominance: This is important for presbyopic patients desiring monovision (e.g., nonspectacle dependence for both near and distance vision by correcting the dominant eye for distance vision and undercorrecting the nondominant eye for near vision).

- Refractive error: Objective (retinoscope determination) and subjective (patient determination) refraction for both near and far. Most importantly, cycloplegic refraction should be done to determine accommodative power.

- Scotopic (dim vision) pupil size: This will determine the width of the ablation zone (which should be larger than the scotopic pupil). To reiterate, if the ablation zone is smaller than the pupil at any point, the patient might experience significant glare or light insensitivity.

- Slit-lamp examination: Confirming absence of anterior segment pathology (particularly dry eyes).

- Dilated funduscopy: Confirming absence of posterior segment pathology.

ANESTHESIA

PRK and LASIK are generally performed under topical anesthesia.

PROCEDURE

Photorefractive keratectomy (PRK) and laser-assisted in situ keratomileusis (LASIK) are the two most commonly performed keratorefractive procedures performed and thus warrant further elaboration. The following narrative illustrates basic principles of these two procedures, which can be abstracted to other cases.

Photorefractive Keratectomy (PRK): (See Tables 3.3.1 Rapid Review of Steps and 3.3.2 Surgical Pearls, and Web Tables 3.3.1, 3.3.2, and 3.3.3 for equipment and medication lists); Ideal treatment range: 8 D of myopia to 3 D of hyperopia.

TABLE 3.3.1 Rapid Review of Steps for Photorefractive Keratectomy (PRK)
(1) Epithelial loosening and removal
(2) Excimer laser ablation
(3) Soft contact lens placement

1. *Position/Preparation:* The patient is positioned under the microscope such that the central cornea is directly perpendicular to the laser beam. Proper cleansing with Betadine is essential to remove all debris prior to laser ablation (reduces risk of laser-induced higher-order corneal aberrations). Careful centration of the eye is exceptionally important; in order to ensure this, an optical zone marker marks off a 7- to 8-mm zone centered on the pupil.

2. *Epithelial removal:* 20% alcohol solution can be used to loosen the epithelium. A blade, spatula, abrasive brush, or excimer laser is then used to remove the epithelium. Uniform epithelial removal is necessary to prevent uneven ablations and irregular astigmatism. After complete removal, the underlying Bowman's membrane is exposed.

TABLE 3.3.2 Surgical Pearls
Preoperative:
• Rule out dry eye disease. Patients with autoimmune conditions are not ideal candidates because of delayed epithelialization.
Intraoperative:
• Alcohol or anesthetic drops can be used to loosen the epithelium. Ensure that the stromal bed is dry before excimer treatment is performed. Mitomycin C (MMC) application reduces the risk of postphotorefractive keratectomy (PRK) haze. Residual MMC should be rinsed with chilled balanced salt solution (BSS) before bandage contact lenses and antibiotic/steroid drops are placed.
Postoperative:
• Remind patients that both eyes will be uncomfortable even with the bandage contact lenses until the epithelium is restored. Remind them that visual acuity will take weeks, perhaps even months before final visual acuity is achieved. Inappropriate use of dilute anesthetic drops to manage postoperative discomfort may cause anesthetic keratopathy.

3. *Excimer laser ablation:* Prior to ablation, centration is rechecked. Based on a previously calculated area of ablation (determined by refractive error), the excimer laser ablates a section of tissue; each pulse of laser removes 25 microns of tissue with minimal damage to surrounding tissue. Even hydration of the cornea is of utmost importance during ablation. A wet sponge with saline can be used to achieve even hydration across Bowman's membrane (e.g., if excessive dryness exists, the cornea thins and overcorrection results; if the cornea is overly hydrated, undercorrection results). Throughout the procedure, fixation by the patient (on a light emanating from the laser) is necessary to ensure centration.

4. *Post-Ablation:* Antibiotics, nonsteroidal anti-inflammatory drugs (NSAIDs), and steroid drops are administered. A soft contact lens is placed to reduce postoperative pain and ensure uniform epithelial healing. Alternatively, a pressure patch can be placed.

www. **Laser-assisted in situ keratomileusis (LASIK):** (See Tables 3.3.3 Rapid Review of Steps and 3.3.4 Surgical Pearls, and WEB TABLES 3.3.4 to 3.3.7 for equipment and medication lists); Larger ideal treatment range than PRK: 12 D of myopia to 4 D of hyperopia.

1. *Position/Preparation:* The patient is positioned under the microscope such that the central cornea is directly perpendicular to the laser beam. The eye is cleaned with Betadine solution and a lid speculum is placed. Using a marker, three landmarks are illustrated: (1) the optical center; (2) a line indicating the orientation of the flap; and (3) a 9-mm optical circle delineating the placement of the suction ring (FIG. 3.3.2).

TABLE 3.3.3	Rapid Review of Steps for Laser-Assisted In Situ Keratomileusis (LASIK)
(1) Flap creation with microkeratome or femtosecond laser	
(2) Flap lifting	
(3) Excimer laser ablation	
(4) Flap replacement	
(5) Interface irrigation with balanced salt solution (BSS)	
(6) Drying of flap gutters and striae test	

TABLE 3.3.4	Surgical Pearls
Preoperative:	
• Evaluate to identify poor candidates (e.g., unrealistic expectations, inconsistent refractions, large pupils, dry eye, thin corneas, risk for trauma)	
Intraoperative:	
• Assuming ideal candidate, review the steps and what the patient would experience to reduce anxiety. Have a low threshold for aborting case if flap creation is complicated. Stabilize head position with left hand on forehead to reduce risk of irregular excimer treatment.	
Postoperative:	
• Have patient close both eyes for 15 to 20 minutes before examining flaps with slit lamp. If the flaps are malpositioned, or if striae are present, relift and reposition the flap under the operating microscope.	

2a. *Creation of the flap with a microkeratome:* A suction ring is placed over the marked circle in order to prevent movement of the eye. Once adequate suction is achieved (measured by an IOP > 65 mm Hg), the microkeratome is inserted and manually advanced via a foot pedal controlled by the ophthalmologist. A spacer separating the suction ring and microkeratome determines the depth of the cut. Once the microkeratome passes to the illustrated line delineating the position of the flap, the blade is reversed to its original location (FIG. 3.3.3).

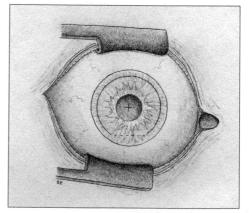

FIGURE 3.3.2 ◆ *LASIK flap setup:* The flap is generally 9 mm in diameter and remains attached to the remainder of the cornea with a "hinge" (dashed line).

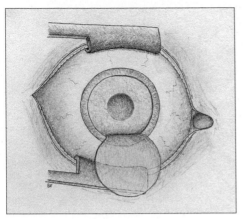

FIGURE 3.3.3 ◆ *Stromal bed ablation:* The flap is lifted to expose the underlying stromal bed, which is then reshaped with an excimer laser.

The vacuum is removed and the suction ring and microkeratome apparatus is removed.

2b. *Alternative flap creation with the femtosecond laser:* Similar to the microkeratome, a suction ring is centered over the cornea. After adequate suction, the femtosecond laser creates a stromal plane to produce the flap. The computer-operated laser has a preprogrammed flap diameter as well as thickness. Proponents of "bladeless" flap creation argue that the femtosecond laser produces a more accurate flap size, shape, and thickness.

3. *Excimer laser ablation:* The flap is lifted and folded over to expose the stromal bed. The patient fixates at a light to ensure appropriate centration. As the ablation extends toward the periphery, a blunt instrument or safety cover is placed over the hinge of the flap in order to prevent inadvertent ablation of the corneal flap.

4. *Repositioning of the flap:* After irrigating the underside of the corneal flap and stromal bed with saline, the flap is placed onto the stromal bed with a blunt instrument. Saline is infused in the interface between the flap and bed to ensure removal of all debris. After the interface is dry, a "stria test" is conducted to determine successful placement of the flap. That is, with peripheral corneal depression, stria, or lines pass onto the flap from all angles.

5. *Closure:* An antibiotic and NSAID drop are administered. The speculum is slowly removed and

the patient is instructed to slowly close his or her eyes. A shield is placed to prevent dislocation of the flap.

COMPLICATIONS

Photorefractive Keratectomy (PRK)

- Undercorrection: Likely due to inadequate surgical ablation, excessive corneal hydration, or excessive wound healing. Postoperative management involves increasing topical steroids to slow wound healing.

- Overcorrection: For the first month, 1 D of overcorrection is necessary to account for the usual 0.5 to 1.0 D regression over the first year postoperatively. Unintended overcorrection is likely due to excessive surgical ablation, inadequate corneal hydration, or poor wound healing.

- Corneal haze/scarring: Typically appears 1–4 months postoperatively with resolution by 1 year. Late-onset haze is less common but occurs 4–14 months postoperatively and is generally more severe, warranting steroids and/or mitomycin C treatment. Late-onset haze is linked to ultraviolet (UV) exposure; patients are advised to wear UV protection for 2 years postoperatively.

- Central islands: Central elevations in the corneal topography likely because of increased central corneal hydration during ablation. Resolution might occur spontaneously or require retreatment.

- Pain: Epithelium is innervated by pain fibers leading to postoperative pain. Topical NSAIDS significantly reduce pain by inhibiting prostaglandin release.

- Decentration: Due to poor preoperative management or poor patient fixation during ablation. Patient reports increased glare and decreased visual acuity (VA) with keratometry indicating irregular astigmatism. Retreatment is generally required.

- Higher-order visual aberrations: Patient reports glare/haloes (mostly at night). These symptoms generally subside within 6 months. With advent of tracking systems and "Wavefront-guided LASIK," these symptoms are reported less frequently.

- Infectious keratitis: Requires appropriate diagnostic workup (Gram stain and culture) and broad spectrum antibiotics. Adverse effects include haze/scarring and decrease in VA.

Laser-assisted in situ keratomileusis (LASIK)

- Microkeratome complications: Include free cap (complete flap dislocation), incomplete flap, thin flap, irregular flap, or buttonhole (blade surfaces in the middle leading to hole in the middle of the flap).
- Undercorrection or overcorrection: Some extent of overcorrection is acceptable immediately postoperative.
- Central islands: See above.
- Decentration: See above.
- Diffuse lamellar keratitis (DLK): An inflammatory response at the flap/stromal bed interface characterized by diffuse, white granular deposits. Etiology is unknown although it is believed to be caused by debris left at the interface producing an inflammatory response. The patient may present with tearing, pain, foreign body sensation, and photophobia within 1 week postoperatively. Treatment involves hourly low-dose topical steroids. If significant granularity is observed, the flap might need to be lifted and the interface adequately irrigated with sterile saline.
- Epithelial ingrowth: Opacification of the flap/stromal interface due to proliferation of epithelial cells. Commonly seen within the first month postoperatively. The patient may present with foreign body sensation, glare, photophobia, and/or decrease in visual acuity. If significant, the flap must be lifted with adequate scraping and irrigation of the interface before resetting the flap.
- Keratoectasia: Randleman et al. identified risk factors for this complication: abnormal topography (primary risk factor), corneal thickness of < 510 microns, residual stromal bed thickness of < 300 microns, age < 30 years, and myopia > 8 D. Risk factors are additive with cumulative score stratifying patients preoperatively into low-, moderate-, and high-risk categories. High-risk patients should not undergo LASIK due to the likelihood of postoperative keratectasia.
- Infectious keratitis: See above.
- Flap striae: Likely due to poor flap alignment, forceful postoperative blinking, or a mismatch between the posterior flap curvature and stromal bed. Vision is affected if the wrinkle or striae

enters the visual field. Lifting the flap and adequately irrigating before resetting is generally necessary if visual acuity is adversely affected.

POSTOPERATIVE CARE

PRK

- Bandage soft contact lens is removed after 3–5 days once adequate epithelial healing has occurred.
- Antibiotics and NSAIDS are discontinued after the epithelium has healed.
- Topical steroids are tapered over 3–6 months based on postoperative refractive correction. Steroid usage is increased if patient is undercorrected and is decreased more rapidly if patient is overcorrected.
- If epithelial haze is increased, topical steroid dosage is increased as well.
- UV protection is advised for 1–2 years to avoid late-onset corneal haze.

LASIK

- Follow-up in clinic the next day to assess proper flap placement, interface debris, and visual acuity (success = better than 20/40).
- Continue prophylactic antibiotics four times per day for the first week. Topical steroids or lubrication are optional (and largely surgeon dependent).
- Normal activity can be resumed after the first day. Patients are advised to avoid contact sports and rubbing their eyes, in order to minimize the chance of flap dislocation. This is a rare complication, however, after the first few days.

Further Reading

Text

Kramarevsky N, Hardten, DR. Excimer laser photorefractive keratectomy (PRK). In: Yanoff M, Duker J, eds. *Ophthalmology*. 3rd ed. Philadelphia, PA: Mosby; 2009:131–145.

Tatsuya M, Azar DT. Current concepts, classification, and history of refractive surgery. In: Yanoff M, Duker J, eds. *Ophthalmology*. 3rd ed. Philadelphia, PA: Mosby; 2009:107–118.

Wilkinson PS, Davis EA, Hardten RD. LASIK complications. In: Yanoff M, Duker J, eds. *Ophthalmology*. 3rd ed. Philadelphia, PA: Mosby; 2009:145–159.

Young JA, Kornmehl EW. Preoperative evaluation for refractive surgery. In: Yanoff M, Duker J, eds. *Ophthalmology*. 3rd ed. Philadelphia, PA: Mosby; 2009:118–122.

Primary Sources

Ditaen K, Anschuetz T, Shroeder E. Photorefractive keratectomy to treat low, medium, and high myopia: a multicenter study. *J Cataract Refract Surg*. 1994;20(suppl): 234–238.

Mrochen M, Kaemmerer M, Seiler T. Wavefront-guided laser in situ keratomileusis: early results in three eyes. *J Refract Surg*. 2000;16(2):116–121.

Puliafito CA, Steinert RF, Deutsch TF, et al. Excimer laser ablation of the cornea and lens: experimental studies. *Ophthalmology*. 1985;92(6):741–748.

Randleman JB, Woodward M, Lynn MJ, et al. Risk assessment for ectasia after corneal refractive surgery. *Ophthalmology*. 2008;115(1):37–50.

Sher NA, Chen V, Bowers RA, et al. The use of the 193-nm excimer laser for myopic photorefractive keratectomy in sighted eyes: a multi-center study. *Arch Ophthalmol*. 1991;109(11): 1525–1530.

3.4 PTERYGIUM REMOVAL

- Surgical excision of a fibrovascular proliferation of bulbar conjunctiva that has grown over the peripheral cornea.

- The most basic procedure entails pterygium excision without conjunctival closure (the *bare scleral technique*). Recurrence rates tend to be high and can be reduced significantly with adjunctive techniques.

INDICATIONS

- Timing of surgical intervention depends on the patient's tolerance of symptoms and interest in cosmetic improvement. He or she must understand that recurrent growth is possible and tends to be more aggressive.

- Indications to operate include visual axis obstruction, irritation unrelieved by medical therapy, irregular astigmatism, and restricted ocular motility/diplopia.

ALTERNATIVES AND ADJUNCTIVE TECHNIQUES

Medical Therapy

- Conservative measures: The likelihood of growth is reduced by using hats and sunglasses for ultraviolet (UV) protection and by avoiding smoky or dusty environments.

- Preservative free lubricants: Frequent application can reduce symptoms of irritation.

- Mild topical steroids/Nonsteroidal anti-inflammatory drugs (NSAIDs): Drops can be applied to control inflammation of the ocular surface.

Adjunctive techniques to reduce recurrence:

- Primary closure: Creation of relaxing incisions permits previously unexposed conjunctiva to be rotated into the palpebral fissure and closed over the defect.

- Autograft: Unexposed conjunctiva from the superotemporal quadrant is harvested and transferred to fill the defect.

- Amniotic membrane transplant (AMT): Preserved allograft is sutured and/or glued over the defect. Use does not require systemic immunosuppression due to low antigenicity.

- Antiproliferative agents: Intraoperative administration of mitomycin C (MMC) to the excision site reduces recurrence but may cause scleral/corneal ulceration, uveitis, and secondary glaucoma at higher doses.

- Beta radiation: Exposure to strontium-90 decreases the replication of vascular cells that permit recurrent growth, but is associated with risk of scleral necrosis, cataract formation, and persistent epithelial defects.

- Excimer laser: A 193-nm wavelength argon-fluoride laser can be used to smooth corneal surface irregularities and encourage wound reepithelialization.

- Anterior lamellar keratoplasty: Transplants can be used to treat extensive scarring or thinning of the cornea, often after multiple surgeries for pterygium recurrence.
- Limbal stem cell transplant: This may restore the potential for reepithelialization if prior pterygium surgery has damaged the limbal stem cells. Donor tissue is taken from the healthy contralateral eye or from donor corneoscleral tissue.

RELEVANT PHYSIOLOGY/ANATOMY

Pterygium Overview

- A fibrovascular proliferation of exposed bulbar conjunctiva that invades the cornea and damages Bowman's membrane.
- Pterygia originates nasally 90% of the time. They are often bilateral and rarely cross the midline of the eye.
- The highest incidence is near the equator; development is associated with prolonged exposure to UV radiation, wind, and dust.
- Prevalence increases with age.
- Growth may stop spontaneously at any stage of development.
- Recurrent lesions tend to grow more aggressively than primary lesions.

Pterygium Anatomy (FIG. 3.4.1)

Three components

- Body: The conjunctival base is thickened and vascular.
- Head: The apex is thinned and firmly adherent to the cornea.
- Cap: A subepithelial "halo" can be seen at the leading edge of the lesion.

Pinguecula Overview

- Exposed bulbar conjunctiva becomes thickened and discolored but does not extend onto the cornea.
- Lesions are histologically identical to pterygia, but without the associated Bowman's membrane defects.
- Incidence increases with age and exposure to UV radiation, wind, and dust. Most people develop pingueculae by 70 years of age.
- They are generally asymptomatic but occasionally become inflamed. Pingueculitis can be treated with mild topical steroids or NSAIDs.

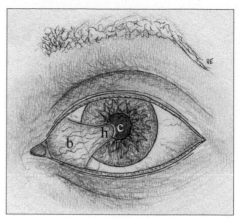

FIGURE 3.4.1 ◆ *Pterygium:* A fibrovascular proliferation of bulbar conjunctiva that has grown over the peripheral cornea. It consists of three zones: A *body* with a thickened, vascular conjunctival base (b), a thinner *head* firmly adherent to the cornea (h), and a *cap*, or subepithelial "halo," at the leading edge of the lesion (c).

PREOPERATIVE SCREENING

- Rule out pseudopterygium.
- Pseudopterygia are fibrovascular extensions of bulbar conjunctiva that adhere to the cornea at sites of prior damage (e.g., inflammation, ulceration, and chemical injury).
- Unlike pterygia, they do not adhere to the limbus. Try passing an instrument behind the body of the lesion to differentiate it from a true pterygium.
- They may arise in atypical locations (i.e., from conjunctiva that has not been exposed within the palpebral fissure) and can be treated with simple lysis.

ANESTHESIA

- Topical or sub-Tenon's anesthesia is sufficient for most patients.
- General anesthesia may be necessary for pediatric and uncooperative patients.

PROCEDURE

1. *Bare Scleral Technique:* The entire pterygium is excised, leaving the underlying bare sclera exposed.

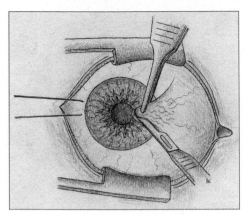

FIGURE 3.4.2 ◆ *Bare scleral technique:* The pterygium head is placed on tension with forceps and dissected off of the cornea with a fine blade.

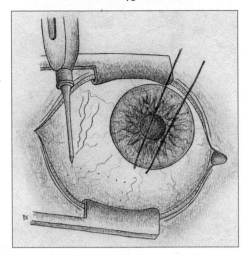

FIGURE 3.4.4 ◆ *Conjunctival autograft:* After pterygium removal, the dimensions of the bare scleral defect are measured. Limbal traction sutures are then used to rotate the globe inferomedially, exposing the superotemporal donor site. A patch of conjunctiva of the appropriate size is then outlined with cautery spots.

First, the globe is abducted with a limbal traction suture. The pterygium head is then placed on tension with forceps and dissected off of the cornea with a fine blade (FIG. 3.4.2). The pterygium body, along with underlying Tenon's capsule, is dissected away from the medial rectus and removed. Finally, the cornea is polished with a diamond bur or laser to create a smooth surface for epithelial migration.

2. *Adjunctive Procedures to Prevent Recurrence*
   • *Primary Closure:* After pterygium excision, relaxing incisions are made to create superior and inferior conjunctival flaps that can be rotated into the palpebral fissure. This permits closure of the defect and provides a smooth surface for tear film distribution (FIG. 3.4.3).

• *Autograft:* After excision, the defect is filled with harvested conjunctiva. First, the bare scleral defect is measured to create a template for the conjunctival autograft. Limbal traction sutures are then used to rotate the globe inferomedially, exposing a superotemporal donor site, which is outlined with cautery spots (FIG. 3.4.4). The conjunctival graft is harvested with scissors (FIG. 3.4.5). It is then sutured over the defect and/or glued

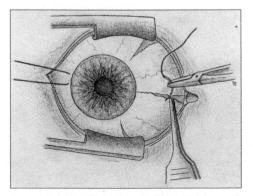

FIGURE 3.4.3 ◆ *Primary closure:* After pterygium excision, relaxing incisions are made, and superior and inferior conjunctival flaps are rotated into the palpebral fissure, permitting closure of the defect.

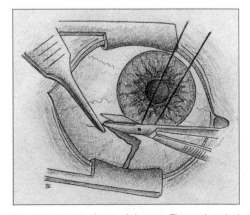

FIGURE 3.4.5 ◆ *Autograft harvest:* The conjunctival autograft is dissected free from underlying layers with scissors. This donor site is generally left open.

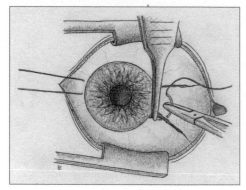

FIGURE 3.4.6 ◆ *Graft placement:* Autograft or amniotic membrane can be sutured over the defect. Amniotic membrane may be glued to the underlying layers for additional security.

with fibrin sealant (FIG. 3.4.6). The donor site is generally left open.

- *Amniotic Membrane Transplant*: A processed amniotic membrane can be used in place of conjunctival autograft and is the preferred adjunct in dry eyes. It provides a substrate for epithelial migration and will ultimately result in greater conjunctival mucin production. As with autograft, it is sutured over the defect and/or glued with fibrin sealant. Initial inflammation can be reduced with topical steroids, but systemic immunosuppression is not required.

COMPLICATIONS

- Medial rectus injury: Cautious dissection is necessary to prevent damage resulting in postoperative diplopia.
- Recurrence:
  - Generally more aggressive, with higher incidence of growth into the visual axis.
  - Usually occurs within a year, often as early as 6 to 8 weeks postoperatively.

POSTOPERATIVE CARE

- Administer antibiotics and oral analgesics.
- Perform regular follow-up to monitor for recurrence.
- The specifics of care depend on which adjunctive technique is used (e.g., topical steroids to reduce the inflammation associated with amniotic membrane transplant).

Further Reading

Text

Ang LP, Chua JL, Tan DT. Current concepts and techniques in pterygium treatment. *Curr Opin Ophthalmol.* 2007;18(4): 308–313.

Lang G. Conjunctiva. In: *Ophthalmology—A Pocket Textbook Atlas.* 2nd ed. New York, NY: Georg Thieme Verlag; 2007:chap 4.

Marten L, Wang MX, Karp CL, et al. Conjunctival surgery. In: Yanoff M, Duker J, eds. *Ophthalmology.* 3rd ed. Philadelphia, PA: Mosby; 2009:363–366.

Todani A, Melki SA. Pterygium: current concepts in pathogenesis and treatment. *Int Ophthalmol Clin.* 2009;49(1): 21–30.

Primary Sources

Farid M, Pirnazar JR. Pterygium recurrence after excision with conjunctival autograft: a comparison of fibrin tissue adhesive to absorbable sutures. *Cornea.* 2009; 28(1):43–45.

Hirst LW. Prospective study of primary pterygium surgery using pterygium extended removal followed by extended conjunctival transplantation. *Ophthalmology.* 2008;115(10):1663–1672.

Küçükerdönmez C, Akova YA, Altınörs DD. Comparison of conjunctival autograft with amniotic membrane transplantation for pterygium surgery: surgical and cosmetic outcome. *Cornea.* 2007;26(4):407–413.

Solomon A, Kaiserman I, Raiskup FD, Landau D, et al. Long-term effects of mitomycin C in pterygium surgery on scleral thickness and the conjunctival epithelium. *Ophthalmology.* 2004;111(8):1522–1527.

CHAPTER 4

General and Comprehensive

Hylton R. Mayer, Susan Forster, and C. Robert Bernardino

4.1   CATARACT EXTRACTION

- Removal of opaque native lens material to restore visual acuity (VA)
- The most common eye operation in the United States and worldwide

INDICATIONS

- Surgery is generally performed when the patient's activities of daily living are affected by decreased vision that is attributable to the cataract. With bilateral cataracts, the eye with worse VA is operated on first.
- While most cataract surgery is elective, mature or hypermature cataracts may require emergent removal to treat phacomorphic or phacolytic glaucoma.
- Extraction may be necessary for thorough assessment of retinal pathology.
- Due to third-party payment, attempts may be made to quantify the threshold for surgery. The American Academy of Ophthalmology recommends best corrected VA less than or equal to 20/50 in dim, ambient light.
- Many ophthalmologists employ "glare testing" to assess VA under conditions that more accurately reflect real-life situations. Impairment can also be assessed with the Visual Function Index, a standardized questionnaire used to screen for cataract symptoms.

ALTERNATIVES

Medical Therapy
- Lifestyle and medical interventions may reduce the incidence of cataract formation (e.g., smoking

cessation, dietary improvement, limitation of ultraviolet (UV) light and steroid exposure, and control of ocular or systemic diseases).
- Once a cataract has formed, there is no effective medical treatment.
- Galactosemic, hyperglycemic, and traumatic cataracts will occasionally resolve with time and/or correction of metabolic abnormalities (e.g., with a galactose-free diet).

SURGICAL TECHNIQUES AND INTRAOCULAR LENSES

Types of Surgery
- Phacoemulsification ("phaco"): The most common extraction technique in the United States. Ultrasonic energy is used to break apart the cataract, which can then be removed with irrigation and aspiration, leaving the lens capsule intact. This is performed through a sub-3-mm limbal incision into the anterior chamber.
- Extracapsular cataract extraction ("ECCE" or "extra-cap"): The historic predecessor to phacoemulsification, now generally reserved for cataracts too dense for ultrasonic removal. The cataractous lens is expressed en bloc through a 5- to 10-mm limbal incision, leaving the lens capsule intact.
- Intracapsular cataract extraction ("ICCE" or "intra-cap"): The predecessor to ECCE, it is now very rare in the United States. After enzymatic or mechanic lysis of the lens zonules, the cataractous lens and capsular bag are removed as a unit through a 10-mm limbal incision.

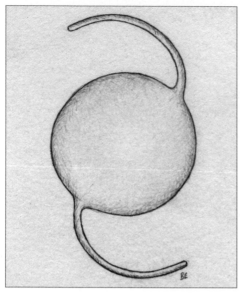

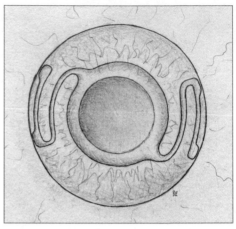

A

B

FIGURE 4.1.1 ◆ *Intraocular lenses:* **(A)** A posterior chamber intraocular lens (PCIOL) consists of a central optic coupled to twin haptics that support the lens in the capsular bag. Haptics are integrated in one-piece IOLs (shown) and distinct in three-piece IOLs. **(B)** An anterior chamber intraocular lens (ACIOL) is seen secured in the angle, anterior to the iris and pupil. In cases with inadequate capsular support, ACIOL placement may be technically simpler than alternative PCIOL placement.

Lens Type/Placement

- Typically, an acrylic or silicone posterior chamber intraocular lens (PCIOL) is placed in the evacuated capsular bag at the time of cataract removal (FIG. 4.1.1A).
- Alternative lens locations and/or types are used in a number of circumstances:
  - Several compromised lens zonules: An endocapsular ring is inserted to stabilize the capsular bag, permitting the use of a standard PCIOL.
  - Many compromised lens zonules: The capsular bag cannot be used, so the PCIOL is inserted in an alternative location or an anterior chamber intraocular lens (ACIOL) is substituted.
  - Alternative PCIOL placement: A PCIOL can be fixed to the iris or sclera with sutures or can be placed in the ciliary sulcus, which lies between the posterior iris and ciliary body. Because the distance between the cornea and lens changes with these techniques, IOL power must be recalculated (see Appendix: Intraocular Lens Calculation).
  - ACIOL placement: An anterior chamber lens can be inserted in the angle (FIG. 4.1.1B) or fixed to the iris.

- IOL optic types: Monofocal lenses are used most commonly, but several "premium lens" alternatives are rapidly growing in popularity.
- Multifocal lenses: The IOL power varies from top to bottom to permit near vision without the use of reading glasses.
- Toric lenses: IOL power varies in different meridians to permit correction of astigmatism. Proper intraoperative positioning is critical to lens function.
- Pseudo-accommodative lenses: The anterior-posterior position of the lens optic changes with ciliary body contraction, permitting mild accommodation for near vision.

- Aphakic spectacles and/or contacts are very rarely used in place of IOLs.

RELEVANT ANATOMY AND PATHOPHYSIOLOGY

Lens Overview (FIG. 4.1.2)

Origin: The lens is formed by embryologic invagination of the surface ectoderm.

Attachments: The equator of the lens capsule is suspended by fibrous zonules that radiate from the ciliary body.

Components:

- Capsule: An acellular, elastic basement membrane that contains the cortex and nucleus of the lens. Capsular integrity is essential for maintaining the lens contents in a relative state of dehydration. Traumatic penetration of the capsule will result in lens swelling and opacity. The anterior capsule is significantly thicker than the posterior capsule.

- Epithelium: A single anterior layer of cells that regulate lens homeostasis and differentiate into new lens fibers.

- Fibers: Thin, densely packed cells that account for most of the lens volume. The newest fibers are found in the cortex, whereas the oldest are contained within the nucleus. When mature, lens fibers do not contain nuclei or organelles.

Function:

- The lens provides between 10 and 20 diopters (D) of refraction, depending on the accommodative state, and helps focus light onto the retina. The curvature of the cornea and its interface with air supplies the majority of refractive power.

- It also protects the retina from UV radiation.

Growth:

- The lens is the only internal organ that grows throughout life. Increasing age predisposes one to angle closure glaucoma due to crowding of the anterior segment structures.

- It is nourished by aqueous diffusion through the lens capsule.

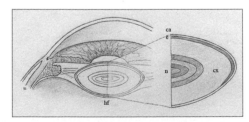

FIGURE 4.1.2 ◆ *Native lens anatomy:* The lens rests in the hyaloid fossa (hf) of the vitreous and is supported circumferentially by zonules anchored to the ciliary body. The nucleus (n), from outside to inside, consists of adult, infantile, fetal, and embryonic layers. It is surrounded by the cortex (cx), anterior lens epithelium (e), and basement membrane capsule (ca).

Age-related changes:

- Water content, metabolic activity, antioxidant synthesis, and elasticity decrease with age.

- The proportion of insoluble to soluble lens proteins increases with age.

- These changes predispose to cataract formation and underlie the development of presbyopia.

Key Terms

- Aphakic: The adjective used to describe an eye after extraction of the native lens without IOL placement (Noun: aphakia).

- Pseudophakic: The adjective used to describe an eye after extraction of the native lens, with IOL placement (Noun: pseudophakia).

Cataract Classification

Acquired

- Age-related ("senile"): The most common form of cataract, seen in patients 50 years of age and older with no apparent precipitating cause.

- Systemic disease-associated: Potential causes include diabetes, galactosemia, and renal insufficiency, which can cause osmotic swelling of the lens.

- Secondary: Due to primary intraocular pathology, such as uveitis.

- Postoperative: Common after vitrectomy with silicone oil or gas tamponade.

- Traumatic: Due to ocular contusion, capsule penetration, electrical injuries, or ionizing radiation.

- Toxic: Caused by exposure to drugs or toxic agents, such as corticosteroids, anticholinergics, phenothiazines, and substances in tobacco smoke.

Congenital

- May be idiopathic, hereditary, or due to transplacental infections, such as rubella, mumps, and hepatitis (remember TORCHES which refers to congenital infections such as **TO**xoplasmosis, **R**ubella, **C**ytomegalovirus, **HE**rpes symplex, and **S**yphilis).

Cataract Morphology

- Nuclear: Accumulation of altered lens proteins causes gradual development of a central, yellow-to-brown cataract (nuclear sclerosis). The nucleus becomes denser, resulting in an increased index of refraction. In presbyopic patients, this produces lenticular myopia or "second sight." Individuals previously dependent on reading glasses may become more comfortable without them.

- Cortical: Degeneration of the peripheral lens fibers, coupled with the development of fluid-filled vacuoles, causes early loss of VA and problems with glare. Cortical cataracts may progress to form white "intumescent" mature cataracts.

- Anterior subcapsular: A plaque of opaque connective tissue is synthesized by the lens epithelial cells. This may occur in response to anterior segment inflammation.

- Posterior subcapsular: Lens epithelial cells, normally found anterior to the equator, migrate posteriorly under the influence of various stimuli. Here they form misshapen, globular fibers called "bladder cells." These cells accumulate, causing glare and rapid onset of visual loss despite occupying only a small volume of the lens. This form of cataract frequently develops with exposure to corticosteroids or radiation.

- Mature: This is the common end-stage of all forms of cataract; VA is generally reduced to Hand Motion or Light Perception.

- Hypermature: Liquefaction of the cortex permits leakage of lens proteins, resulting in a flaccid capsular bag. Macrophages ingest these proteins and may obstruct the trabecular meshwork, elevating intraocular pressure (phacolytic glaucoma). Emergent cataract extraction is indicated to preserve the retinal nerve fiber layer.

PREOPERATIVE SCREENING

- Exclude other potential causes of decreased vision with a careful exam of the anterior chamber and fundus. Test for the presence of a relative afferent pupillary defect (APD), which could indicate damage to the retina or optic nerve. Be sure to rule out refractive error, corneal disease, glaucoma, macular degeneration, optic nerve atrophy, and so forth.

- Perform biometry to calculate the ideal refractive power of the intraocular lens (see Appendix: Intraocular Lens Calculation for details).

- Use A-scan ultrasound to measure the axial length, anterior chamber depth, and lens thickness.

- Use keratometry to evaluate the corneal curvature and refractive power.

- Use B-scan ultrasound to assess the posterior segment if a mature cataract prevents adequate visualization of the fundus by routine ophthalmoscopy.

TABLE 4.1.1 Rapid Review of Steps
(1) Premedication
(2) Paracentesis incision
(3) Vital dye injection (optional for dense cataracts)
(4) Viscoelastic injection
(5) Creation of main incision
(6) Capsulorrhexis
(7) Hydrodissection
(8) Hydrodelineation (optional: surgeon preference)
(9) Nuclear phacoemulsification
(10) Cortex cleanup
(11) Inflation of capsular bag
(12) Lens injection
(13) Evaluate wound (hydration or suture placement as necessary)
(14) Postmedication and shield

ANESTHESIA

Retrobulbar, peribulbar, or topical anesthesia is sufficient for most patients (see Appendix: Local Anesthesia in Ophthalmology for details).

- Retrobulbar block: Injection of local anesthetic inside the muscle cone produces reliable, rapid-onset anesthesia and akinesia, but has the highest rate of complications (e.g., globe perforation, optic nerve damage, and retrobulbar hemorrhage).

- Peribulbar block: A higher volume of anesthesia is injected outside of the muscle cone, resulting in a slower onset of anesthesia but minimizing the risk of optic nerve damage.

- Topical anesthesia: Has a rapid onset of action with few complications but does not provide akinesia, resulting in a more technically challenging case.

General anesthesia is required for children and may be necessary in rare circumstances for anxious or uncooperative adults.

PROCEDURE

 SEE TABLES 4.1.1 Rapid Review of Steps and 4.1.2 Surgical Pearls, and WEB TABLES 4.1.1 to 4.1.4 for equipment and medication lists. For information on phacoemulsification techniques and settings, please refer to Appendix: Phacoemulsification Principles and Techniques.

TABLE 4.1.2 Surgical Pearls

Preoperative:
- Patient selection, identification of existing ocular pathology, and preoperative planning are critical for successful cataract surgery.
- Obtain a history of previous trauma, ocular inflammation or serious infection (such as herpetic keratitis), use (or previous use) of α-adrenergic agonists such as tamsulosin (Flomax), and other significant ocular disease.
- Surgeons should note and correct ocular adnexal problems such as blepharitis, lagophthalmos, nasolacrimal duct obstruction, or lid malposition prior to surgery, as many of these disorders can increase the risk of endophthalmitis.
- Record anterior chamber depth, pupil dilation, presence of pseudoexfoliation, phacodonesis (movement of the lens), or zonular loss, grade of cataract, and quality of red reflex.
- Perform a thorough exam looking for any systemic or ocular pathology that may complicate the perioperative experience or limit the final visual outcome. Common ocular comorbidities one may encounter include corneal scars or irregular astigmatism, retinal tears or detachments, epiretinal membranes, macular degeneration or other macular pathology, and glaucoma or other optic neuropathies.
- Identify nonocular patient factors that may complicate the intraoperative experience such as significant anxiety, hearing loss, kyphosis, or chronic obstructive pulmonary disease (COPD).
- Set realistic patient expectations, especially in the setting of significant ocular comorbidities.

Intraoperative Pearls:
- It is often useful to position the patient under the microscope prior to scrubbing and prepping the patient, as it can confirm the appropriate position and/or allow easier manipulation of the patient, bed, and microscope to an ideal surgical position. Evaluation of the patient and eye under the microscope can also help identify the quality of the red reflex or other ocular pathologies that may have not been noticed during (or changed since) the initial surgical consultation.
- The patient's forehead and maxilla should be parallel with the floor.
- The bed height should be adjusted to allow the surgeon's legs to fit comfortably under the headrest, while maintaining the surgeon's arms at a natural angle (90 to 100 degrees).
- If the patient has significant kyphosis or back pain, the neck and back rests should be positioned to allow the patient to lie comfortably. Once the patient is comfortable, it is often possible to elevate the entire bed and lower the cranial portion of the bed (Trendelenburg position).
- General anesthesia should be considered if a comfortable position for the patient and/or a safe position for the surgeon are not obtained.
- Taping the patient's head can serve as a reminder to the patient and help prevent significant intraoperative head movements.
- Anesthesia should be tapered to the patient's comfort and level of anxiety. Too much anesthesia can result in disinhibition and excess patient movement or disorientation.
- Retrobulbar blocks (50:50 mix of 2% lidocaine and 0.75% Marcaine) are most appropriate for early surgeons as a successful block results in excellent anesthesia and paralysis. Peribulbar blocks also allow excellent anesthesia and variable degrees of paralysis. Blocks have higher risk of damage to the globe or retrobulbar structures, often require more significant anesthesia and preoperative manipulation, and can result in undesirable periocular ecchymosis.
- Topical anesthesia are typically only appropriate for cooperative patients and experienced, efficient surgeons. Generally for successful topical anesthesia, a surgeon should be able to perform a fast and controlled capsulorrhexis (under 30 seconds), and the entire case should not exceed 30 minutes.
- One factor that has been definitively shown to reduce the risk of endophthalmitis include treatment of preexisting adnexal disease and the use of 5% Betadine in the fornices and 10% Betadine to scrub lashes and prep the skin. Preoperative and postoperative antibiotics have not been shown to change rates of endophthalmitis, but they have become commonplace, do not seem to hurt the patient, and may provide a benefit.
- Fast intraoperative times should be a result of efficient movements, early identification of intraoperative situations, and appropriate use of techniques and maneuvers. Large, fast movements in an effort to reduce surgical times often results in more complications and longer surgical times. *Be efficient, not fast.*

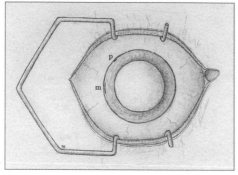

FIGURE 4.1.3 ◆ *Incision placement:* A view of the dilated left eye, demonstrating typical locations of the paracentesis (p) and main (m) corneal incisions for a right-handed surgeon. The temporal main incision is used to introduce the capsulorrhexis forceps, phacoemulsification probe, and lens injection system.

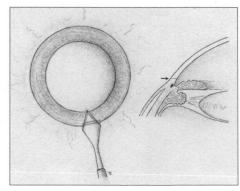

FIGURE 4.1.4 ◆ *Clear corneal tunnel:* A specialized blade is used to create a self-sealing incision in the temporal cornea. The cross-section demonstrates the location of a uniplanar incision with respect to anterior chamber anatomy. Some surgeons elect to make multiplanar incisions.

The exact sequence varies depending on surgeon preference and the requirements of a particular case. Outlined below are the general steps that you are likely to encounter in cataract phacoemulsification with PCIOL placement.

1. *Preoperative Medication:* Pupillary dilation permits exposure of the anterior lens capsule, and is usually achieved by combining a topical sympathomimetic (e.g., phenylephrine) with a parasympatholytic (e.g., tropicamide). Nonsteroidal anti-inflammatory drugs (NSAIDs) can be added to decrease operative inflammation and help to inhibit miosis through blockage of PGE_2 production. Antibiotic prophylaxis is given to cover conjunctival and skin flora that can cause endophthalmitis.

2. *Paracentesis Incision/Viscoelastic Injection:* A 1-mm paracentesis port is made in the peripheral cornea with a fine blade, permitting injection of viscoelastic media (FIG. 4.1.3). This incision should be oriented for easy access with the surgeon's nondominant hand. Viscoelastics are thick, jelly-like polymers that stabilize the anterior chamber while protecting the corneal endothelium and posterior lens capsule during cataract emulsification.

3. *Main Incision:* A 2.2- to 2.8-mm incision in the temporal limbus or clear cornea is then made with a specialized blade that forms a self-sealing tunnel into the anterior chamber (FIG. 4.1.4). Some surgeons manipulate the blade to create a multiplanar tunnel, which may reduce the

likelihood of wound leakage, but is not essential for a sutureless closure. Wider incisions should be made more peripherally to permit astigmatic neutrality and may require sutures for adequate closure. Although clear corneal incisions are popular, some surgeons prefer to create a scleral tunnel, initiating the incision approximately 1 mm posterior to the limbus. Some also place their incisions at specific clock-hour locations to achieve a predictable effect on preoperative corneal astigmatism.

4. *Vital Dye Injection:* A good red reflex aids visualization of the capsulorrhexis. Since dense cataracts may obscure this reflex, a vital dye such as trypan blue can be injected to stain the lens capsule and help differentiate it from underlying lens material.

5. *Capsulorrhexis:* A cystotome or pair of fine forceps is introduced through the main incision to make a controlled, circular tear in the anterior lens capsule, permitting access to the underlying cortex and nucleus (FIG. 4.1.5). To preserve capsular integrity and ensure IOL stability, it is essential to prevent the advancing edge of the capsulorrhexis from straying too far peripherally. This can be avoided by perpendicular application of force, and by frequent regrasping of the free capsular edge. In the event that it does occur, the capsulorrhexis can be rescued by redirecting with a series of short "can opener" incisions.

6. *Hydrodissection:* Balanced salt solution (BSS) is injected between the posterior lens capsule and

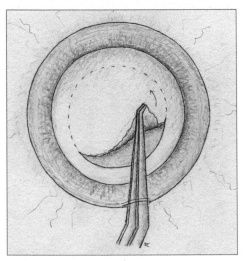

FIGURE 4.1.5 ◆ *Continuous curvilinear capsulor-rhexis:* The anterior capsule is removed with fine forceps to expose the underlying lens material for phacoemulsification.

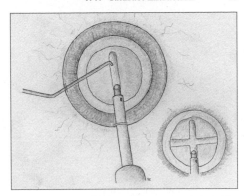

FIGURE 4.1.6 ◆ *Divide and conquer technique:* The phacoemulsification probe is used to divide the lens nucleus into pie-shaped segments **(see inset)**, which can be vacuum aspirated after ultrasound emulsification.

the cortex using a narrow cannula. The cortex is circumferentially adherent to the capsule at the lens equator, and depression of the nucleus will cause a wave of solution to dissect through these connections. The lens can then be rotated freely within the capsular bag, permitting easier fractioning and removal.

7. *Hydrodelineation:* Some surgeons also inject fluid directly into the nucleus to separate the softer epinucleus from the harder endonucleus, facilitating subsequent phacoemulsification.

8. *Phacoemulsification:* Numerous techniques have been developed to disassemble the nuclear component of the cataract for removal. "Chopping" is commonly employed for routine cases. The phaco tip is used to crack the nucleus into several pie-shaped segments with the assistance of a second instrument introduced through the paracentesis port. In the "divide and conquer" technique, the phaco handpiece is used to create two perpendicular grooves in a nuclear cataract. Instruments are subsequently used to crack it into quadrants (FIG. 4.1.6). After disassembly, the remaining lens fragments are emulsified and vacuum aspirated. See Appendix: Phacoemulsification Techniques for greater detail.

9. *Cortex Removal:* The residual cortex is then removed with an irrigating and aspirating handpiece that does not require ultrasonic energy.

10. *Lens Implantation:* The empty capsular bag is inflated with viscoelastic prior to insertion of a foldable IOL. This lens is implanted either with forceps or with a specialized injection system (FIG. 4.1.7). The advantage of an injection system

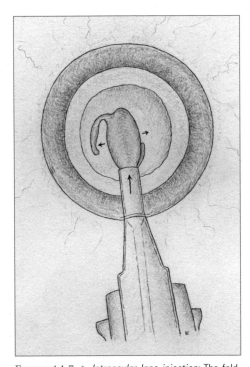

FIGURE 4.1.7 ◆ *Intraocular lens injection:* The foldable lens is deployed into the capsular bag using a specialized injector system. This permits use of a smaller main incision and isolates the lens from potential contaminants in the operative field.

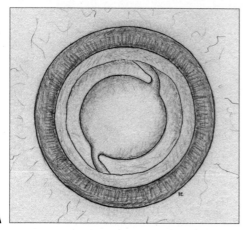

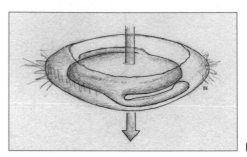

A ⋯ B

FIGURE 4.1.8 ◆ *Correct intraocular lens placement:* **(A)** An anterior view of a PCIOL with haptics properly aligned in the capsular bag beneath a dilated pupil. Note how the lens resembles a backward "S." **(B)** An oblique view of the capsular bag demonstrating its relationship to the IOL optic and haptics.

is that it uses a smaller incision and isolates the lens from potential contaminants in the surgical field. After the lens unfolds and the haptics are properly positioned (FIG. 4.1.8A-B), viscoelastic is evacuated and replaced with BSS, which resembles aqueous in composition and pH. The main incision should be self-sealing if it was properly constructed and instrument insertion during the case was atraumatic (FIG. 4.1.9). Some surgeons "hydrate" the incision with the goal of achieving tighter closure. This entails using an instrument to induce local stromal edema within the walls of the tunnel.

11. *Postoperative Medication:* Most surgeons instill antibiotic and steroid drops at the completion of surgery.

Special Considerations: Intraoperative floppy iris syndrome (IFIS) is linked to tamsulosin and other selective α-1 adrenergic receptor antagonists used to treat benign prostatic hyperplasia (BPH). These medications affect the pupillary dilator, causing the iris to billow with anterior chamber irrigation, prolapse through incisions, and progressively constrict during surgery. Routine premedication may be

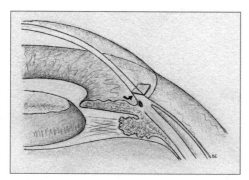

FIGURE 4.1.9 ◆ *Sutureless incision:* If the clear corneal incision was correctly made, and instrumentation was atraumatic, then it should be self-sealing. The pressure of the aqueous (arrow) pushes the tunnel closed. Depending on surgeon preference, the incision may be uniplanar (shown) or multiplanar.

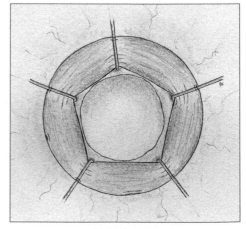

FIGURE 4.1.10 ◆ *Iris hooks:* Pictured here after capsulorrhexis, they may be used with IFIS to prevent the iris from obscuring the operative field, prolapsing through the main incision, or constricting inappropriately.

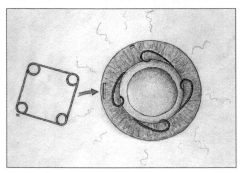

FIGURE 4.1.11 ◆ *Malyugin ring:* For cases with poor pupillary dilation, some surgeons prefer the Malyugin ring system, which does not require multiple paracentesis incisions. It is inserted into the anterior chamber with a specialized injector system.

insufficient to produce adequate mydriasis. In such cases, IFIS can be addressed with intracameral phenylephrine, iris hook placement (FIG. 4.1.10), or a combination of these techniques. Some surgeons prefer the Malyugin ring system to iris hooks, as it does not require the creation of multiple paracentesis incisions (FIG. 4.1.11).

COMPLICATIONS

Intraoperative

1. *Broken posterior capsule* (FIG. 4.1.12): This is the most common serious complication of cataract phacoemulsification. It increases the risk of endophthalmitis, cystoid macular edema, vitreous loss, and retinal detachments. Excellent visual results can still be obtained with identification of the broken capsule, appropriate anterior vitrectomy, and alternative lens placement. Posterior

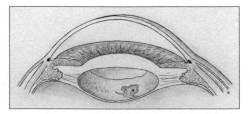

FIGURE 4.1.12 ◆ *Vitreous prolapse:* Strands of vitreous are seen passing into the evacuated capsular bag through a posterior capsular tear. With early recognition, anterior vitrectomy, and alternate lens placement, good visual outcomes are usually still achieved.

vitrectomy may be necessary if nuclear material drops through the capsular break.

2. *Uncontrolled or traumatic capsulorrhexis tears:* These compromise capsule stability and may require alternative lens placement if the bag is severely damaged.

3. *Thermal burns to the corneal incision or endothelium:* Burns may result if the phacoemulsification tip irrigation becomes blocked, preventing heat dissipation. Incision burns heal with time, but may necessitate suture placement for adequate tunnel closure. Endothelial cells cannot regenerate, so significant burns increase the risk of corneal decompensation.

4. *Zonular dehiscence or rupture:* Broken zonules can cause the entire native or artificial lens to sublux or dislocate. This is more common in patients with pseudoexfoliation, Marfan syndrome, homocystinuria, or a history of ocular trauma.

5. *Descemet's detachment:* Traumatic instrumentation of the anterior chamber can create a defect in Descemet's membrane, resulting in stromal edema.

6. *Anterior segment hemorrhage:* Damage to small vessels breaks down the blood-ocular barrier, causing intraocular inflammation and increasing the risk of subsequent synechia formation.

7. *Pupil constriction:* Most commonly seen with IFIS, this impairs visualization and surgical access, increasing the likelihood of other complications.

8. *Iris prolapse:* Caused by the herniation of the iris through the anterior chamber tunnel due to improper incision location, acute intraocular pressure (IOP) elevation, or IFIS.

9. *Tunnel perforation:* A rare complication that arises from traumatic instrument passage. It can compromise anterior chamber stability and may require sutured closure of the main incision.

10. *Hemorrhagic choroidal detachment:* Accumulation of blood in the suprachoroidal space is rarely seen, but can occur in the setting of hypotony at the time of cataract extraction, usually in patients with uncontrolled hypertension and generalized atherosclerotic vasculopathy. In mild cases, a small dome-shaped retinal elevation forms, but may resolve with time. The worst-case scenario is a hemorrhage so massive that intraocular contents prolapse through the cataract incision, resulting in devastating visual loss.

Postoperative

1. *Cystoid macular edema:* Cytokine release from activated inflammatory cells is thought to trigger breakdown of the blood-retinal barrier, leading to fluid accumulation in the outer plexiform layer of the macula. This distorts central vision and produces cystic spaces visible on optical coherence tomography (OCT). It is the most common cause of unexpected vision loss following cataract surgery, but usually resolves with administration of corticosteroids and NSAIDs.

2. *Posterior capsule opacification:* Following phacoemulsification, a "secondary cataract" often develops due to proliferation and migration of residual lens epithelial cells. If VA is significantly affected, this is treated with laser capsulotomy (see Chapter 4.2 Nd:YAG Laser Capsulotomy for details).

3. *Wound dehiscence/leakage:* Leakage of aqueous through an inadequately sealed surgical incision increases the risk of hypotony and intraocular infection. This complication can be identified by performing a Seidel test with topical fluorescein.

4. *Intraocular pressure elevation:* This may occur due to occlusion of the trabecular meshwork by incompletely evacuated viscoelastic, hyphema, or inflammatory debris. Pressure lowering medications, and occasionally anterior chamber washout, may be merited.

5. *Capsular block syndrome:* Residual viscoelastic may become trapped between the IOL and posterior capsule. It can subsequently push the lens forward, producing an unexpected myopic shift.

6. *Endocapsular hematoma:* Blood may become trapped between the IOL and posterior capsule, decreasing VA.

7. *Corneal edema/bullous keratopathy:* Stromal swelling and cystic fluid accumulation between the basal epithelial cells may be caused by endothelial damage that results from intraoperative trauma, inflammation, or prolonged IOP elevation. This complication is more commonly seen in patients with intrinsic endothelial cell dysfunction such as Fuchs dystrophy.

8. *IOL dislocation:* Causes include asymmetric haptic placement, loss of zonular support, and pupillary capture (part of the pupil margin is displaced behind the IOL).

9. *Endophthalmitis:* Intraocular infection due to introduction of pathogens through the surgical wounds; a rare but devastating complication treated with intracameral antibiotics (see Intravitreal Injections).

10. *Refractive error:* Potential causes include improper biometry measurements resulting in inaccurate IOL selection, placement of the wrong lens due to clerical error, and induced astigmatism from tight sutures or large primary incisions.

POSTOPERATIVE CARE

- Apply topical corticosteroids and antibiotics for 1 month in uncomplicated cases.

- Consider use of mydriatics, IOP-lowering drops, or a prolonged course of steroids in complicated, traumatic cases.

- Follow up:
  - At 24 hours: Check vision, IOP, wound stability, anterior chamber depth, and rule out infection or significant inflammation.
  - Week 1 to 2: Check vision, IOP, and wound stability; rule out signs of infection, and titrate medications.
  - Week 4 to 6: The eye should be stable. Assess the need for new corrective lenses or refractive surgery.

Routine follow-up should occur 3 to 6 months after surgery, then annually.

Suggested Reading

Text

Abdel-Aziz S, Mamalis N. Intraoperative floppy iris syndrome. *Curr Opin Ophthalmol.* 2009;20(1):37–41.

Allen D. Phacoemulsification. In: Yanoff M, Duker J, eds. *Ophthalmology.* 3rd ed. Philadelphia, PA: Mosby; 2009:447–451.

Awasthi N, Guo S, Wagner BJ. Posterior capsular opacification: a problem reduced but not yet eradicated. *Arch Ophthalmol.* 2009;127(4):555–562.

Bollinger KE, Langston RH. What can patients expect from cataract surgery? *Cleve Clin J Med.* 2008;75(3):193–196, 199–200.

Devgan U. Surgical techniques in phacoemulsification. *Curr Opin Ophthalmol.* 2007;18(1):19–22.

Eagle RC Jr, ed. Lens. In: *Eye Pathology: An Atlas and Basic Text.* Philadelphia, PA: W. B. Saunders;1999:101–115.

Hasanee K, Ahmed II. Capsular tension rings: update on endocapsular support devices. *Ophthalmol Clin North Am.* 2006;19(4):507–519.

Lang G, ed. Lens. In: *Ophthalmology: A Pocket Textbook Atlas*. 2nd ed. New York, NY: Georg Thieme Verlag; 2007:169–202.

Talley-Rostov A. Patient-centered care and refractive cataract surgery. *Curr Opin Ophthalmol*. 2008;19(1):5–9.

Primary Sources

Al-Mezaine HS, Kangave D, Al-Assiri A, Al-Rajhi AA. Acute-onset nosocomial endophthalmitis after cataract surgery: incidence, clinical features, causative organisms, and visual outcomes. *J Cataract Refract Surg*. 2009; 35(4):643–649.

Cho YK. Early intraocular pressure and anterior chamber depth changes after phacoemulsification and intraocular lens implantation in nonglaucomatous eyes. Comparison of groups stratified by axial length. *J Cataract Refract Surg*. 2008;34(7):1104–1109.

Ishii K, Kabata T, Oshika T. The impact of cataract surgery on cognitive impairment and depressive mental status in elderly patients. *Am J Ophthalmol*. 2008;146(3):404–409.

4.2 ND:YAG LASER CAPSULOTOMY

- Pulses from a neodymium-doped yttrium aluminum garnet (Nd:YAG) laser are used to remove an opacified posterior lens capsule from the visual axis after cataract surgery.

INDICATIONS

- Development of a visually significant posterior capsular opacity (PCO), or "secondary cataract," after phacoemulsification has been performed. Symptoms resemble those of a primary cataract and include decreased contrast, visual acuity, and color sensitivity, as well as increased glare.

- Posterior capsular striae (wrinkles) may form if the IOL haptics stretch and distort the evacuated capsular bag. The patient may initially experience streaking around lights, which usually resolves with capsular contraction. Laser capsulotomy may be undertaken in the rare event that symptoms are severe and persistent.

ALTERNATIVES

Medical Therapy
- There are no medical interventions available to treat PCOs once they have formed.

Surgery
- Since popularization of the Nd:YAG laser, surgical capsulotomy is very rarely performed. While effective, incisional procedures increases the risk of endophthalmitis and other potential complications.

RELEVANT ANATOMY AND PATHOPHYSIOLOGY

Lens Anatomy (Fig. 4.2.1)
Posterior Capsular Opacities
- Secondary cataract formation is one of the most common complications of cataract phacoemulsification.

- Opacification develops in up to 50% of adult patients within 5 years of surgery, although the incidence is decreasing with improvements in surgical instruments and intraocular lens design.

- Even with optimal surgical technique, some residual lens epithelial cells remain adherent to the anterior lens capsule and equator.

- Following cataract extraction, these cells can proliferate, differentiate, and migrate behind the IOL, obstructing the visual axis (Fig. 4.2.2).

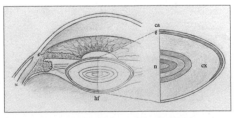

FIGURE 4.2.1 ◆ *Native lens anatomy:* The lens rests in the hyaloid fossa of the vitreous (hf) and is supported circumferentially by zonules anchored to the ciliary body. The nucleus (n), from outside to inside, consists of adult, infantile, fetal, and embryonic layers. It is surrounded by the cortex (cx), anterior lens epithelium (e), and basement membrane capsule (ca).

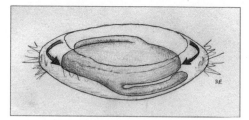

FIGURE 4.2.2 ◆ *PCO formation:* Following cataract extraction, residual lens epithelial cells can proliferate, differentiate, and migrate behind the IOL, obstructing the visual axis.

- There are two basic types of PCOs, which may coexist:
  1. *Fibrous membranes:* Residual cells differentiate into myofibroblasts and deposit extracellular matrix, which forms opaque plaques on the posterior capsule. Furthermore, myofibroblast contraction may lead to capsular wrinkling and distortion.
  2. *Elschnig pearls:* Residual epithelial cells differentiate into lens fibers, but remain globular because there are no surrounding layers of cortex to influence their morphology and growth pattern. Clusters of these pearls can accumulate and obstruct the visual axis.

Innovations to Decrease PCO Formation
- Improvements in phacoemulsification instruments and technique have permitted more complete evacuation of lens epithelial cells during cleanup.
- The posterior surfaces of many intraocular lenses are now designed to sit flush with the posterior capsule, impeding aberrant epithelial cell migration.
- Some artificial lens materials, such as polyacrylic, appear to inhibit PCO formation better than others.

PREOPERATIVE ASSESSMENT

- Slit lamp exam: Look for thickened, irregular posterior capsule in the visual axis.
- Dilated fundus exam: Rule out other potential causes of decreased visual acuity, such as age-related macular degeneration, diabetic retinopathy, cystoid macular edema, and retinal detachment. Most cataract extractions are

performed in older patients, who are at a greater risk of developing these disease processes.
- Additional studies, such as macular OCT and fluorescein angiography, may be useful for evaluating retinal pathology.

ANESTHESIA

- Topical drops are sufficient to anesthetize the cornea prior to capsulotomy.

PROCEDURE

1. *Premedication:* A topical alpha-2 adrenergic agonist (e.g., apraclonidine, brimonidine) is

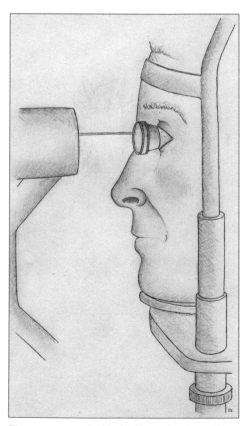

FIGURE 4.2.3 ◆ *Positioning:* The patient is seated opposite the ophthalmologist. His or her chin and forehead are positioned in the laser headrest and secured with a Velcro strap. A contact lens may be placed on the anesthetized cornea to magnify the posterior capsule.

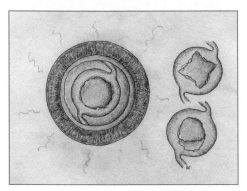

FIGURE 4.2.4 ♦ *Capsulotomy technique:* Depending on ophthalmologist preference, the posterior capsular defect can be made in the shape of a circle, cross, or inverted "U."

administered to prevent intraocular pressure elevation following laser use. Depending on ophthalmologist preference, the pupil may also be dilated using a topical mydriatic (e.g., tropicamide).

2. *Positioning:* The patient is seated opposite the ophthalmologist. His or her chin and forehead are positioned in the laser headrest and secured with a Velcro strap. A contact lens may be placed on the anesthetized cornea to magnify the posterior capsule (Fig. 4.2.3).

3. *Laser application:* It is essential to focus the laser on the capsule rather than on the IOL or posterior segment of the eye. Laser application is begun at low-power settings and gradually increased as necessary to penetrate the posterior capsule. Depending on operator preference, the capsular defect can be made in the shape of a circle, cross, or inverted "U" (Fig. 4.2.4). The ultimate goal is to produce an opening with a diameter slightly larger than that of the pupil (generally 3 to 4 mm). This removes the opacity from the visual axis while preserving the strength of the remaining capsular bag.

COMPLICATIONS

1. *IOL pitting or subluxation:* If focused in the incorrect plane, the laser may damage or dislodge the artificial lens, causing visual disturbances.

2. *Increased IOP:* Significant pressure elevation is rare with α-blocker pretreatment. Ocular

hypotensive medications can be administered as necessary.

3. *Retinal detachment:* This is most often seen in eyes with a long axial dimension (e.g., high myopia) or preexisting retinal pathology. See *Scleral Buckle* and *Pars Plana Vitrectomy* for treatment options.

4. *Cystoid macular edema:* Cytokine release from activated inflammatory cells is thought to trigger breakdown of the blood-retinal barrier, leading to fluid accumulation in the outer plexiform layer of the macula. This causes distortion of the central vision, which usually resolves when treated with corticosteroids and NSAIDs.

5. *Uveitis:* Laser application can precipitate or worsen intraocular inflammation.

POSTOPERATIVE CARE

- Check postoperative IOP and administer a pressure-lowering medication if persistent elevation is detected.

- After an IOP spike, follow up the next day in the clinic. Otherwise, schedule an office visit 1 week after the procedure.

- Some ophthalmologists prescribe a 4- to 7-day course of topical corticosteroids to limit intraocular inflammation.

Further Reading

Text

Aslam TM, Devlin H, Dhillon B. Use of Nd:YAG laser capsulotomy. *Surv Ophthalmol.* 2003;48(6):594–612.

Cheng JW, Wei RL, Cai JP, et al. Efficacy of different intraocular lens materials and optic edge designs in preventing posterior capsular opacification: a meta-analysis. *Am J Ophthalmol.* 2007;143(3):428–436.

Werner L. Secondary cataract. In: Yanoff M, Duker J, eds. *Ophthalmology.* 3rd ed. Philadelphia, PA: Mosby; 2009:497–503.

Primary Sources

Cleary G, Spalton DJ, Koch DD. Effect of square-edged intraocular lenses on neodymium:YAG laser capsulotomy rates in the United States. *J Cataract Refract Surg.* 2007;33(11):1899–1906.

Pollack IP, Brown RH, Crandall AS, et al. Effectiveness of apraclonidine in preventing the rise in intraocular pressure after neodymium:YAG posterior capsulotomy. *Trans Am Ophthalmol Soc.* 1988;86:461–472.

Steinert RF, Puliafito CA, Kumar SR, Dudak SD, Patel S. Cystoid macular edema, retinal detachment, and glaucoma after Nd:YAG laser posterior capsulotomy. *Am J Ophthalmol.* 1991;112(4):373–380.

Vock L, Menapace R, Stifter E, Georgopoulos M, Sacu S, Bühl W. Posterior capsule opacification and neodymium:YAG laser capsulotomy rates with a round-edged silicone and a sharp-edged hydrophobic acrylic intraocular lens 10 years after surgery. *J Cataract Refract Surg.* 2009;35(3):459–465.

4.3 TEMPORAL ARTERY BIOPSY

Temporal artery biopsy is the gold standard for diagnosing temporal arteritis (i.e., giant cell arteritis).

INDICATIONS

- Sudden, painless visual loss accompanied with symptoms of temporal arteritis (see the following).

RELEVANT PHYSIOLOGY AND ANATOMY

Forehead Anatomy (FIGURE 4.3.1)

Temporal Arteritis

Temporal arteritis is a systemic vasculitis that affects small to medium-sized vessels. Commonly affected vessels include branches off of the external carotid (i.e., temporal, ophthalmic, and posterior ciliary arteries).

This disease generally occurs in patients over 50 years of age and is rarely seen in younger patients.

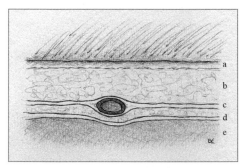

FIGURE 4.3.1 ◆ *Temporal forehead:* Layers include skin (a), connective tissue (b), superficial temporal fascia (c), which invests the temporal artery, deep temporal fascia (d), and temporalis muscle (e).

Symptoms include visual loss (usually unilateral but can progress quickly to bilateral if not promptly treated), headache (unilateral), jaw claudication (pain with opening and closing of mouth), tenderness over the inflamed artery, proximal myalgias, fever, and/or weight loss.

- Laboratory Findings: erythrocyte sedimentation rate (ESR), C-reactive protein (CRP), and platelet count may be normal or elevated. Temporal artery biopsy remains the gold standard for diagnosis.

- *Arteritic Ischemic Optic Neuropathy (AION):* This is the primary ocular manifestation of temporal arteritis due to occlusion of vessels feeding the retina or choroid. This presents as significant, rapid-onset visual loss (hand motion or finger counting) and an APD.

- Less common ocular manifestations: central retinal artery occlusion (CRAO) or cranial nerve palsy (the sixth nerve most commonly affected) leading to diplopia.

- Temporal artery biopsy pathology: Diffuse mononuclear infiltrate with multinucleated giant cells (characteristic aggregate of mononuclear cells), destruction of the internal elastic lamina, and possible occlusion of the lumen.

Differential Diagnosis

Although temporal arteritis is accompanied by a temporal headache and/or temporal forehead tenderness, vision loss is not accompanied by ocular pain. The following differential should be considered in cases of painless vision loss:

- Nonarteritic anterior ischemic optic neuropathy (NAION): sudden, painless visual loss with APD. This generally occurs in younger patients (<50 years of age) and does not have accompanying systemic symptoms of temporal arteritis. Funduscopic exam is indistinguishable from AION.

- Central retinal artery occlusion (CRAO): sudden, monocular painless vision loss with APD. Funduscopic exam reveals no disc edema, a pale retina (due to retinal nerve fiber edema), and possible cherry-red spot over the macula.
- Central retinal vein occlusion (CRVO): sudden, monocular painless vision loss with APD. Funduscopic exam reveals diffuse retinal hemorrhages, dilated and tortuous veins, and/or cotton wool spots. These cumulative findings have been referred to as a "blood and thunder" fundus.
- Inflammatory optic neuritis: Less severe and less sudden visual loss. Generally affects patients under 50 years of age. Pain may occur with eye movements. Funduscopic exam reveals disc swelling with more diffuse hemorrhage.

PREOPERATIVE SCREENING

History: age, onset of visual symptoms (monocular or binocular, sudden or gradual), jaw claudication, headache (unilateral vs. bilateral), facial or scalp tenderness, muscle and/or joint pains, fever, anorexia, and weight loss. Ask about previous history of facelift or browplasty; the temporal artery is often obliterated in these instances and alternative vessels (e.g., occipital artery) are required for diagnosis.

Exam: palpate temporal artery (assessing tenderness, pulsatile vs. nonpulsatile), VA, pupillary reflexes (looking for APD), visual fields, extraocular movements (cranial nerve [CN] palsy), dilated funduscopic exam (looking for disc edema and pallor, retinal hemorrhages; rule out CRVO, CRAO)

Laboratory test: ESR, CRP, and platelets

Fluorescein angiogram: may show delayed choroidal filling suggestive of AION

EMPIRIC TREATMENT

If there is a strong clinical suspicion of temporal arteritis, high-dose oral or intravenous steroids are started immediately (prior to biopsy).

Oral steroids: Administer 80- to 100-mg prednisone daily until biopsy results come back.

IV steroids: Administer 250-mg methylprednisolone every 6 hours while inpatient. Switch to oral steroids once outpatient.

Steroids are implemented prior to definitive diagnosis in order to preserve (and potentially restore)

visual acuity in the affected eye and to prevent the spread of visual symptoms to the contralateral eye. If treatment is delayed, the contralateral eye may be affected within a day of symptom onset in the presenting eye.

Biopsy must be performed within 1 week after the initiation of steroids for accurate diagnosis.

ANESTHESIA

Local infiltrative anesthesia with epinephrine to aid hemostasis.

Mark the skin incision prior to anesthetic infiltration as subcutaneous fluid may distort the contour of the temporal forehead.

PROCEDURE

 SEE TABLES 4.3.1 Rapid Review of Steps and 4.3.2 Surgical Pearls, and WEB TABLES 4.3.1 to 4.3.4 for equipment and medication lists.

1. *Artery identification:* A pulse is palpated and the artery is marked, creating a "pulse line" overlying the temporal artery (FIG. 4.3.2). In more advanced disease, a pulse may not be felt, requiring use of Doppler ultrasound to identify the position of the artery. In severe disease, the artery may be palpable as a nonpulsatile fibrotic cord.

2. *Surgical exposure:* The hair over the pulse line is shaved; minimal hair is removed to preserve cosmesis (FIG. 4.3.3). A 2- to 3-cm curvilinear skin incision is then made posterior and parallel to the pulse line (FIG. 4.3.4). This prevents inadvertent injury to the artery. Using either blunt or

TABLE 4.3.1 Rapid Review of Steps
(1) Prep and drape
(2) Palpation and marking of "pulse line"
(3) Shaving of hair in surgical field
(4) Curvilinear incision (posterior and parallel to "pulse line")
(5) Blunt dissection of fascia and adventitia away from vessel
(6) Vessel ligation (2-cm strip)
(7) Vessel removal
(8) Closure of subcutaneous tissue
(9) Closure of skin

TABLE 4.3.2 Surgical Pearls

Preoperative:
- Prescreening patients for previous eyebrow or scalp surgery is key. A history of facial surgery may mean the temporal arteries have been obliterated.
- If multiple branches of the temporal artery are identified, a branch in the scalp is ideal to hide the postoperative of scar.

Intraoperative:
- Being aware of anatomy is key. It is easy to dissect too deep and miss the temporal artery.
- Once the temporal artery is identified, it is not essential to dissect it carefully from surrounding adventitia. First, suture ligate the artery to control bleeding, then dissect the artery out.
- At least 2-cm length is essential due to skip lesions of inflammation.

Postoperative:
- A pressure dressing may be desired to prevent postoperative hematoma in the scalp.
- Careful coordination with pathology, internist, rheumatologist, and/or neurologist is key in managing steroid treatment based on the histopathologic findings.

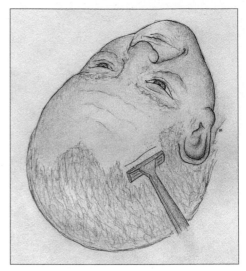

FIGURE 4.3.3 ◆ *Hair removal:* If the pulse line of the temporal artery is posterior to the hairline, the overlying hair is removed with a razor.

sharp dissection, the incision is continued to the depth of the superficial temporalis fascia (FIGS. 4.3.5 and 4.3.6). The fascia is opened with scissors to visualize the temporal artery. Using blunt dissection, the vessel is freed from the surrounding adventitia for a length of approximately 2 cm. Before proceeding, the feeder vessels are cauterized to ensure adequate hemostasis.

3. *Vessel ligation:* A 2-cm strip of vessel is identified and the inferior and superior margins to be excised are arbitrarily set. At the inferior margin, a silk suture is passed just deep to the vessel and tied securely. Care is taken not to nick the vessel while passing the needle. Likewise, at the superior margin, a silk suture is passed just deep to the vessel and tied off. The biopsy site is now devoid of flowing blood. An optional third suture can be placed in the middle of the two original sutures to "tag" the vessel for specimen collection; the additional advantage is improved hemostasis (FIG. 4.3.7). (Note: Some surgeons use cauterization as an alternative to suture ligation.)

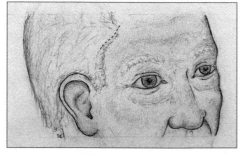

FIGURE 4.3.2 ◆ *Artery location:* The pulse of the temporal artery (**dotted line**) is identified by palpation. In more advanced disease, Doppler ultrasound may be required to locate the artery. In severe disease, the artery may be palpable as a nonpulsatile fibrotic cord.

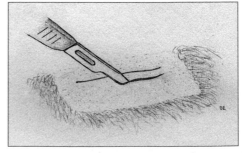

FIGURE 4.3.4 ◆ *Skin incision:* A 2- to 3-cm curvilinear skin incision is made posterior and parallel to the pulse line. This prevents inadvertent injury to the artery.

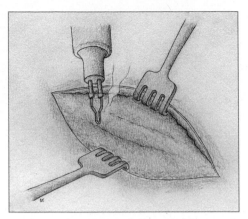

FIGURE 4.3.5 ✦ *Hemostasis:* Wound bed hemostasis is achieved with cautery.

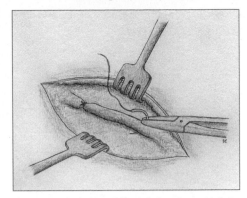

FIGURE 4.3.7 ✦ *Vessel ligature:* Superior and inferior sutures are passed deep to the vessel and tied securely. A central suture may be placed to "tag" the vessel for specimen collection.

4. *Vessel removal:* Using sharp scissors, the vessel is cut at the superior and inferior margins delineated by the suture ties. Care should be taken to cut internal to the knots to maintain hemostasis (FIG. 4.3.8). Temporal arteritis can present with "skip lesions," meaning the inflammation may only be present in certain sections of vessel. Therefore, an adequate length of the vessel is required for correct diagnosis. Connective tissue surrounding the tissue may occasionally be inflamed and is often included with the biopsy specimen.

5. *Closure:* The subcutaneous tissue is reapproximated with buried, interrupted sutures. The skin incision is then closed with a fine running suture.

COMPLICATIONS

- Failure to identify the temporal artery (more common in advanced disease with a nonpulsatile artery)
- Hematoma: inadequate hemostasis prior to closure

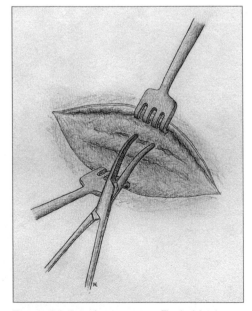

FIGURE 4.3.6 ✦ *Artery exposure:* The incision is continued to the depth of the superficial temporalis fascia using blunt dissection. This exposes the temporal artery.

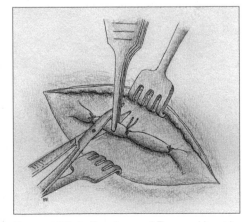

FIGURE 4.3.8 ✦ *Vessel removal:* The vessel is cut inside of the sutures to maintain hemostasis. The intervening segment of artery, which should be at least 2 cm long, is then sent to pathology for histologic processing.

- Cellulitis: may develop around incision site; risk is significantly reduced with appropriate topical antibiotic application
- Damage to facial nerve branches
- Scalp necrosis (rare)

POSTOPERATIVE CARE

- Topical antibiotic ointment is applied to incision site for up to 1 week.
- Sutures are removed at 1 week to prevent excessive scarring.
- High-dose prednisone is continued until biopsy results return.

If the pathology report is negative for a 2-cm biopsy specimen, the likelihood of temporal arteritis is minimal. Steroids may be stopped or quickly tapered. If clinical suspicion remains high, the surgeon may opt to biopsy the contralateral temporal artery as well.

If the pathology report reveals temporal arteritis, the patient must remain on high-dose oral prednisone. The tapering of dosage is based on periodic (monthly) ESR checks and the resolution of clinical symptoms. If symptoms recur or the ESR increases, the steroid dosage must be increased. Optimal therapy minimizes steroid dose while adequately controlling the symptoms or ESR level. Steroid treatment may be required for 1 to 2 years before discontinuation is possible.

Further Reading

Text

Guercio JC, Balcer LJ. Inflammatory optic neuropathies and neuroretinitis. In: Yanoff M, Duker J, eds. *Ophthalmology.* 3rd ed. Philadelphia, PA: Mosby; 2009:964–970.

Whitcher J, Riordan-Eva P, eds. Ocular disorders associated with systemic diseases. In: *Vaughan and Asbury's General Ophthalmology.* Columbus, OH: Lange Medical Books/McGraw-Hill; 2004:212–228.

Primary Sources

Albert DM, Ruchman MC, Keltner JL. Skip areas in temporal arteritis. *Arch Ophthalmol.* 1976;94:2072.

Allsop CJ, Gallagher PJ. Temporal artery biopsy in giant cell arteritis. *Am J Surg Pathol.* 1981;5:317.

Hedges TR, Gieger GL, Albert DM. The clinical value of negative temporal artery biopsy specimens. *Arch Ophthalmol.* 1983;101:1251.

Glaucoma

Hylton R. Mayer, M. Bruce Shields, and James C. Tsai

5.1 GLAUCOMA DRAINAGE IMPLANTS

Implants lower intraocular pressure (IOP) by supplementing or replacing the trabecular meshwork outflow with drainage through a silicone tube that channels aqueous to a plate beneath the bulbar conjunctiva.

This plate is analogous to a trabeculectomy bleb (see Chapter 5.4 Trabeculectomy). It gradually dissipates the drained aqueous, which then is absorbed into the blood, lymph, and tear film.

INDICATIONS

Historically, drainage implants have been used when a trabeculectomy is not likely to survive due to the presence of significant conjunctival scarring or an ocular condition that promotes conjunctival fibrosis. Currently, glaucoma drainage implants are gaining popularity as primary surgeries, though trabeculectomies remain more common.

Neovascular glaucoma (NVG) is a common indication for drainage implants. Trabeculectomy is likely to fail because the sclerectomy becomes occluded by fibrovascular tissue and the release of growth factors causes the trabeculectomy bleb to scar down.

Uveitic glaucoma, aphakic or pseudophakic glaucoma, and iridocorneal endothelial (ICE) syndromes can cause angle scarring that leads to trabeculectomy failure.

Refractory glaucoma that has failed a trabeculectomy with adjunctive mitomycin C (MMC) is unlikely to respond to repeat filtering surgery.

Glaucoma that is accompanied by extensive conjunctival scarring due to prior perilimbal surgery (e.g., a scleral buckle for retinal detachment) or rheumatoid arthritis, for example, makes trabeculectomy far more difficult to perform and unlikely to survive.

Drainage implants may be indicated for patient who are unlikely to comply with the complex medication and follow-up regiment necessary for a successful trabeculectomy.

In addition, drainage implants may be beneficial for patient with significant lid disease or lifestyle activities (e.g., swimming or gardening) that increase the risk of bleb-related ocular infections.

DRAINAGE IMPLANT BASICS

Implant Mechanism

The balance between aqueous production and drainage determines intraocular pressure. Drainage implants reduce pressure by supplementing aqueous outflow from the anterior chamber.

The drainage tube opening is directed toward the middle of the anterior chamber so that it will not damage the cornea or occlude with ocular tissues or fibrovascular membranes.

The tube is connected to a drainage plate and fixed to the sclera, which dissipates the aqueous. In the weeks following implantation, this plate becomes encapsulated by fibrous tissue. This capsule prevents hypotony by limiting the rate of aqueous drainage, but can also cause implant failure if it thickens to the point of significantly limiting the diffusion and reabsorption of aqueous.

Prior to capsule formation, aqueous outflow must be controlled by another mechanism. Some implants contain mechanical valves that limit flow. Implants without such valves must be temporarily occluded until the fibrous capsule can form.

Implant Types

Implant design varies based on the surface area and several drainage plates, as well as on the presence of a mechanical valve to limit aqueous outflow.

The IOP-lowering potential of a given implant roughly correlates with drainage plate surface area. Larger devices, however, become progressively harder to implant and may take longer to encapsulate and begin functioning.

In general, valved and nonvalved implants are equally effective at lowering pressure, but valved implants require more topical IOP-lowering therapy, while nonvalved implants are more frequently associated with postoperative hypotony.

Valved Implants

Ahmed: A 184-mm^2 single plate or 364-mm^2 double plate, made of rigid polypropylene or pliable silicone. It incorporates a unidirectional valve that limits aqueous outflow, preventing early hypotony (FIG. 5.1.1A). The valve must be primed with saline solution prior to placement and is more easily occluded by blood or fibrin.

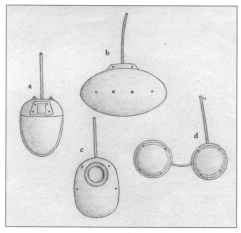

FIGURE 5.1.1 ✦ *Drainage implants:* **(a)** *Ahmed:* A 184-mm^2 single plate or 364-mm^2 double plate, made of rigid polypropylene or pliable silicone. It incorporates a unidirectional valve that limits aqueous outflow, preventing early hypotony. **(b)** *Baerveldt:* A pliable silicone reservoir with lateral "wings" that are placed beneath the adjacent rectus muscles. It is available in 250-mm^2 and 350-mm^2 sizes. *Molteno:* A modification of the first drainage device, now available as a 175-mm^2 or 230-mm^2 single plate **(c)** or as a 270-mm^2 double plate, made of rigid polypropylene **(d)**.

Nonvalved Implants

Molteno: The original drainage device, introduced in 1969. A third-generation model is available as a 175-mm^2 or 230-mm^2 single plate, made of rigid polypropylene (FIG. 5.1.1C). Older models are still available, including a double plate implant (FIG. 5.1.1D).

Baerveldt: A pliable silicone reservoir with lateral "wings" that must be tucked beneath the lateral and superior rectus muscles. It is available in 250-mm^2 and 350-mm^2 sizes (FIG. 5.1.1B).

Tube Placement

Tubes are most commonly placed in the anterior chamber, but can also be introduced through the ciliary sulcus or pars plana in aphakic or pseudophakic eyes.

Pars plana placement requires vitrectomy because strands of vitreous would otherwise obstruct the tube and prevent drainage.

ALTERNATIVES

Medical/Laser Therapy

Maximum topical IOP-lowering therapy is typically pursued prior to considering incisional surgery. In some cases, topical therapy may be ineffective in lowering IOP, may cause adverse side effects, or the patient may be unable to afford medications or comply with their administration.

Laser trabeculoplasty (argon laser trabeculoplasty [ALT] or selective laser trabeculoplasty [SLT]): Application of laser spots to the pigmented trabecular meshwork stimulates trabecular meshwork function and increases aqueous drainage, lowering the IOP. This procedure should be used with caution in uveitic eyes and may not lower pressures sufficiently in glaucoma with low or average IOP.

Timely intraocular anti-VEGF (vascular endothelial growth factor) injections (bevacizumab or ranibizumab) or panretinal photocoagulation (see Chapter 8.3 Retinal Laser Photocoagulation) can inhibit or reverse the development of anterior chamber neovascularization and scarring. This may prevent the onset of NVG.

Surgery

- *Trabeculectomy:* A guarded fistula is created between the anterior chamber and sub-Tenon space, reducing IOP by permitting the aqueous to drain beneath the scleral flap, filter into a conjunctival bleb, and reabsorb into the blood, lymph, and tear film or evaporate after transudation.

- *Canaloplasty:* A "nonpenetrating" glaucoma surgery that reduces IOP by dilating Schlemm's canal to increase outflow through the trabecular meshwork. After injection of viscoelastic, a Prolene suture is threaded through the canal and tightened to stent open the meshwork and increase its porosity. This procedure is generally not effective in neovascular, inflammatory, or chronic angle closure glaucomas.

- *Trabectome* (i.e., *ab interno trabeculotomy*): A specialized bipolar electro-ablation device is introduced into the anterior chamber through a clear corneal incision to remove a segment of the trabecular meshwork and "unroof" the underlying Schlemm's canal. This lowers pressure by permitting more direct outflow through the collector channels and episcleral veins.

- *Ex-PRESS Mini Glaucoma Shunt:* A 3-mm stainless steel drainage tube is inserted in the anterior chamber angle to bypass the trabecular meshwork. The implant is placed beneath a partial-thickness scleral flap to regulate outflow and create a trabeculectomy-like filtration bleb.

- *iStent:* Using a clear corneal incision, a 1-mm heparin-coated titanium drainage tube is inserted through the trabecular meshwork and into Schlemm's canal, reducing the resistance to aqueous outflow.

- *Cyclodestruction:* Diode laser cyclophotocoagulation or cryotherapy (which has fallen out of favor as too destructive and inflammatory) can reduce aqueous production by ablating a portion of the ciliary body, either transsclerally or via an endoscopic approach. Ciliary body destruction is generally irreversible, although the aqueous humor producing nonpigmented epithelium may partially regenerate (*Note:* This is more common in children, but can occur in adults as well). The IOP response is not immediate and repeat administration may be required to achieve satisfactory results.

NOTE: *Low IOPs can be irreversible and may lead to phthisis, so the procedure is generally reserved for patients with poor preoperative vision or for those who are not good surgical candidates.*

RELEVANT ANATOMY AND PATHOPHYSIOLOGY

Anatomy of Aqueous Drainage (Fig. 5.1.2)
Neovascular Glaucoma (NVG)
Ischemic retinal disorders (e.g., diabetic retinopathy or central retinal vein occlusion) can cause neovascularization of the iris and anterior chamber angle due to VEGF release (also known as rubeosis iridis).

This initially causes secondary open angle glaucoma due to obstruction of the trabecular meshwork by a fibrovascular membrane. In later stages, it leads to secondary angle closure as formation of anterior synechiae pulls the peripheral iris toward the cornea.

Anti-VEGF agents (bevacizumab and ranibizumab) and PRP are the most effective initial therapy because they reduce the stimulus for neovascularization. Once NVG has developed, drainage implants become the therapy of choice.

Uveitic Glaucoma
Protein and inflammatory cells accumulate due to the breakdown of the blood-ocular barrier.

Inflammation within the anterior chamber leads to formation of synechiae between the peripheral iris and cornea.

As with NVG, this causes angle closure and increased intraocular pressure.

Iridocorneal Endothelial (ICE) Syndrome
A group of disorders characterized by abnormal corneal endothelium.

These disorders cause iris atrophy, corneal edema, and secondary angle closure due to the formation of peripheral anterior synechiae.

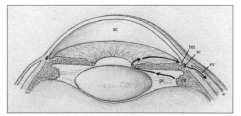

FIGURE 5.1.2 ◆ *Aqueous flow:* Produced by the nonpigmented ciliary body epithelium (cb), enters the posterior chamber (pc), passes through the pupil into the anterior chamber (ac), drains via the trabecular meshwork (tm), enters Schlemm's canal (sc), and returns to circulation via the episcleral veins (ev).

PREOPERATIVE SCREENING

Establish whether current glaucoma therapy is adequate using serial IOP measurements. Determine the rate of disease progression and the target IOP with serial evaluation of optic disc morphology and visual fields.

Conduct a careful external exam to determine whether there is conjunctival scarring from prior surgery or inflammation.

Perform a full slit-lamp exam with gonioscopy to examine the angle morphology and to check for signs of anterior chamber neovascularization or inflammation (e.g., cell and flare).

ANESTHESIA

Retrobulbar, peribulbar or topical/subconjunctival anesthesia is sufficient for most patients, and it can be supplemented by local infiltration of the tissues that are dissected during plate placement.

General anesthesia may be necessary for pediatric and uncooperative patients.

PROCEDURE

See Tables 5.1.1 Rapid Review of Steps and 5.1.2 Surgical Pearls, and Web Tables 5.1.1 to 5.1.4 for equipment and medication lists.

1. *Preoperative Medication:* If IOP is greater than 35 mm Hg, the patient can be pretreated with IV mannitol or other pressure-lowering medications.

2. *Conjunctival Incision:* The conjunctiva is generally incised at the limbus to create a fornix-based flap. If there is extensive conjunctival scarring or a history of prior filtration surgery, a limbus-based flap may be substituted (Fig. 5.1.3). It is important to avoid prior trabeculectomy sites as disruption may result in overfiltration and hypotony. Single-plate implants require dissection in only one quadrant and can be placed through a shorter conjunctival incision. The superotemporal quadrant is preferred, but any quadrant can be used if necessary. Double plate implants require dissection of two quadrants (most often the superotemporal and supranasal), and therefore require a longer incision. Relaxing incisions are often made in the

TABLE 5.1.1 Rapid Review of Steps
(1) Premedication +/− retrobulbar block
(2) Conjunctival dissection (limbus- or fornix-based approach)
(3) Scleral bed exposure
(4) Muscle isolation
(5) Prepare implant
- Suture occlusion and venting slit placement in drainage tube of valveless implants (Molteno and Baerveldt)
- Prime Ahmed valve
(6) Secure plate to sclera
(7) Cauterize site of sclerostomy
(8) Creation of sclerostomy
(9) Anterior chamber tube insertion
(10) Paracentesis
(11) Patch graft placement
(12) Conjunctival closure
(13) Postmedication, patch and shield

conjunctiva to prevent tearing of the flap during manipulation. The free corners can be tagged with sutures for easy identification and to aid in exposure (Fig. 5.1.4).

3. *Scleral Bed Exposure:* Conjunctiva and Tenon's capsule are elevated from the underlying sclera

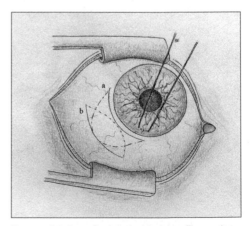

Figure 5.1.3 ◆ *Conjunctival incision:* The conjunctiva can be incised at the limbus to create a "fornix-based" flap (a) or ~ 5 mm posteriorly to create a "limbus-based" flap (b). The corresponding dashed lines outline the sub-Tenon's pocket that will be dissected in conjunction with each incision for drainage plate placement.

TABLE 5.1.2 Surgical Pearls

Preoperative:

- Inform patients that they will likely require intraocular pressure (IOP)-lowering drops even after surgery, and may require further surgery.
- Communicate with patient that you may use cadaverous donor tissue. Rarely, some patients have religious or other reasons for avoiding such tissue.
- Use a Q-tip or small sponge to evaluate the surgical quadrant with the least postoperative scarring. Normal conjunctiva freely moves over the underlying sclera.
- Evaluate anterior chamber depth and potential placement of the tube in the anterior chamber at the slit lamp. Consider sulcus tube placement or concomitant pars plana vitrectomy and pars plana tube placement for eyes with very shallow anterior chambers.
- Preoperative anti-VEGF agents can significantly decrease anterior chamber (AC) neovascularization. Waiting a few days to place a glaucoma implant after an intraocular anti-VEGF injection may decrease the risk for intraoperative hemorrhage (hyphema).

Intraoperative:

- A traction suture can facilitate conjunctival exposure and can serve as a guide for appropriate sectoral placement of the tube.
- Use calipers and a marking pen to indicate on the sclera the anticipated location of the anterior edge of the plate. The marking pen can also be used to note the insertions of the muscle.
- Rotate the knots of the plate securing sutures to avoid a nidus for conjunctival erosion.
- Cauterize at the location of the sclerostomy to avoid blood tracking into the anterior chamber. Firmly grasp the sclera prior to the passage of the needle used to create the sclerostomy. Pass the needle in the plane of the iris and visualize that the needle is in the appropriate position (the tube will typically exactly follow the needle's path).
- A long bevel on the tube can facilitate the passage of the tube into the anterior chamber. Occasionally, it can be helpful to use a viscoelastic to dilate and lubricate the sclerostomy.
- Evaluate the tube position with the eye inflated with balanced salt solution (BSS) to its normal physiologic depth. An ideal position is to have the tube just above and in the plane of the iris. A posterior tube that is just touching the iris is much preferred to an anterior tube that may be touching the cornea.
- If the tube position is not ideal, remove the tube and create a new sclerostomy. Occasionally, a suture is necessary to close the previous sclerostomy.
- Trim or bevel the scleral reinforcement graft so that the anterior edge of the graft provides appropriate coverage of the tube, but is not too thick or prominent at the limbal edge.
- Release the traction suture and rotate the eye to its natural position, prior to closure of the conjunctiva. Occasionally, it is necessary to create relaxing incisions and rotate conjunctiva over to allow coverage of the implant and surgical site.

Postoperative:

- Titrate steroids based on intraocular inflammation
- Aqueous suppression may decrease inflammatory mediators that reach the bleb, possibly decreasing the risk for excessive encapsulation and failure of the bleb.
- Postoperatively, confirm the appropriate position of the tube and coverage of the implant (look for exposure of the plate or tube).

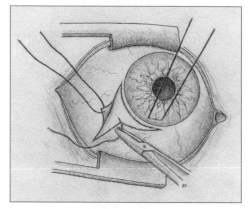

FIGURE 5.1.4 ◆ *Relaxing incisions:* The superotemporal quadrant is the preferred position for most drainage implants, but they may be placed in any quadrant. Relaxing incisions are often made in the conjunctiva, either centrally (as shown) or at the ends of the incision, to prevent tearing of the flap during manipulation. The free corners can be tagged with sutures for easy identification and exposure.

with blunt dissection (FIG. 5.1.5). This creates a pocket for plate placement.

4. *Muscle Isolation:* The scleral insertions of the adjacent rectus muscles are identified and captured with muscle hooks. The muscle bodies are dissected free of surrounding fascial tissue.

Thick sutures can then be passed beneath the muscles to facilitate their manipulation during plate placement.

5. *Plate Placement:* Implants are generally secured to the sclera about 8 mm from the limbus by passing partial-thickness sutures through anterior holes in the plate(s). This position offers protection while still allowing implant visualization through the conjunctiva on downgaze. Each device also has specific placement guidelines, depending on the number and shape of drainage plates.

Ahmed: This valved device requires priming prior to implantation; forced irrigation through the drainage tube separates the valve leaflets and ensures their subsequent function. Because of its longer anterior–posterior dimension and narrow horizontal dimension, the plate does not overlap with the adjacent rectus muscles.

Baerveldt: This valveless implant requires temporary suture occlusion to prevent hypotony (see *Suture Occlusion*). It is significantly wider than the Ahmed, and the adjacent rectus muscles must be manipulated to permit placement. When positioned in the superotemporal quadrant, one "wing" of the plate is tucked under the superior rectus and the other is tucked under the lateral rectus (FIG. 5.1.6).

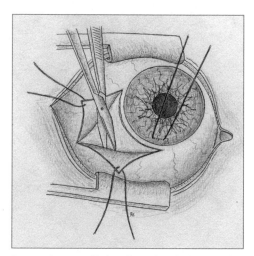

FIGURE 5.1.5 ◆ *Pocket dissection:* Conjunctiva and Tenon's capsule are elevated from the underlying sclera with blunt dissection. This creates a pocket for plate placement.

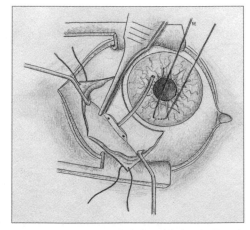

FIGURE 5.1.6 ◆ *Baerveldt implant placement:* The adjacent rectus muscles must be manipulated to permit placement. When positioned in the superotemporal quadrant, one "wing" of the plate is tucked under the superior rectus and the other is tucked under the lateral rectus.

Double Plate Molteno: Like the Baerveldt, this
valveless device requires temporary suture
occlusion to prevent hypotony (see *Suture
Occlusion*). Usually, one plate is positioned in
each superior quadrant. The plates are
joined with a connecting tube that is routed
above the superior rectus.

6. *Suture Occlusion (Molteno and Baerveldt Only):*
A nonabsorbable 3-0 suture is passed into the
drainage tube lumen. A second absorbable suture is then tied around the tube to secure the occluding suture. This prevents hypotony while a
fibrous capsule is still forming around the plate.
The surgeon can then remove the nonabsorbable
suture, or the absorbable suture will generally
dissolve after 4 to 6 weeks, restoring flow into the
capsule. Slits are often made in the drainage tube
with a fine blade. These act as release valves to
prevent an IOP spike (FIG. 5.1.7). The Ahmed
does not require an occluding suture as the valve
mechanism sets the IOP at approximately
10 mm Hg.

7. *Anterior Chamber Tube Insertion:* The drainage
implant tube is cut obliquely at a length that
permits it to approach the center of the anterior
chamber but not to obstruct the visual axis.

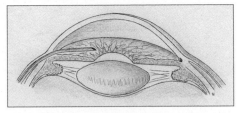

FIGURE 5.1.8 ✦ *Anterior chamber tube:* The
drainage tube is cut obliquely at a length that permits
it to approach the center of the anterior chamber (AC)
but not to obstruct the visual axis. This cut is oriented
so that the bevel faces upward to avoid occlusion by
iris tissue.

This cut is oriented so that the bevel faces
upward to avoid occlusion by iris tissue. The
tube is then inserted through a narrow sclerostomy tunnel made with a 23-gauge needle
(FIG. 5.1.8).

8. *Patch Graft:* A square of processed donor tissue
(e.g., pericardium or sclera) is used to cover the
silicone tube as it passes over bare sclera between
the plate and corneal limbus. This patch decreases the likelihood that the tube will erode
through the conjunctiva postoperatively. Its corners are secured with partial-thickness 8-0 scleral sutures (FIG. 5.1.9).

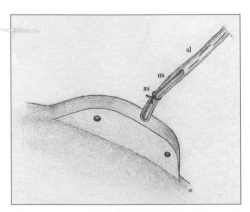

FIGURE 5.1.7 ✦ *Nonvalved (Molteno and Baerveldt)
implant suture occlusion:* A nonabsorbable 3-0 suture is
passed into the drainage tube lumen (ns). A second absorbable suture is then tied around the tube to secure
the occluding suture (as). This prevents hypotony while
a fibrous capsule is still forming around the plate. Slits
are often made in the drainage tube with a fine blade
(sl). These act as release valves to prevent an IOP spike.
By contrast, the Ahmed implant does not require ligature
sutures because it incorporates a valve that sets intraocular pressure (IOP) at around 10 mm Hg.

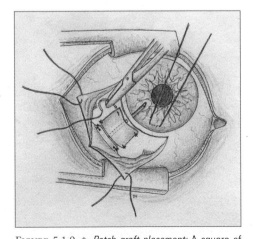

FIGURE 5.1.9 ✦ *Patch graft placement:* A square of
processed donor tissue (often sclera or pericardium) is
used to cover the silicone tube as it passes over bare
sclera between the plate and limbus. This patch decreases the risk of postoperative tube erosion through
the conjunctiva. The corners of the patch are secured
with 8-0 partial-thickness scleral sutures.

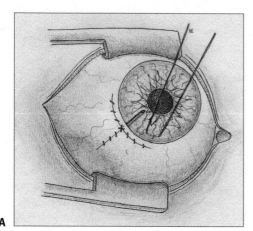

A

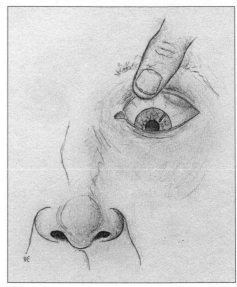

B

FIGURE 5.1.10 ◆ *Drainage implant in situ:* **(A)** The conjunctival flap is tacked to the limbus with running or interrupted sutures and the relaxing incision is closed. **(B)** The tube can be seen in the superotemporal quadrant following surgery.

9. *Conjunctival Closure:* The conjunctival flap is then tacked to the limbus with running or interrupted sutures (FIG. 5.1.10A,B). With valveless implants, the free end of the occluding suture is brought forward beneath the conjunctiva for easy postoperative access.

COMPLICATIONS

Intraoperative

- Bleeding: This occurs frequently with NVG due to disruption of fibrovascular membranes in the anterior chamber. Significant hyphema should be evacuated to prevent occlusion of the drainage tube.

- Tube misdirection: If the tube is directed anteriorly, it may abrade the corneal endothelium, causing edema. If the tube is directed posteriorly, it may occlude with iris tissue, induce traumatic cataract formation, or inadvertently enter the posterior chamber.

- Anterior chamber loss: This may occur due to aqueous leakage during sclerostomy creation, inadequate suture ligation of a nonvalved implant, or a faulty Ahmed valve mechanism. It can be reversed with viscoelastic injection.

- Suture perforation of the globe: This can occur when the drainage plate is anchored to the sclera. The risk is increased in patients with thin sclera. Perforations often close without significant repercussions, but they occasionally cause retinal detachment or vitreous hemorrhage.

Early Postoperative

- Hypotony: Low IOP due to rapid aqueous drainage, which is usually seen prior to maturation of the plate capsule. It is treated by injecting viscoelastic or temporarily reoccluding the tube with a suture ligature.

- Increased IOP: There are many potential causes of increased intraocular pressure in the early postoperative period. These include tube blockage by iris tissue, vitreous, blood clots, fibrin or retained viscoelastic, and Ahmed valve failure.

- Choroidal effusion: Fluid accumulates in the choroid, often as a complication of hypotony. Small effusions often resolve spontaneously, but larger effusions may require evacuation.

Late Postoperative

- Increased IOP: The "hypertensive phase" occurs 4 to 6 weeks after tube placement due to excess deposition of fibrous tissue in the drainage plate capsule. Fibrous tissue growth can occasionally be controlled with IOP lowering agents, capsule aspiration, antimetabolites, or corticosteroids. Other late causes of increased pressure include occlusion of the tube lumen, which is sometimes treated with Nd:YAG (neodymium-doped yttrium aluminum garnet) laser application or tube replacement.

- IOP decrease: Sudden drops in intraocular pressure are generally due to wound dehiscence or drainage plate extrusion.

- Corneal decompensation: Close proximity of, or contact between, the drainage tube and endothelial cells increases the risk of corneal edema.

- Diplopia: This is most common with larger, high-profile implants, but is often self-limiting.

- Plate migration: This can occur if scleral fixation is disrupted prior to complete encapsulation of the drainage plate.

- Tube erosion: The tube can wear through the underlying sclera or overlying patch and conjunctiva, potentially leading to endophthalmitis and/or implant extrusion. If the eroded site is not infected, the patch can be replaced. If it is infected, the tube may require removal.

POSTOPERATIVE CARE

Administer topical corticosteroids for up to 2 months.

Stop antibiotics after 1 week if there is no evidence of wound leakage and the corneal epithelium is intact on slit lamp examination.

With valveless implants, remove the occluding suture 4 to 6 weeks after the operation. At this point, a fibrous capsule has started to form over the drainage plate and the IOP should begin to rise gradually.

A small conjunctival incision is made over the tail of the occluding suture, and it is removed with gentle traction. Absorbable sutures will spontaneously dissolve at a relatively predictable rate (about 6 weeks post-op for a 7-0 polygalactin suture). Ligation release prior to capsule formation can result in severe hypotony and must be avoided.

Further Reading

Text

Freedman J, Trope GE. Drainage implants. In: Yanoff M, Duker J, eds. *Ophthalmology.* 3rd ed. Philadelphia, PA: Mosby; 2009:1277–1283.

Kahook MY. Neovascular glaucoma. In: Yanoff M, Duker J, eds. *Ophthalmology.* 3rd ed. Philadelphia, PA: Mosby; 2009:1178–1182.

Lang GK. Glaucoma. In: *Ophthalmology: A Pocket Textbook Atlas.* 2nd ed. New York, NY: Georg Thieme Verlag; 2007:chap 10.

Minckler DS, Francis BA, Hodapp EA, et al. Aqueous shunts in glaucoma: a report by the American Academy of Ophthalmology. *Ophthalmology.* 2008;115(6):1089–1098.

Sarkisian SR Jr. Tube shunt complications and their prevention. *Curr Opin Ophthalmol.* 2009;20(2):126–130.

Schwartz KS, Lee RK, Gedde SJ. Glaucoma drainage implants: a critical comparison of types. *Curr Opin Ophthalmol.* 2006;17(2):181–189.

Primary Sources

Gedde SJ, Schiffman JC, Feuer WJ, et al. Treatment outcomes in the tube versus trabeculectomy study after one year of follow-up. *Am J Ophthalmol.* 2007;143(1):9–22.

Nguyen QH. Primary surgical management refractory glaucoma: tubes as initial surgery. *Curr Opin Ophthalmol.* 2009;20(2):122–125.

Tsai JC, Johnson CC, Kammer JA, et al. The Ahmed shunt versus the Baerveldt shunt for refractory glaucoma II: longer-term outcomes from a single surgeon. *Ophthalmology.* 2006;113(6):913–917.

5.2   LASER IRIDOTOMY

- Creation of a full-thickness defect in the peripheral iris with a Nd:YAG (neodymium-doped yttrium aluminum garnet) or argon laser equalizes the anterior and posterior chamber pressures, eliminating pupillary block and opening the angle to promote aqueous outflow.

INDICATIONS

- Most often used to treat acute or chronic angle closure associated with a pupillary block mechanism.

- Considered as a prophylactic treatment for patients with history of angle closure in the fellow eye, family history of angle closure, or an angle that occludes with provocative testing (e.g., administration of a mydriatic).

- May be used prior to laser trabeculoplasty (argon laser trabeculoplasty [ALT] or selective laser trabeculoplasty [SLT]) to deepen the angle and provide better access to the trabecular meshwork.

- Occasionally used to treat pigmentary glaucoma, though this remains controversial. The presumed pathophysiology is that backward bowing of the iris causes chafing of the posterior pigmented epithelium against the lens zonules. This releases pigment granules that can occlude the trabecular meshwork. Iridotomy is thought to eliminate pigment release by equalizing the anterior and posterior chamber pressures, thus inducing a forward shift of the iris.

NOTE: *Iridotomy is not effective in cases of angle closure due to a mechanism other than pupillary block (e.g., neovascular glaucoma leads to formation of peripheral anterior synechiae, which will occlude the angle even after a successful iridotomy).*

LASER SELECTION

- Argon laser iridotomy: The argon laser uses thermal burns to coagulate blood vessels and destroy iris tissue. This minimizes the risk of subsequent bleeding.

- Nd:YAG laser iridotomy: The Nd:YAG laser uses a photodisruptive process that results in higher rates of iridotomy patency, but does not effectively coagulate bleeding vessels.

- Combined treatment: Iridotomy patients who have known bleeding disorders or who are receiving anticoagulation should not be treated by Nd:YAG laser alone. Often, an argon laser is used to thin the iris and coagulate adjacent vessels before it is definitively penetrated with a Nd:YAG laser. This technique is also helpful in patients with dark irides and thick stroma.

ALTERNATIVES AND ADJUNCTS

Medical Therapy

- Intraoperative pressure (IOP) reduction with a combination of PO ("by mouth") or IV

(intravenous) carbonic anhydrase inhibitors and topical medications (e.g., beta blockers, alpha agonists) is the first line of therapy in acute angle closure. Pilocarpine is then given to constrict the pupil and open the angle (it cannot be used initially because high intraocular pressures induce iris muscle ischemia, blunting the response to miotics).

- Pharmacologic IOP reduction is often used prior to laser iridotomy to decrease corneal edema, permitting better laser focus and visualization of the underlying iris stroma.

- Compression of the central cornea with a cotton-tipped applicator may help to deepen the peripheral anterior chamber and lower intraocular pressure.

Surgery

- Surgical iridectomy: This procedure is occasionally performed when poor iris visibility precludes laser iridotomy (e.g., extensive corneal scarring or stromal edema that does not respond to medical therapy). Or in patients who are unable to hold still or cooperate during the laser procedure.

RELEVANT PATHOPHYSIOLOGY AND ANATOMY

Aqueous Humor Flow (FIG. 5.2.1)

Pupillary Block Mechanism

- Posterior chamber pressure exceeds anterior chamber pressure because close apposition of the iris and lens impedes aqueous flow.

- This blockage may be due to fixed obstructions, such as posterior synechiae or inflammatory membranes, or merely to the close proximity of anatomic structures (the lens grows with age, increasing the risk of pupillary block angle closure).

- The pressure differential between chambers causes the iris to balloon forward, narrowing the angle and preventing outflow of aqueous through the trabecular meshwork (FIG. 5.2.2).

- Iridotomy equalizes the pressure between chambers and deepens the angle, restoring aqueous outflow (FIG. 5.2.3).

PREOPERATIVE ASSESSMENT

- Evaluate the cornea for edema and scars to ensure that the underlying iris is clearly visible.

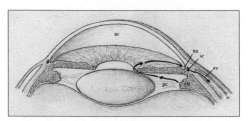

FIGURE 5.2.1 ✦ *Aqueous flow:* Produced by the non-pigmented ciliary body epithelium (cb), enters the posterior chamber (pc), passes through the pupil into the anterior chamber (ac), drains via the trabecular meshwork (tm), enters Schlemm's canal (sc), and returns to circulation via the episcleral veins (ev).

- Perform gonioscopy to assess the angle for the extent of peripheral anterior synechiae (PAS) and/or neovascularization. Iridotomy generally will not deepen the angle if these conditions are advanced.

ANESTHESIA

- Topical anesthetics can be administered bilaterally to decrease blinking and patient discomfort.

PROCEDURE

1. *Premedication:* Topical pilocarpine is administered to induce miosis, thinning the iris for easier laser penetration. An alpha-2 agonist (e.g., apraclonidine, brimonidine) should also be given 30 to 60 minutes prior to iridotomy to reduce the risk of a postoperative IOP spike.
2. *Positioning:* The patient is seated opposite the ophthalmologist. His or her chin and forehead

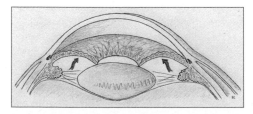

FIGURE 5.2.2 ✦ *Pupillary block angle closure:* Posterior chamber pressure exceeds anterior chamber pressure because increased apposition between the iris and lens impedes aqueous flow. The pressure differential between chambers causes the iris to balloon forward, narrowing the angle and preventing outflow of aqueous through the trabecular meshwork.

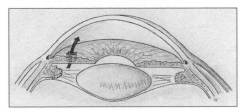

FIGURE 5.2.3 ✦ *Iridotomy:* Creation of a full-thickness defect in the peripheral iris equalizes the pressure between chambers and deepens the angle, restoring aqueous outflow.

are positioned in the laser headrest and secured with a Velcro strap. An Abraham or Wise contact lens, with methylcellulose gel on the optic, is then placed on the cornea to magnify the iris and concentrate the laser energy (FIG. 5.2.4).

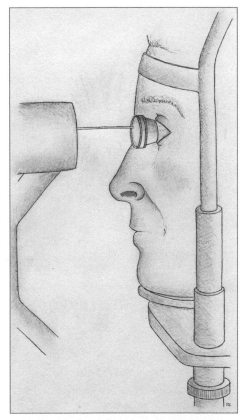

FIGURE 5.2.4 ✦ *Positioning:* The patient is seated opposite the ophthalmologist with his or her chin and forehead in the laser headrest. An Abraham or Wise contact lens, coated with methylcellulose gel, is then placed on the cornea.

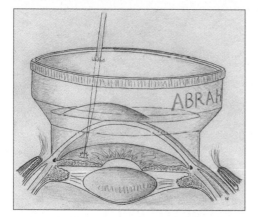

FIGURE 5.2.5 ◆ *Laser application:* The iris crypts are often targeted with the laser because there is less tissue to penetrate. Care is taken to avoid major peripheral blood vessels. An iridotomy size of 100 to 200 microns is generally adequate to equalize pressure and prevent reocclusion.

3. *Iridotomy:* The iridotomy is generally placed between the 11 and 1 o'clock positions, as far peripherally as possible. This position permits coverage by the upper lid and decreases the risk of postoperative diplopia. The iris crypts are often targeted with the laser because there is less tissue to penetrate. Care is taken to avoid major peripheral blood vessels. An iridotomy size of 100 to 200 microns is generally adequate to equalize pressure and prevent reocclusion (FIG. 5.2.5). With successful iris perforation, displaced pigment can often be seen entering the anterior chamber. The peripheral anterior chamber (AC) should also deepen, and the anterior lens capsule may be visible through the newly created defect.

COMPLICATIONS

- Anterior chamber bleeding: This is usually minimal and self-limited even with Nd:YAG laser iridotomy. Corneal pressure is applied with the Abraham or Wise lens to tamponade the bleeding.
- IOP pressure spike: This may occur due to temporary occlusion of the meshwork by displaced pigment and inflammatory debris. Pressure usually peaks within 1 hour and can be dampened by preoperative administration of an alpha-2 adrenergic agonist.

- Laser-induced iritis: This occurs due to localized breakdown of the blood-aqueous barrier. It is seen transiently in all patients and may be treated with topical steroids.
- Corneal burns: The impact of these lesions is generally transient and they do not require specific treatment.
- Iridotomy failure: This may occur if the iridotomy is too small, if it is blocked by a residual layer of iris pigment epithelium, or if it reoccludes due to pigment proliferation. Retreatment is often necessary.
- Diplopia: Double images may result from the creation of an exposed optical aperture in the iris. They may also occur if the iridotomy site is near the lid margin due to a prism effect of the tear meniscus. If symptoms disturb the patient, a cosmetic contact lens can be used to prevent light from reaching the fundus through the iridotomy.
- Lens opacity: This can present acutely due to direct laser damage or insidiously due to the alteration of aqueous flow. Opacities from direct damage tends to remain localized and usually does not obstruct the visual axis.
- Persistent uveitis, malignant glaucoma, and retinal burns are all rare.

POSTOPERATIVE CARE

- Check IOP 1 hour after the procedure and administer pressure-lowering medications as needed. Repeat measurements in clinic the following day if a pressure spike occurs.
- Apply topical steroids QID ("four times a day") for 4 to 7 days to reduce inflammation. Short-term administration of miotics can help maintain iridotomy patency.
- Perform postoperative gonioscopy between 1 week and 1 month to assess the effect of the iridotomy on angle configuration and to rule out the development of peripheral anterior synechiae.
- Consider prophylactic treatment of the fellow eye at the 1-week follow-up.
- Check the iridotomy again at 4 to 6 weeks. If patent at this point, it is unlikely to occlude unless significant neovascularization or uveitis develops.

Further Reading

Text

Damji KF. Argon laser trabeculoplasty and peripheral iridectomy. In: Yanoff M, Duker J, eds. *Ophthalmology.* 3rd ed. Philadelphia, PA: Mosby; 2009:1227–1233.

Lang G. Glaucoma. In: *Ophthalmology: A Pocket Textbook Atlas.* 2nd ed. New York, NY: Georg Thieme Verlag; 2007:chap 10.

Liebmann JM, Ritch R. Laser iridotomy. *Ophthalmic Surg Lasers.* 1996;27(3):209–227.

Ng WS, Ang GS, Azuara-Blanco A. Laser peripheral iridoplasty for angle-closure. *Cochrane Database Syst Rev.* 2008;16(3):CD006746.

Riedel PJ, Samuelson TW. Angle closure glaucoma. In: Yanoff M, Duker J, eds. *Ophthalmology.* 3rd ed. Philadelphia, PA: Mosby; 2009:1172–1175.

Primary Sources

He M, Friedman DS, Ge J, et al. Laser peripheral iridotomy in eyes with narrow drainage angles: ultrasound biomicroscopy outcomes. The Liwan Eye Study. *Ophthalmology.* 2007;114(8):1513–1519.

Lai JS, Tham CC, Chua JK, et al. To compare argon laser peripheral iridoplasty (ALPI) against systemic medications in treatment of acute primary angle-closure: midterm results. *Eye.* 2006;20(3):309–314.

5.3 LASER TRABECULOPLASTY (ARGON LASER TRABECULOPLASTY, SELECTIVE LASER TRABECULOPLASTY)

- Application of laser spots to the pigmented trabecular meshwork increases aqueous drainage, lowering intraocular pressure (IOP).

- Argon laser trabeculoplasty (ALT) uses thermal energy to create focal contraction burns in the meshwork.

- Selective laser trabeculoplasty (SLT) employs a newer Nd:YAG (neodymium-doped yttrium aluminum garnet) technology that can ablate pigmented cells without damage to surrounding tissues.

INDICATIONS

- Open-angle glaucoma that does not adequately responsive to medical therapy
- Pigmentary or pseudoexfoliative glaucoma
- Augmentation of aqueous outflow in eyes with narrow angles or angle closure after laser iridotomy or iridoplasty has been performed
- Patients who are unhappy with or intolerant of medications or non-compliant with medication use or follow up

NOTE: *ALT generally cannot be repeated due to poor therapeutic response and increased risk of sustained IOP elevation. Conversely, SLT is thought to be effective and safe in most eyes with one prior ALT or SLT application.*

CONTRAINDICATIONS

- Laser trabeculoplasty can exacerbate preexisting ocular inflammation or increase IOP in active uveitis.

- Chronic angle closure inhibits visualization of the trabecular meshwork and increases the risk of peripheral anterior synechiae formation.

ADJUNCTIVE TECHNIQUES

- Laser iridotomy: This technique reverses acute angle closure due to a pupillary block mechanism by equalizing the anterior and posterior chamber pressures (see Chapter 5.2 Laser Iridotomy).
- Iridoplasty: Nonpenetrating laser burns are applied to the peripheral iris in a circumferential

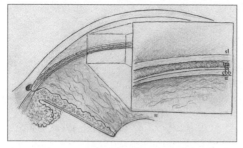

FIGURE 5.3.1 ✦ *Angle Anatomy: Schwalbe's line* (sl): The outer limit of Descemet's membrane, which marks the anterior border of the trabecular meshwork. *Trabecular meshwork* (tm): Spongy tissue that permits transport of aqueous into Schlemm's canal. *Scleral spur* (ss): A ridge of protruding sclera, anterior to the root of the iris, that anchors the trabecular meshwork and provides points of insertion for the longitudinal ciliary muscle fibers. *Ciliary body band* (cbb): A sliver of the anterior ciliary body, visible in a wide-open angle. *Iris root* (ir): The thinnest portion of the iris, which inserts into the ciliary body.

pattern. The resulting tissue contraction widens the angle, providing access to the trabecular meshwork.

ALTERNATIVES

Medical Therapy

- Glaucoma medications reduce IOP by two primary mechanisms and can be combined synergistically.
  - Suppression of aqueous production: Beta-blockers, alpha-2 adrenergic agonists, and carbonic anhydrase inhibitors (CAIs)
  - Facilitation of aqueous outflow: Prostaglandin analogs and parasympathomimetics

Surgery

- Trabeculectomy: This filtration surgery is considered if a patient's target IOP is unlikely to be achieved with trabeculoplasty (see Chapter 5.4 Trabeculectomy).
- Glaucoma drainage implants: These devices are often used for uveitic or neovascular glaucomas as well as for eyes with failed trabeculectomy, which do not respond well to trabeculoplasty or repeat trabeculectomy. These implants are also being used more frequently for the initial surgical management of primary open angle

glaucoma (see Chapter 5.1 Glaucoma Drainage Implants).

- Other surgical strategies gaining in popularity include the Ex-PRESS Mini Glaucoma Shunt, Trabectome, iStent, and suture canaloplasty (see 5.4 Trabeculectomy, Alternatives to Trabeculectomy, Surgery section for further details).

RELEVANT PHYSIOLOGY AND ANATOMY

Angle Anatomy (FIG. 5.3.1)

- Schwalbe's line: The outer limit of Descemet's membrane. On gonioscopy, this marks the anterior border of the trabecular meshwork.
- Trabecular meshwork: Spongy tissue, lined by trabeculocytes, that permits drainage of aqueous into Schlemm's canal.
- Scleral spur: A ridge of protruding sclera, anterior to the root of the iris, that anchors the trabecular meshwork and permits insertion of the longitudinal ciliary muscle fibers.
- Ciliary body band (CBB): A rim of the ciliary body that can be seen between the scleral spur and insertion of the iris if the angle is fully open.

Aqueous Humor Flow (FIG. 5.3.2)

Trabeculoplasty Mechanisms

- ALT: Laser burns are thought to increase aqueous outflow by physically opening channels in the meshwork and by encouraging proliferation of the trabecular endothelial cells.
- SLT: Laser photodisruption may increase aqueous outflow by removing pigment and debris from the meshwork and by stimulating

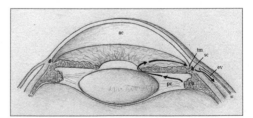

FIGURE 5.3.2 ✦ *Aqueous flow:* Produced by the non-pigmented ciliary body epithelium (cb), enters the posterior chamber (pc), passes through the pupil into the anterior chamber (ac), drains via the trabecular meshwork (tm), enters Schlemm's canal (sc), and returns to circulation via the episcleral veins (ev).

the trabecular endothelial cells. The exact mechanism, however, is not well understood.

PREOPERATIVE ASSESSMENT

- Determine the adequacy of current glaucoma therapy with serial IOP measurements (most often using Goldmann applanation tonometry at the slit lamp).
- Determine the target IOP by evaluating the rate of disease progression, as well as the patient's optic disc morphology and visual fields.
- Carefully examine the trabecular meshwork and angle anatomy with gonioscopy. Rule out peripheral synechiae and angle configurations that are not conducive to primary trabeculoplasty.

ANESTHESIA

Administration of topical anesthesia decreases corneal discomfort.

PROCEDURE

1. *Premedication and Positioning:* A topical alpha-2 adrenergic agonist (e.g., apraclonidine, trade name: Iopidine) can be administered to decrease the risk of postoperative IOP elevation. The patient is then seated opposite the ophthalmologist, with his or her chin and forehead firmly positioned in the laser headrest. A three-mirror Goldmann goniolens or one-mirror Latino SLT lens, with methylcellulose gel on the optic, is placed on the cornea (FIG. 5.3.3). A light adjacent to the laser source provides the patient with a fixation target for his or her fellow eye.

2. *Laser Application:* After key angle landmarks are identified, laser application begins at the 12 o'clock position of the goniolens (the reflected laser will hit the meshwork at 6 o'clock) and progresses clockwise (FIG. 5.3.4).
   - ALT: Up to 360 degrees of ALT can be performed after pretreatment with apraclonidine, provided that the patient does not have advanced nerve fiber damage and is not routinely taking an alpha agonist (the pressure-lowering effect will be blunted in this case). Twenty to twenty-five laser spots, each

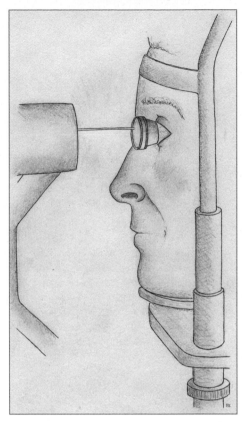

FIGURE 5.3.3 ◆ *Positioning:* The patient is seated opposite the ophthalmologist, with his or her chin and forehead firmly against the laser headrest. A three-mirror Goldmann goniolens, coated with methylcellulose gel, is then placed on the cornea.

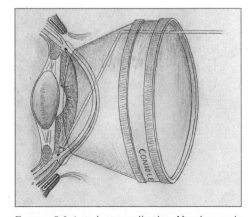

FIGURE 5.3.4 ◆ *Laser application:* After key angle landmarks are identified, laser application begins at the 12 o'clock position of the goniolens (the reflected laser will hit the meshwork at 6 o'clock) and progresses clockwise.

50 microns in diameter, are generally applied per quadrant. Care is taken to avoid placing the spots too close to the scleral spur, because this increases the likelihood of peripheral anterior synechiae (PAS) formation.

- SLT: Up to 360 degrees of SLT can be administered per eye in a single session, since there is a lower risk of postoperative IOP elevation (*Note:* Eyes with pigment dispersion may still undergo significant IOP elevation). Nearly confluent laser spots, 400 microns in diameter, are applied to the meshwork. This procedure induces less intraocular inflammation and has a lower risk of PAS formation.

3. *Retreatment Considerations:* While full 360 degrees laser application provides the maximum pressure reduction, 180 degrees ALT permits delayed treatment of the other half of the meshwork, either when the initial IOP-lowering effect wears off or after postoperative inflammation has subsided. Of note, retreatment with 360 degrees SLT is possible after 360 degrees of initial treatment.

COMPLICATIONS

- Vasovagal syncope: This can occur when activation of the oculocardiac reflex triggers a significant reduction in heart rate. It should be treated by halting ocular manipulation and providing supportive care.

- IOP spike: This is most commonly seen within 24 hours of trabeculoplasty and is treated with pressure-lowering medications. In the rare instances that IOP elevation is severe and prolonged, it may require emergent filtering surgery.

- Anterior chamber reaction: Argon laser application generates a mild inflammatory response in most eyes, which can be treated with steroids or NSAIDs. The Nd:YAG laser generally induces far less inflammation.

- Corneal burns: These generally heal within a few days without specific intervention.

POSTOPERATIVE CARE

- Check the IOP 1 hour after laser application to rule out a pressure spike. If the pressure is

significantly elevated, acetazolamide or glycerol is administered and tonometry is repeated at regular intervals.

- If the IOP spikes in the immediate postoperative period, see the patient in clinic the following day for further measurements. Otherwise, the next visit may take place 1 week after the procedure.

- In general, give a week of topical steroids following ALT. Steroids are not routinely required after SLT, but topical NSAIDs are sometimes prescribed.

- Continue all glaucoma medications in the postoperative period. While doses may be adjusted or the drug regimen simplified, medications usually cannot be eliminated altogether.

- The full effect of the procedure is usually not apparent immediately after treatment. Definitive assessment of the therapeutic response is possible by 4 to 6 weeks. After this, efficacy gradually decreases over the course of months to years.

Further Reading

Text

Barkana Y, Belkin M. Selective laser trabeculoplasty. *Surv Ophthalmol.* 2007;52(6):634–654.

Damji KF. Argon laser trabeculoplasty and peripheral iridectomy. In: Yanoff M, Duker J, eds. *Ophthalmology.* 3rd ed. Philadelphia, PA: Mosby; 2009: 1227–1233.

Lang G. Glaucoma. In: *Ophthalmology: A Pocket Textbook Atlas.* 2nd ed. New York, NY: Georg Thieme Verlag; 2007:chap 10.

Realini T. Selective laser trabeculoplasty: a review. *J Glaucoma.* 2008;17(6):497–502.

Rolim de Moura C, Paranhos A Jr, Wormald R. Laser trabeculoplasty for open angle glaucoma. *Cochrane Database Syst Rev.* 2007;17(4):CD003919.

Primary Sources

Damji KF, Bovell AM, Hodge WG, et al. Selective laser trabeculoplasty versus argon laser trabeculoplasty: results from a 1-year randomised clinical trial. *Br J Ophthalmol.* 2006;90(12):1490–1494.

Hong BK, Winer JC, Martone JF, et al. Repeat selective laser trabeculoplasty. *J Glaucoma.* 2009;18(3): 180–183.

Pham H, Mansberger S, Brandt JD, et al. Argon laser trabeculoplasty versus selective laser trabeculoplasty. *Surv Ophthalmol.* 2008;53(6):641–646.

5.4 TRABECULECTOMY

A partial-thickness filtration procedure decreases intraocular pressure (IOP) by creating a limbal fistula, allowing aqueous to filter across the conjunctival bleb and wash away in the tear film.

INDICATIONS

- Most glaucoma patients who have failed maximal-tolerated medical and laser therapy (i.e., have progressive disease likely to result in further visual impairment)
- Occasionally performed earlier in the disease course in good surgical candidates.

RELEVANT ANATOMY AND PHYSIOLOGY

Aqueous Physiology

IOP determined by rate of aqueous production versus resistance to outflow (primarily due to trabecular meshwork).

Total volume ~250 μl and rate of production ~2.5 μl/minute.

Aqueous Flow (FIG. 5.4.1)
Corneoscleral Block (FIG. 5.4.2)

ALTERNATIVES TO TRABECULECTOMY

Medical Therapy

1. Suppression of aqueous production:
    - Topical beta-blockers (e.g., timolol, betaxolol, levobunolol, carteolol)
    - Alpha-adrenergic agonists (e.g., brimonidine, apraclonidine)
    - Carbonic anhydrase inhibitors (e.g., dorzolamide, brinzolamide = topical; acetazolamide = systemic)

2. Facilitation of aqueous outflow:
    - Prostaglandin analogs (e.g., latanoprost, travoprost, bimatoprost)
    - Parasympathomimetic agents (e.g., pilocarpine, carbachol, echothiophate)
    - Epinephrine

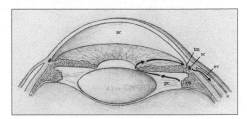

FIGURE 5.4.1 ◆ *Aqueous flow:* Produced by the non-pigmented ciliary body epithelium (cb), enters the posterior chamber (pc), passes through the pupil into the anterior chamber (ac), drains via the trabecular meshwork (tm), enters Schlemm's canal (sc), and returns to circulation via the episcleral veins (ev).

Lasers
- Laser Trabeculoplasty (argon laser trabeculoplasty [ALT] vs. selective laser trabeculoplasty [SLT])

Surgery
- Ex-PRESS Mini Glaucoma Shunt: A 3-mm stainless steel drainage tube that is inserted in the anterior chamber to lower IOP. Unlike traditional

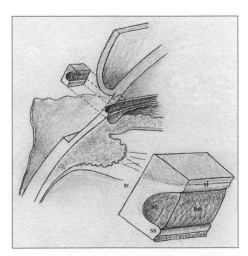

FIGURE 5.4.2 ◆ *Corneoscleral block anatomy:* Removal creates an alternate route (fistula) for aqueous drainage from the anterior chamber. The scleral spur (ss) anchors the trabecular meshwork (tm) and is the insertion of the longitudinal ciliary muscle fibers. Schwalbe's line (sl) marks the peripheral limits of Descemet's membrane.

implants, it does not have a drainage plate. Instead, aqueous outflow is controlled by placing the end of the tube beneath a scleral flap. (*Note:* This procedure is very similar to trabeculectomy, but does not require sclerectomy creation.)

- Canaloplasty: A "nonpenetrating" glaucoma surgery that reduces IOP by dilating Schlemm's canal to increase outflow through the trabecular meshwork. Cannula insertion permits injection of viscoelastic to dilate the canal. The cannula is then used to thread a radial Prolene suture through the canal. When tightened, the suture maintains canal dilation. This procedure is generally not effective in neovascular, inflammatory, or chronic angle closure glaucomas.

- Trabectome: Bipolar electrocautery is used to ablate the internal portion of the trabecular meshwork while maintaining patency of the collector channels that drain aqueous from Schlemm's canal to the episcleral veins.

- Cyclodestruction: Diode laser cyclophotocoagulation or cryotherapy (not commonly used) can reduce aqueous production by ablating a portion of the ciliary body, either transsclerally or via an endoscopic approach. This is generally irreversible, although children tend to have a more resilient ciliary body epithelium. IOP response can be unpredictable, so the procedure is generally reserved for patients with poor preoperative vision or for those who are not good surgical candidates.

ANESTHESIA

Local anesthesia (e.g., retrobulbar, peribulbar, or topical) with monitored anesthetic care (MAC) is preferable for most patients.

General anesthesia is avoided when possible because of increased risk of postoperative suprachoroidal effusion and hemorrhage associated with coughing.

PROCEDURE

SEE TABLES 5.4.1 Rapid Review of Steps and 5.4.2 Surgical Pearls, and WEB TABLES 5.4.1 to 5.4.4 for equipment and medication lists.

TABLE **5.4.1**   Rapid Review of Steps
(1) Conjunctival exposure
(2) Subconjunctival dissection (limbus- or fornix-based approach)
(3) Scleral flap creation
(4) Mitomycin C (MMC) application (optional)
(5) Paracentesis
(6) Removal of corneoscleral block
(7) Iridectomy (optional)
(8) Scleral flap closure
(9) Tenon's and conjunctival closure
(10) Evaluation of bleb

1. *Conjunctival Exposure:* A corneal traction suture is placed near the limbus between 11 and 1 o'clock (FIG. 5.4.3). It penetrates only two-thirds of the corneal thickness. Suture ends are then clipped to the surgical drape at the 6 o'clock position, allowing infraduction of the globe for maximum exposure of the superior conjunctiva.

2. *Conjunctival Incision and Flap:* The primary incision may be limbus- or fornix-based (FIG. 5.4.3). The limbus-based incision may be used in eyes without previous surgical intervention, whereas the fornix-based technique permits excision of scarred limbal tissue. (Surgeon preference

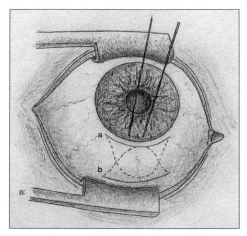

FIGURE 5.4.3 ◆ *Incision:* Conjunctival exposure with a traction suture permits creation of a fornix-based (a) or limbus-based (b) incision. The following figures depict the limbus-based incision, used in eyes without prior surgical intervention or perilimbal scarring.

TABLE **5.4.2** Surgical Pearls

Preoperative:

- Communicate with the patient that the postoperative course is variable and that it may take a few weeks (rarely a month or two) to return to baseline vision.
- Communicate that there may still be a need for intraocular pressure (IOP)-lowering drops or more surgery in the future.
- Include in the consent the increased possibility for late bleb-related endophthalmitis.

Intraoperative:

- Select incision location based on local vascularity and scarring. Consider the future need for the performance of additional surgery, such as repeat trabeculectomy or glaucoma drainage implant surgery.
- Create as small a conjunctival incision as possible to improve wound closure. Once the underlying Tenon's is incised, the conjunctival incision typically stretches and enlarges much more readily.
- Avoid overcauterizing the scleral bed, as this can cause unnecessary inflammation and may cause the sclera to contract, complicating wound closure.
- Create steep, straight-walled scleral flap edges. This will facilitate flap closure and control of aqueous filtration. A thin, oblique-walled flap can occasionally be very difficult to close and increases the risk for postoperative hypotony.
- Carry the flap dissection anteriorly into the clear cornea. This will create a valve-like closure that can further decrease the risk of hypotony and will help avoid iris incarceration into the sclerectomy.
- Prior to entering the anterior chamber under the flap, and creation of the sclerectomy, check with your surgical scrub technician that you have the appropriate instruments ready to enable smooth subsequent surgical maneuvers without unnecessary delays (e.g., Kelly punch, Vannas scissors, 10-0 nylon). After the sclerectomy has been created and when the flap is open but unsutured, the eye is hypotonus and at greatest risk for expulsive choroidal hemorrhage.
- Consider preplacing sutures in the flaps to facilitate closure of the scleral flap.
- If the sclerectomy is created too far posterior, the ciliary body or iris root may be damaged resulting in significant intraocular bleeding. The 23-gauge cautery can be used to control intraocular bleeding, but use with care to avoid collateral damage to other structures such as the crystalline lens.
- Once the scleral flap is secured with sutures, use balanced saline solution (BSS) to reinflate the anterior chamber. The chamber should deepen prior to filtration of aqueous under the flap. Use sponges to assess filtration, check IOP and chamber depth/stability prior to conjunctival closure. Add sutures to reduce flow, or loosen or replace sutures in a flap that is not slowing filtering.
- Avoid unnecessary or excessive manipulation of the conjunctiva. Avoid inadvertent damage to the conjunctiva with the suture needle. Meticulous closure and evaluation for wound leaks during the first surgery can reduce the need for reoperation and increase the chances for surgical success.

Postoperative:

- Carefully check for wound leaks. Small wound leaks will often close spontaneously. Larger wound leaks may require interventions such as bandage contact lens or surgical revision. The presence of a large, elevated bleb is a good indicator that the wound leak is small and will close spontaneously.
- Communicate with the patient that they should not bend, strain, or lift heavy objects until cleared by the primary surgeon.
- Monitor for excessive postoperative inflammation. Consider oral or periocular depot steroids to control excessive inflammation.
- Aim for IOPs around 10 mm Hg and remove sutures one visit at a time. Removing too many sutures too quickly can result in overfiltration and hypotony.
- Consider postoperative subconjunctival 5-fluorouracil (5-FU) if there is excessive vascularity to the bleb or elevated IOP.
- A shallow anterior chamber in a hypotonus eye often corrects with time. A flat anterior chamber rarely corrects without intervention. In the setting of a flat anterior chamber, consider reformation of the anterior chamber with viscoelastic or revision and tighter closure of the flap. If there is hypotony but a flat bleb, look for a wound leak, or consider aqueous hyposecretion due to inflammation or choroidal detachment.
- A flat anterior chamber with moderately or significantly elevated IOP may be due to aqueous misdirection. This can be treated with cycloplegics (atropine) and aqueous suppressants (dorzolamide). Definitive treatment of aqueous misdirection includes Nd:YAG (neodymium-doped yttrium aluminum garnet) capsulotomy/anterior hyaloidotomy or pars plana vitrectomy with irido-zonular-hyloidectomy to create a unicameral eye (complete and open communication between the anterior and posterior chambers).

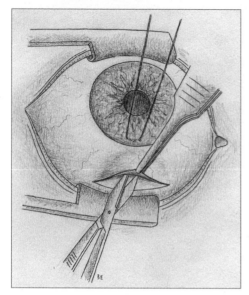

FIGURE 5.4.4 ◆ *Scleral exposure:* Blunt dissection of the limbus-based conjunctival flap with scissors permits exposure of underlying sclera.

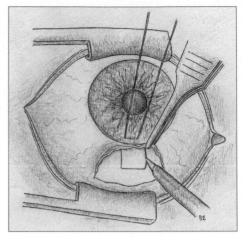

FIGURE 5.4.5 ◆ *Scleral flap creation:* Creation of a partial thickness scleral flap permits exposure of the corneoscleral junction for fistula creation.

combined with clinical scenario largely determines which incision is made.) For a limbus-based approach, sharp scissors are used to make an 8- to 10-mm incision through the conjunctiva and Tenon's capsule that parallels the fornix. The flap is then created with blunt dissection, resulting in scleral exposure (FIG. 5.4.4).

3. *Scleral Flap:* A scleral flap (usually 4 × 4 mm and two-thirds thickness) is outlined at the 12 o'clock position using a fine scalpel (FIG. 5.4.5). The posterior margin of the incision is then raised with blunt forceps and the flap is created with a blade exposing the site of the corneoscleral block.

4. *Mitomycin C (MMC) Application* (optional step): Topical administration of this antimetabolite, if performed, is generally applied after the corneoscleral block is adequately exposed.

5. *Paracentesis:* A fine blade is used to create a temporary self-sealing tract through the cornea and into the anterior chamber. This permits injection of fluid to gauge flow through the trabeculectomy site.

6. *Corneoscleral Block:* A fine blade or a corneoscleral punch (e.g., Kelly Punch) is used to make a 2 × 3-mm full-thickness incision into the anterior chamber just posterior to the hinge of the scleral

flap. The block is then removed using scissors or a punch (FIG. 5.4.6). If the block is too large, the result is overfiltration and hypotony (IOP < 5); if too small, adequate flow will not be achieved.

7. *Iridectomy:* After the corneoscleral block is removed, the iris may obstruct the fistula and aqueous outflow. The peripheral iris can be lifted through the block opening with forceps and a small section is removed with scissors. After this

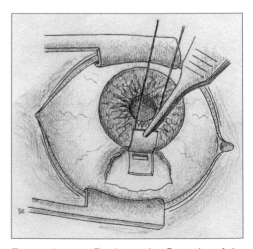

FIGURE 5.4.6 ◆ *Fistula creation:* Retraction of the scleral flap permits removal of the corneoscleral block. Peripheral iris is then removed to avoid obstruction of the newly created fistula (peripheral iridectomy).

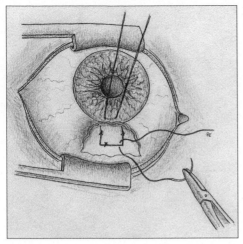

FIGURE 5.4.7 ✦ *Scleral flap closure:* This is accomplished with fine sutures (9-0 or 10-0 nylon). Aqueous exits through the fistula, drains between the flap sutures, and enters the subconjunctival space, creating the filtering bleb.

cut is made, aqueous from the posterior chamber may pour out through the iridectomy.

8. *Scleral Flap Closure:* Two to five scleral flap sutures are then placed and tied (FIG. 5.4.7), and the anterior chamber is insufflated through the paracentesis tract. If the flap is closed too tightly, no flow occurs and IOP increases; if the flap is closed too loosely, overfiltration occurs. These sutures will be removed as needed postoperatively by laser suture lysis or by removal of releasable sutures with forceps under the slit lamp.

9. *Tenon's/Conjunctival Closure:* A single- or double-layer closure is generally done. For double-layer closure, a locking suture is used to close Tenon's capsule, followed by a running suture to close the conjunctiva. After closure, the anterior chamber is insufflated to inflate the bleb and check it for leaks (Bleb Test).

FURTHER CONSIDERATIONS

Antimetabolites

Episcleral fibrosis is the number one cause of trabeculectomy failure.

Antiproliferative agents (5-fluorouracil [5-FU], MMC) increase the success rate of complicated cases by inhibiting fibroblast proliferation at the filtration site.

MMC is applied topically intraoperatively while 5-FU is given by postoperative subconjunctival injection.

Low Risk: No metabolite necessary

Medium and High Risk: Low and high doses of antimetabolites used, respectively

> **NOTE:** *If concentration of these agents are too high or are used in low risk eyes, long-term hypotony and bleb breakdown are likely.*

COMPLICATIONS

Intraoperative

- Conjunctival buttonhole (part of conjunctival flap tears)
- Scleral flap tear/disinsertion
- Vitreous loss postiridectomy (vitreous will plug filtration pathway); common in aphakic eyes
- Bleeding from iris or ciliary body after iridectomy (can lead to blockage)
- Suprachoroidal hemorrhage

Early Postoperative

- Underdrainage: Increased IOP; managed by digital pressure followed by sequential release of scleral flap sutures
- Overdrainage: Shallow anterior chamber, hypotony, hypotony maculopathy; usually the result of poor scleral flap closure, occasionally due to a missed conjunctival buttonhole
- Choroidal effusion

Late Postoperative

- Episcleral fibrosis: May result from heavy vascularization and healing/scarring around the bleb, with failure of procedure
- Tenon's cyst formation
- Chronic hypotony from bleb leaks (particularly if overtreated with antimetabolites)
- Endophthalmitis

POSTOPERATIVE CARE

- Topical steroids: Given to prevent inflammation and scarring (variable taper based on bleb appearance)

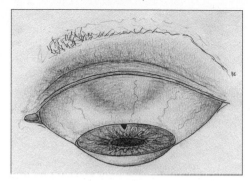

FIGURE 5.4.8 ◆ *Filtration bleb:* A healthy filtration bleb is seen as a bulge in the superior conjunctiva when eye is depressed. Also depicted is a patent peripheral iridotomy at 12 o'clock, which prevents occlusion of the corneoscleral block by iris tissue.

- Topical antibiotic and mydriatic/cycloplegic (e.g., atropine)

First 2 weeks: The bleb is followed carefully for leaks and vascularity (FIG. 5.4.8), the anterior chamber (AC) is examined for inflammation (flare/cells) and depth, and the posterior segment is examined for choroidal effusions. If the bleb is failing due to fibrosis or vascularization, subconjunctival 5-FU may be administered.

The timing for suture release or laser suture lysis is critical and varies by the individual; early lysis may result in hypotony, and late lysis may result in bleb failure.

Further Reading

Text

Allingham R, Damji K, Freedman S, et al., eds. *Shields' Textbook of Glaucoma.* 5th ed. Philadelphia, PA: Lippincott Williams and Wilkins; 2004.

Salmon JF. Glaucoma. In: Whitcher, J, Riordan-Eva P, eds. *Vaughan and Asbury's General Ophthalmology.* New York, NY: McGraw-Hill; 2004:212–228.

Yanoff M, Duker J. Trabeculectomy. In: *Ophthalmology.* St. Louis, MO: Mosby; 2004:1586–1595.

Primary Sources

AGIS (Advanced Glaucoma Intervention Study) Investigators. The Advanced Glaucoma Intervention Study (AGIS): 7. The relationship between control of intraocular pressure and visual field deterioration. *Am J Ophthalmol.* 2000;130(4):429–440.

Dastur YK. The role of early trabeculectomy in the control of chronic simple glaucoma. *J Postgrad Med.* 1994;40(2): 74–77.

Rothman RF, Liebmann JM, Ritch R. Low-dose 5-fluorouracil trabeculectomy as initial surgery in uncomplicated glaucoma: long-term follow-up. *Ophthalmology.* 2000;107(6):1184–1190.

Singh K, Mehta KAAA, Shaikh NM, et al. Trabeculectomy with intraoperative mitomycin C versus 5-fluorouracil. Prospective randomized clinical trial. *Ophthalmology.* 2000;107(12): 2305–2309.

White T. Hypotonous maculopathy after trabeculectomy with subconjunctival 5-fluorouracil. *Am J Ophthalmol.* 1993;115(4):547–548.

CHAPTER 6

Pediatrics

Daniel J. Salchow

6.1 STRABISMUS SURGERY

- Restores ocular alignment by changing the length or scleral insertion of targeted extraocular muscles.
- Horizontal deviations:
  - These are commonly corrected by performing a resection, or shortening, of one horizontal muscle (medial or lateral rectus) accompanied by a recession, or more posterior reinsertion, of its antagonist in the same eye.
  - Such deviations can also be addressed with bilateral recessions or resections. Transecting muscle during a resection is painful; bilateral recessions, therefore, reduce postoperative analgesic requirements as compared to alternative management strategies.
- Repair of vertical and torsional deviations is more complex because the affected muscles all have secondary functions.

INDICATIONS

- In cases of infantile strabismus, binocular vision is still developing. Correction is therefore undertaken in patients as young as 6 months, in order to permit normal maturation of visual functions (e.g., stereopsis). Amblyopia is also aggressively treated.
- When strabismus emerges later in childhood, surgery is urgently indicated to preserve consolidating binocular vision.
- In adult patients, binocular vision is usually well established. Therefore, surgery is less urgent and usually takes place after stability of the observed deviations has been confirmed.

ALTERNATIVES AND ADJUNCTS

Medical Therapy

NOTE: *These therapies usually do not eliminate the ultimate need for eye muscle surgery and are used as adjuncts to surgical management.*

- Prisms: Simulate changes in eye position by altering the path of incident light. They can be attached to existing spectacles with adhesive (Fresnel prisms) or incorporated into newly ground lenses for longer term use.
- Orthoptics: Exercises to strengthen the eye movements that would restore ocular alignment (known as vergence movements). Convergence exercises, which are used to treat convergence insufficiency, have been shown to be effective.
- Botox injections: Temporarily paralyze the targeted muscles, permitting the unopposed action of their antagonists to restore ocular alignment.
- Sector occlusion: Strategically placed spectacle lens covers reduce diplopia in incomitant strabismus by blocking regions of the visual field associated with diplopia.
- Patching: Complete occlusion of the less affected eye prevents or reverses amblyopia, often in preparation for surgical realignment.

RELEVANT PATHOPHYSIOLOGY AND ANATOMY

Strabismus Essentials

- Due to ocular misalignment, object images are projected to noncorresponding points of the retina.

- Children less than 6 to 8 years of age readily suppress the image of one eye in strabismus. They may rapidly develop amblyopia and lose stereopsis.

- Older children and adults have greater difficulty suppressing conflicting images and experience diplopia.

- At any given time, only one eye (the fixating eye) is able to focus on the target of interest, while the other eye is deviated.

Strabismus Classification

Comitant

- The strabismus angle is constant in all directions of gaze.

- This can be monocular (the patient has a consistent "fixation preference") or alternating (the fixating eye switches).

- Esotropia is most frequent in infancy, whereas exotropia is more common in childhood.

- Vertical deviations, such as hypertropia or hypotropia, are less common in all age groups.

- Potential etiologies include: Congenital/genetic causes, unilateral vision impairment, prior orbital surgery (e.g., decompression for thyroid eye disease), insufficient image fusion (e.g., anisometropia or aniseikonia), and uncorrected hyperopia, which can cause esotropia due to the link between convergence and accommodation.

Incomitant

- The angle of deviation varies depending on gaze position, due to paralysis or mechanical restriction of one or more extraocular muscles.

- Etiologies include cranial nerve palsies (CN III, IV, or VI) and entrapment resulting from orbital floor fracture, Graves disease, and prior surgery.

- Potential paralytic lesion locations include:
  - Internuclear ophthalmoplegia: The lesion is within the medial longitudinal fasciculus (MLF), a pair of brainstem tracts that helps synchronize the action of cranial nerves on opposing sides.
  - Nuclear: The lesion lies within the brainstem nucleus of a specific cranial nerve.
  - Supranuclear: The lesion is in a higher order tract, such as the paramedian pontine reticular formation (PPRF), which coordinates conjugate eye movements.

- Differential diagnosis for paralytic lesions include:
  - Congenital: Includes encephalitis, aplasia, and birth trauma (e.g., aggressive forceps delivery).
  - Acquired: Includes diabetes, vascular disease, trauma, mass effect from space occupying lesions, infections, increased intracranial pressure, multiple sclerosis, and, rarely, HIV/AIDS.

Extraocular Muscle Anatomy (FIG. 6.1.1)

- Muscle origins:
  - All four rectus muscles originate from the Annulus of Zinn, a fibrous ring that

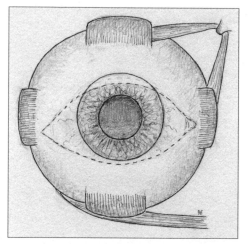

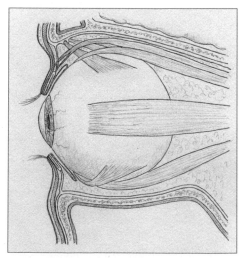

A **B**

FIGURE 6.1.1 ◆ *Extraocular muscle anatomy:* **(A)** Anterior view of the globe with superimposed palpebral fissure outline, and **(B)** lateral view. The borders of the rectus and oblique muscles merge with Tenon's capsule, a thin fascial layer between the conjunctiva and sclera (not pictured).

	Primary Function	Secondary Functions	Cranial Nerve Innervation	Strabismus Classification (If paralyzed)
Lateral Rectus	Abduction	—	Abducens (VI)	Esotropia
Medial Rectus	Adduction	—	Oculomotor (III)	Exotropia
Superior Rectus	Elevation	Incyclotorsion, adduction	Oculomotor (III)	Hypotropia
Inferior Rectus	Depression	Excyclotorsion, adduction	Oculomotor (III)	Hypertropia
Superior Oblique	Depression	Incyclotorsion, abduction	Trochlear (IV)	Hypertropia, excyclotorsion
Inferior Oblique	Elevation	Excyclotorsion, abduction	Oculomotor (III)	Hypotropia, incyclotorsion

encloses the optic canal and nerve at the orbital apex.

- The superior oblique and levator palpebrae superioris arise from the sphenoid bone, just outside of the annulus.
- The inferior oblique arises just deep to the medial orbital rim.

- Muscle insertions:
  - The distance between the corneal limbus and scleral insertions of the rectus muscles is described by the Spiral of Tillaux:
    ○ Medial rectus: 5.5 mm
    ○ Inferior rectus: 6.5 mm
    ○ Lateral rectus: 6.9 mm
    ○ Superior rectus: 7.7 mm
  - After passing through the trochlea, the superior oblique fans out to insert beneath the superior rectus, posterior to the axis of rotation.
  - The inferior oblique passes beneath the inferior rectus and inserts in the inferior temporal quadrant of the posterior globe.
- Vascular supply:
  - Each rectus muscle is accompanied by two anterior ciliary arteries, except for the lateral rectus, which usually has just one.
  - These muscular branches arise from the ophthalmic artery and contribute to an anastomotic circle at the root of the iris.
  - Disruption of multiple arteries can produce anterior segment ischemia. Surgery on extraocular muscles, therefore, is usually limited to two rectus muscles per eye and session.
- Key anatomic associations:
  - The sclera is thinnest just posterior to the rectus muscle insertions (~300 microns vs. ~700 microns elsewhere).

- Near their insertions, the oblique muscles travel below the corresponding rectus muscles.
- The inferior oblique inserts over the macula.

Extraocular Muscle Function

See table above.

PREOPERATIVE ASSESSMENT

- Stability of ocular deviation is usually confirmed by at least two sets of measurements prior to surgical intervention, commonly performed 4 to 6 weeks apart.
- Ocular alignment is assessed for distance and near vision in the nine diagnostic gaze positions (straight, left, up/left, up, up/right, right, down/right, down, and down/left; these are measured in 30 degrees excentric gaze).
- Forced ductions are used to rule out external impingements on ocular motility. They are tested by moving the eye with forceps, either in the operating room under general anesthesia or in clinic under topical anesthesia (if the patient is able to cooperate). A cotton-tip applicator can also be used to move the eye but is less accurate.

ANESTHESIA

- General anesthesia produces the best globe akinesia and is typically required in younger patients.
- Retrobulbar anesthesia is occasionally used in older, cooperative patients.

PROCEDURE

SEE TABLES 6.1.1 Rapid Review of Steps and 6.1.2 Surgical Pearls, and WEB TABLES 6.1.1 to 6.1.4 for equipment and medication lists.

The following narrative describes correction of right exotropia with a combined lateral rectus recession and medial rectus resection. It is intended to illustrate basic principles of strabismus surgery, which can be abstracted to other cases.

1. *Conjunctival Incision:* The eye is elevated and adducted using perilimbal traction sutures or forceps. The exposed conjunctiva is then lifted and incised with scissors approximately 8 mm from the limbus, exposing the underlying Tenon's capsule (FIG. 6.1.2).

2. *Tenon's Incision:* The Tenon's capsule is elevated with forceps and incised with scissors to expose the sclera (FIG. 6.1.3A).

TABLE 6.1.1 Rapid Review of Steps

(1) Muscle isolation:
 - Conjunctival incision
 - Tenon's incision
 - Muscle hook placement
 - Blunt/sharp dissection and removal of conjunctiva and fascia over rectus muscle
(2) Recession:
 - Suture placement and disinsertion
 - Caliper measurement and reinsertion at predetermined recessed location
(3) Resection:
 - Suture placement at predetermined distance from its scleral insertion
 - Cross-clamping of muscle anterior to suture
 - Muscle transection anterior to clamp and cautery over clamp
 - Removal of muscle stump from insertion
 - Reinsertion of muscle to original insertion point
(4) Conjunctival closure

TABLE 6.1.2 Surgical Pearls

Preoperative:
- Meticulous and reproducible measurements of ocular misalignment and motility are necessary before surgery can be planned. This requires a customized approach in which the chief complaint of each patient is addressed.
- Primary position (straight ahead) and reading position (looking down) are most important; in complicated cases, alignment in these positions is the goal.

Intraoperative:
- Forced-duction testing may be needed to identify tight muscles.
- Identify scar tissue to choose best approach.
- Be aware of previous eye surgery (particularly prior muscle surgeries), as the muscles may not be in the expected location.
- A limbal incision is easier and anatomically more straightforward.
- A fornix incision is more comfortable for the patient (as the incision is away from the cornea).
- Avoid extensive dissection.
- Avoid violating orbital fat. It can adhere to ocular structures, which can disrupt ocular mobility.
- When operating on the inferior oblique, visualize the vortex vein in order to minimize the risk of bleeding.
- Patients with thyroid eye disease may have very tight muscles.
- Make sure the muscle is securely suspended on the suture in order to avoid retraction and loss of the muscle.
- Hold needle short (e.g., half way) for partial thickness scleral pass. This maximizes control and helps to avoid scleral perforations.
- Handle conjunctiva gently, especially in elderly patients. A limbal incision can help to prevent tears.

Postoperative:
- Assess patient within 1 to 3 days after surgery to make sure the eye moves in the direction of the operated muscle(s). If unexpected motility deficit is seen, suspect slipped muscle.
- Patients with marked scarring (e.g., previous eye muscle surgery) may have more pain. Consider prescribing a stronger pain medication.
- Avoid blood-thinning pain medications (e.g., aspirin) postoperatively.

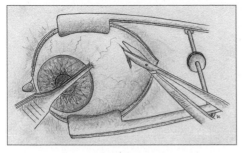

FIGURE 6.1.2 ◆ *Conjunctival incision:* The eye is elevated and adducted with locking forceps, exposing the peripheral conjunctiva, which is then incised with scissors approximately 8 mm from the corneal limbus.

3. *Muscle Hook Placement:* A muscle hook is then inserted between the bare sclera and lateral rectus in order to capture the full width of the muscle. The hook is then pulled toward the limbus to identify the scleral insertion of the rectus (FIG. 6.1.3B).

4. *Conjunctival/Fascial Dissection:* A smaller tenotomy hook is used to retract the overlying conjunctiva and fascia superiorly over the tip of the muscle hook, which can be visualized as a bulge beneath Tenon's capsule (FIG. 6.1.4A,B).

5. *Rectus Muscle Isolation:* The buried tip of the muscle hook is used to guide placement of an incision between the superior margin of the rectus muscle and adjacent Tenon's capsule (FIG. 6.1.4B). The muscle is then fully exposed with a combination of blunt and sharp dissection.

6. *Suture Placement/Muscle Disinsertion:* Once the lateral rectus has been isolated, a double-armed 6-0 Vicryl suture with S-29 needles is placed through the body of the muscle 1 mm distal to its insertion. Locking bites are taken at the superior and inferior muscle margins to ensure suture retention (FIG. 6.1.5). The tendon is then cut at the insertion, leaving the muscle suspended on the suture.

7. *Muscle Reinsertion:* Calipers are used to mark the location of a new scleral insertion based on the recession length calculated in clinic (FIG. 6.1.6). The needles are passed through sclera using partial-thickness bites and the suture is securely tied. Great care must be taken to control needle depth as the sclera is quite thin and there is no transmitted sensation to indicate scleral perforation, which may cause retinal holes and other complications.

8. *Conjunctival Closure:* The conjunctiva is then closed with interrupted 8-0 Vicryl sutures (FIG. 6.1.7). Independent closure of Tenon's capsule is not required.

9. *Resection:* The medial rectus muscle is isolated and elevated with muscle hooks as described previously. A locking double-armed suture is then passed through the rectus at the desired distance

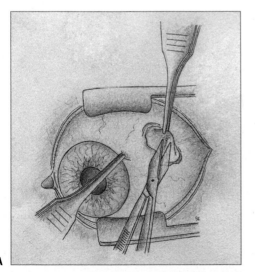
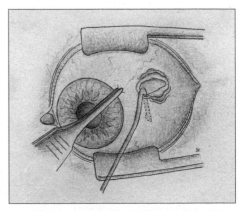

A **B**

FIGURE 6.1.3 ◆ *Tenon's incision:* **(A)** Tenon's capsule is incised inferiorly to the lateral rectus muscle. *Muscle hook placement:* **(B)** A muscle hook is then placed between the rectus muscle and underlying bare sclera. The hook (buried tip shown with a dashed line) should capture the entire width of the muscle.

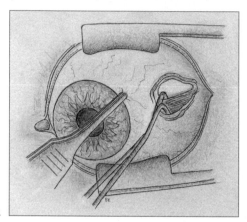

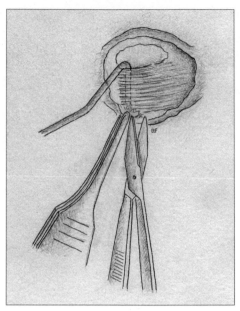

A

B

FIGURE 6.1.4 ✦ *Conjunctival/fascial dissection:* **(A)** Fascia and conjunctiva overlying the lateral rectus muscle are retracted with a small tenotomy hook. *Rectus muscle isolation:* **(B)** The superior margin of the muscle is continuous with Tenon's capsule. The tip of the muscle hook can be seen as a bulge beneath the capsule and is used to guide incision placement.

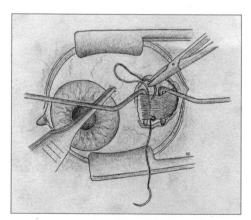

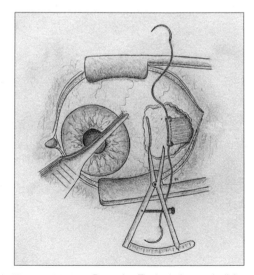

FIGURE 6.1.5 ✦ *Suture placement:* The lateral rectus is seen isolated from surrounding fascia and elevated with muscle hooks. A double-armed suture is then passed through the muscle just distal to its insertion and secured with locking bites.

FIGURE 6.1.6 ✦ *Recession:* The lateral rectus is disinserted and remains suspended on the double-armed suture. Calipers are then used to mark the location of the new insertion point based on a recession length calculated in clinic.

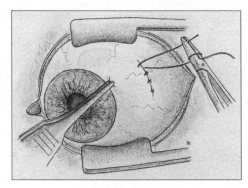

FIGURE 6.1.7 ◆ *Conjunctival closure:* Superficial closure is accomplished with interrupted sutures.

from its insertion. The muscle is cross-clamped just proximal to this suture and transected anterior to the clamp (FIG. 6.1.8A). The cut rectus muscle must be carefully cauterized or it will bleed (Fig. 6.1.8B). After removing the muscle stump, the suspended free end of the rectus is securely sutured to the original insertion, and the overlying conjunctiva is closed.

COMPLICATIONS

Intraoperative

1. *Overcorrection or undercorrection:* This may require reoperation after a period of observation (usually at least 6 weeks) and nonsurgical treatment.

2. *Hemorrhage:* This arises due to inadequate cauterization of the anterior ciliary arteries or to accidental perforation of the vortex veins (most common in oblique muscle surgery).

3. *Globe perforation:* This occurs when scleral suture bites are too deep and can cause retinal detachment, vitreous leakage, or intraocular hemorrhage and infection.

4. *Posterior Tenon's capsule violation:* This can result in prolapse of orbital fat.

Postoperative

1. *Anterior segment ischemia:* The risk increases when surgery is performed on multiple rectus muscles or in older patients with systemic disease.

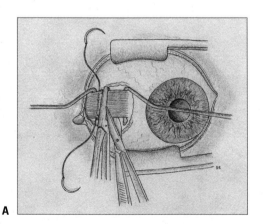

A

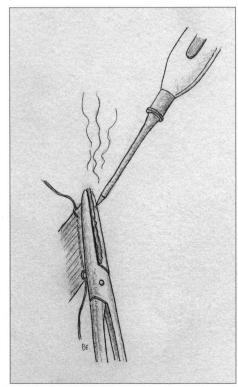

B

FIGURE 6.1.8 ◆ *Medial rectus recession:* **(A)** A double-armed suture is passed through the rectus, which is then cross-clamped and transected proximally to the hemostat. **(B)** The cut end is cauterized to prevent anterior ciliary artery hemorrhage.

2. *Epithelial cysts:* These lesions form when the conjunctiva folds under itself at the incision site. The risk is minimized by careful approximation during closure.

3. *Slipped muscle:* Disinsertion, most commonly of the medial or inferior rectus, can occur if the sutures break or pull through the muscle. It will then retract into orbit, necessitating immediate reoperation to prevent significant long-term complications.

POSTOPERATIVE CARE

- Administer topical steroids and antibiotics.

- Prescribe mild analgesics for postoperative pain (increased by muscle resections).

- Follow up in clinic to measure the attained correction and to screen for potential complications.

- Stable ocular alignment is usually achieved by 4 to 6 weeks.

Further Reading

Text

Crouch ER. Use of botulinum toxin in strabismus. *Curr Opin Ophthalmol.* 2006;17(5):435–440.

Lang G. Ocular motility and strabismus. In: *Ophthalmology: A Pocket Textbook Atlas.* 2nd ed. New York, NY: Georg Thieme Verlag; 2007:chap 17.

Lingua RW, Diamond GR. Techniques of strabismus surgery. In: Yanoff M, Duker J, eds. *Ophthalmology.* 3rd ed. Philadelphia, PA: Mosby; 2009:1370–1379.

Mills MD, Coats DK, Donahue SP, Wheeler DT. Strabismus surgery for adults: a report by the American Academy of Ophthalmology. *Ophthalmology.* 2004; 111(6):1255–1262.

Phillips PH. Strabismus surgery in the treatment of paralytic strabismus. *Curr Opin Ophthalmol.* 2001;12(6): 408–418.

Wong AM. Timing of surgery for infantile esotropia: sensory and motor outcomes. *Can J Ophthalmol.* 2008; 43(6):643–651.

Primary Sources

Jackson S, Harrad RA, Morris M, Rumsey N. The psychosocial benefits of corrective surgery for adults with strabismus. *Br J Ophthalmol.* 2006;90(7):883–888.

Jeoung JW, Lee MJ, Hwang JM. Bilateral lateral rectus recession versus unilateral recess-resect procedure for exotropia with a dominant eye. *Am J Ophthalmol.* 2006; 141(4):683–688.

CHAPTER 7

Oculoplastics

C. Robert Bernardino

7.1 UPPER LID BLEPHAROPLASTY

- Surgical excision of redundant upper lid skin and prolapsed orbital fat to improve visual function and/or cosmetic appearance.

INDICATIONS

- Dermatochalasis (upper lid skin redundancy) and steatoblepharon (bulging of orbital fat through a weakened orbital septum) are common age-related changes that can be addressed with blepharoplasty (Fig. 7.1.1).
- Functional procedures improve vision when lid tissue redundancy is severe enough to partially obstruct the visual axis.
- Cosmetic procedures improve lid appearance in the absence of obstruction.

ALTERNATIVES

Medical Therapy

- Laser skin resurfacing reduces periorbital wrinkling but cannot address significant tissue redundancy or prolapse.

Surgery

- Browplasty: Brow ptosis (age-related sagging of the brows) may contribute significantly to sagging of the upper lid skin. Simultaneous lifting of forehead skin is therefore essential to a satisfactory surgical outcome in select cases.
- Ptosis repair: If significant blepharoptosis accompanies the lid tissue redundancy, simultaneous anterior levator advancement is advisable (see Chapter 7.7 Ptosis Repair).

RELEVANT ANATOMY/PATHOPHYSIOLOGY

Upper Lid Anatomy (Fig. 7.1.2)

- Layers (superficial to deep): skin, minimal subcutaneous connective tissue, orbicularis, orbital septum, fat pads, aponeurosis of levator palpebrae superioris, Müller's muscle, conjunctival fornix
- Eyelid crease: generally 8 to 10 mm above the lid margin in the mid-pupillary axis, though often lower or absent in Asians. It represents the most inferior extent of the orbital septum and fat pads as well as the insertion of levator aponeurosis fibers on the lid skin.
- Fat pads: There are two main upper lid fat pads—the nasal and the central. The nasal pad lies between the medial rectus and superior oblique, and is paler and firmer. The central pad overlies the levator aponeurosis and is separated from the nasal pad by fascial attachments to the trochlea.

Blepharochalasis

- A familial angioneurotic edema syndrome that causes periodic lid inflammation, especially in younger females. This leads to thinning and wrinkling of the periorbital skin.
- Important to distinguish from age-related changes, as it may recur after blepharoplasty.

PREOPERATIVE ASSESSMENT

- Photograph preoperative appearance and document current visual acuity.
- Functional blepharoplasty: Document visual fields before and after taping of the redundant skin (a demonstrable change is key to insurance reimbursement).

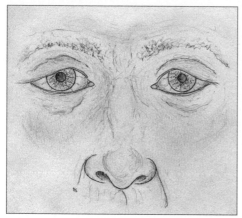

FIGURE 7.1.1 ◆ *A patient with dermatochalasis:* Redundant upper lid skin can be seen overhanging the lateral lid margins and superior irides. These skin folds may progress to obstruct the visual axis, restricting the supertemporal visual fields.

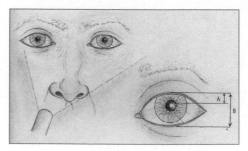

FIGURE 7.1.3 ◆ *Demonstration of the pupillary light reflex in primary gaze.* The marginal reflex distance (MRD) is the distance between the pupillary light reflex and the upper lid margin (A). The palpebral fissure (PF) width is the distance between the upper and lower lid margins in the midpupillary axis (B).

- Periorbital evaluation: Assess lid skin quality and degree of excess, amount and location of prolapsed orbital fat, lid crease position and symmetry, and lacrimal gland location.

- Since surgery can increase corneal exposure, evaluate for lagophthalmos, keratopathy, and adequacy of the tear film (check tear breakup time and perform the Schirmer's test).

- Assess for blepharoptosis by measuring the palpebral fissure width and marginal reflex distance in primary gaze (FIG. 7.1.3).

- Assess for brow ptosis with a manual lift of the forehead skin. Significant improvement of lid skin redundancy may suggest the need for simultaneous browplasty.

- If conducting browplasty, assess forehead skin quality, as well as the position and shape of the brows, brow furrows, orbital rim, and hairline. These factors are important in selecting an appropriate surgical technique.

ANESTHESIA

- Mark the skin incisions prior to anesthetic infiltration as subcutaneous fluid will distort the lid contour.

- Infiltrate local anesthetic with epinephrine to aid hemostasis. It is critical to aspirate prior to injecting to preclude inadvertent intravascular release. Slow injection will limit the pain from lid distension.

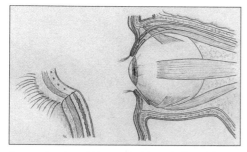

FIGURE 7.1.2 ◆ *Lid anatomy:* The anterior lid lamella consists of the skin and orbicularis; the posterior lamella consists of the tarsus, lid retractors, and palpebral conjunctiva. Orbicularis fibers exit the lid margin to form the gray line, which is posterior to the eyelash line and anterior to the meibomian gland orifices and mucocutaneous line.

TABLE 7.1.1 Rapid Review of Steps
(1) Mark lid crease and determine amount of skin to remove.
(2) Inject local anesthetic and allow for tie to work (5 minutes).
(3) Prep and drape.
(4) Excise skin/orbicularis.
(5) Dissect orbital fat pads.
(6) Reform lid crease (optional).
(7) Close skin incision.

TABLE 7.1.2 Surgical Pearls

Preoperative:
- Marking amount of tissue to be removed prior to infiltrating anesthesia is ideal. Local anesthetic will distort the tissues and, therefore, accuracy will be difficult to attain if marking is performed after infiltration of anesthetic.
- Determining the amount of tissue to be removed is a balance of enough to improve function and cosmesis and not too much to limit closure of the eyelid. Using forceps to pinch the excess skin to ensure that the eyelid can still close is a helpful technique prior to marking.
- A preoperative determination of whether debulking of orbital fat pads is important.
- Injection of anesthetic and allow for adequate time for onset.

Intraoperative:
- If only skin is excised, the orbital septum can be left intact. Skin closure can be performed in whatever technique the surgeon is comfortable, interrupted, running, or subcuticular. At 1 week, a subcuticular closure may appear better than other techniques, but by 6 weeks they are all comparable.
- If fat pad debunking is performed, careful hemostasis is essential. Clamping fat pads, cauterizing, and grasping residual fat before releasing the hemostat to ensure an actively bleeding vessel does not retract into the orbit is a must. Retrobulbar hemorrhage is a serious complication of blepharoplasty.

Postoperative:
- Remember that at the 1-week postoperative visit, it is hard to predict the ultimate postoperative result due to ecchymosis and edema. Therefore, reassuring a patient and holding off on revision surgery until healing is complete is important.

PROCEDURE

 See Tables 7.1.1 Rapid Review of Steps and 7.1.2 Surgical Pearls, and Web Tables 7.1.1 to 7.1.4 for equipment and medication lists.

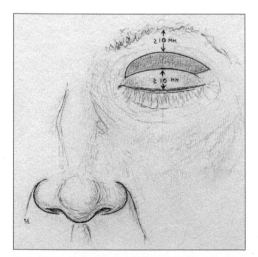

Figure 7.1.4 ◆ *Skin excision outline:* The ellipse of upper lid skin to be excised during blepharoplasty has been outlined. The inferior margin of the ellipse is defined by the anatomic eyelid crease. Note that at least 20 mm of skin should generally remain between the lower margin of the eyebrow and the upper lid lash line to prevent eyelid retraction.

1. *Marking:* An ellipse of upper lid skin is marked for removal. The lower margin of the ellipse is defined by the lid crease, which is typically 8 to 10 mm above the lash line in the midpupillary axis and 4 to 6 mm above it at the medial and lateral canthi. Redundant skin is overlapped with forceps to determine an appropriate upper resection margin. As a rule, at least 20 mm of skin should remain between the lower margin of the eyebrow and the lash line in order to prevent postoperative lid retraction (Fig. 7.1.4).

2. *Incision:* After appropriate demarcation, the skin is incised to the level of the dermis while gentle traction is applied to the lid (Fig. 7.1.5). This can be

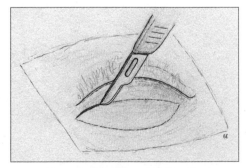

Figure 7.1.5 ◆ *Lid incision:* A scalpel is used to cut the skin while gentle traction is applied to the lid to eliminate wrinkling and ensure an even incision.

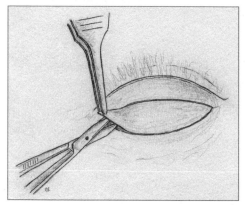

FIGURE 7.1.6 ✦ *Skin removal:* The ellipse of skin is then dissected free with scissors or a blade, leaving the underlying orbicularis intact.

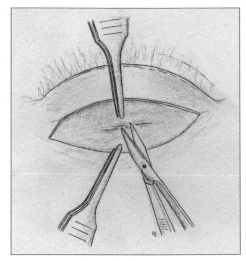

FIGURE 7.1.8 ✦ *Fat pad exposure:* The orbicularis is divided and the underlying orbital septum is incised, exposing the central and nasal fat pads.

accomplished with a traditional, laser, or radiofrequency scalpel. Beginning medially, the ellipse of skin is then dissected free with scissors or the scalpel, leaving the underlying orbicularis intact (FIG. 7.1.6). Careful hemostasis of the raw tissue bed is achieved with a bipolar cautery (FIG. 7.1.7).

3. *Fat Pad Excision:* The orbicularis is then divided just above the inferior margin of the elliptical incision, and the underlying orbital septum is incised, exposing the central and nasal fat pads (FIG. 7.1.8). Each pad is cross-clamped and divided while avoiding excessive traction, which can avulse vessels or damage adjacent orbital structures (FIG. 7.1.9). Meticulous hemostasis is maintained with electrocautery (FIG. 7.1.10). When excising

the central fat pad, care is taken to prevent injury to the underlying levator aponeurosis.

4. *Closure:* The lid crease is reformed by tacking the skin to the levator aponeurosis with interrupted sutures placed at regular intervals (FIG. 7.1.11). Incorporation of the orbital septum is avoided, as this can result in postoperative lid retraction. The skin incision is then closed with a running nylon suture. A subcuticular stitch provides the best short-term cosmetic results, but the difference becomes less noticeable with time.

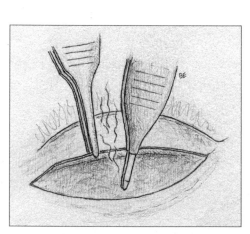

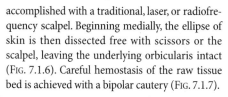

FIGURE 7.1.7 ✦ *Hemostasis:* Careful hemostasis of the raw tissue bed is achieved using a bipolar electrocautery.

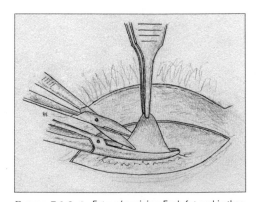

FIGURE 7.1.9 ✦ *Fat pad excision:* Each fat pad is then cross-clamped with a hemostat and divided with scissors or a scalpel. Excessive traction on the pads must be avoided since this can cause vessel avulsion or damage to adjacent orbital structures.

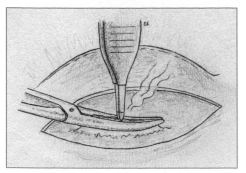

FIGURE 7.1.10 ✦ Fat pad hemostasis is then achieved with the bipolar cautery.

Additional Considerations: A browplasty requires the addition of supraorbital and supratrochlear regional blocks for adequate anesthesia. In general, an ellipse of skin is removed and the incision margins are reapproximated after they have been undermined to aid mobility. This results in vertical shortening of the forehead, eliminating brow ptosis. Several approaches are possible. See table below.

COMPLICATIONS

1. *Retrobulbar hemorrhage:* Occurs from inadequate hemostasis or vessel avulsion due to excessive traction on the fat pads; can progress to permanent vision loss. Check visual acuity and pupillary responses to rule out optic nerve dysfunction. Also, evaluate the fundus for central retinal artery occlusion (CRAO), which can be precipitated by IOP increase due to compressive force of the hematoma. Perform an emergent lateral canthotomy/cantholysis for orbital decompression.

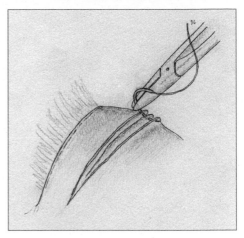

FIGURE 7.1.11 ✦ *Lid crease formation:* Tacking the skin to the levator aponeurosis with interrupted sutures placed at regular intervals reforms the lid crease. Skin closure is then achieved with a running suture.

2. *Central retinal artery avulsion:* A catastrophic complication due to excessive fat pad manipulation, which can produce retinal traction and vessel damage.

3. *Lid retraction:* Excess skin removal can result in lagophthalmos and ocular exposure. Initially treat with lid massage and lubrication; surgical correction is necessary if significant exposure keratopathy develops.

4. *Superior oblique injury:* The muscle is vulnerable to surgical trauma as it passes through the trochlea between the nasal and central fat pads.

5. *Lid bruising and discoloration:* This is anticipated in all patients, but fades with time.

6. *Lid telangiectasias:* May develop due to skin manipulation, but tend to fade with time.

	Incision Location	Amount of Correction	Risk of Nerve Damage and Hematoma	Comments
Direct	Above each eyebrow	+++	+	Permits unilateral correction, if desired. A powerful approach, but produces the most noticeable scars.
Midfrontal	In mid-forehead furrow	++	++	Good with deep furrows or frontal baldness.
Bicoronal	Posterior to hairline	+++	+++	Good with low-to-normal hairline.
Endoscopic	Small incisions posterior to hairline	++	+	Permits faster recovery.

7. *Lid hollowing:* Fat pad resection changes the lid contour, so excessive removal of tissue should be avoided.

8. *Cysts/suture tracts:* This can often be prevented with careful suture placement and early removal.

9. *Infection:* This is rare because the lid is highly vascular with minimal soft tissue, so immune mediators are easily delivered.

POSTOPERATIVE CARE

• Periodically apply antibiotic ointment to the surgical wound.

• Give mild oral analgesics since uncomplicated lid surgery should cause only minor discomfort.

• Counsel the patient to report severe pain immediately. This may be a sign of retrobulbar hemorrhage or corneal abrasion.

• Apply cold packs for the first 48 hours, then heat until the swelling resolves.

• Remove the skin sutures at 5 to 7 days for optimal cosmetic results.

• Avoid anticoagulants for 1 to 2 weeks, control blood pressure, and caution the patient to avoid straining (e.g., heavy lifting, Valsalva).

Further Reading

Text

Ben Simon GJ, McCann JD. Cosmetic eyelid and facial surgery. *Surv Ophthalmol.* 2008;53(5):426–442.

Codere F, Tucker N. Cosmetic blepharoplasty and browplasty. In: Yanoff M, Duker J, eds. Ophthalmology. 3rd ed. Philadelphia, PA: Mosby; 2009:1488–1495.

Gentile RD. Upper lid blepharoplasty. *Facial Plast Surg Clin North Am.* 2005;13(4):511–524, v–vi.

Patrocinio LG, Patrocinio JA. Forehead-lift: a 10-year review. *Arch Facial Plast Surg.* 2008;10(6):391–394.

Purewal BK, Bosniak S. Theories of upper eyelid blepharoplasty. *Ophthalmol Clin North Am.* 2005;18(2):271–398, vi.

Tasman W, Jaeger E, eds. Blepharoplasty. In: *Duane's Clinical Ophthalmology.* Vol 5. Philadelphia, PA: Lippincott Williams & Wilkins; 2008:chap 74.

Wagner P, Lang GK. The eyelids. In: *Ophthalmology: A Pocket Textbook Atlas.* 2nd ed. New York, NY: Georg Thieme Verlag; 2007:17–49.

Primary Sources

Kashkouli MB, Kaghazkanai R, Mirzaie AZ, et al. Clinico-pathologic comparison of radiofrequency versus scalpel incision for upper blepharoplasty. *Ophthal Plast Reconstr Surg.* 2008;24(6):450–453.

Kim HH, De Paiva CS, Yen MT. Effects of upper eyelid blepharoplasty on ocular surface sensation and tear production. *J Ophthalmol.* 2007;42(5):739–742.

7.2 DACRYOCYSTORHINOSTOMY (DCR)

• An occluded nasolacrimal duct is bypassed by creating an alternative drainage route between the lacrimal sac and nasal mucosa.

• This is most often performed through a skin incision, which permits the creation of an epithelium-lined tract. Nasal endoscopic alternatives are also available.

INDICATIONS

• Persistent obstruction of the nasolacrimal duct after an adequate trial of conservative therapy

• Bony obstruction of the duct, which cannot be ameliorated by medical therapy

ALTERNATIVES

Medical Therapy

Congenital Obstruction

• In the first year of life, 90% resolve spontaneously and are managed conservatively with lacrimal sac massage. If necessary, persistent membranes can be perforated with lacrimal drainage system probing.

Acquired Obstruction

• Dacryocystitis with obstruction is initially treated with antistaphylococcal antibiotics. Transcutaneous aspiration of the lacrimal sac to obtain culture specimens ensures adequate coverage of resistant organisms. Postinfectious epiphora can often be ameliorated with a trial of drainage system probing and syringing.

- Sympathomimetic vasoconstrictors (e.g., naphazoline) temporarily shrink the nasal mucosa and free mucus plugs, if present.

- Balloon dacryoplasty with placement of bicanalicular silicon tubing is an effective short-term management strategy, but stenosis generally recurs.

- Etiology-specific treatments are given (e.g., corticosteroids for sarcoidosis).

Surgery

Endoscopic nasal procedures do not require external incisions, but create drainage tracts that are smaller than those created via an external approach. Restenosis rates are consequently higher, but continue to improve with refinements in technique.

RELEVANT PHYSIOLOGY/ANATOMY

Nasolacrimal Physiology/Anatomy

- Disruption of the balance between tear production and drainage leads to a dry or watery eye (epiphora).
- Tear production:
  - Lacrimal gland:
    - Located in the supertemporal orbit beneath the orbital rim
    - Divided into orbital and palpebral segments by the levator aponeurosis
    - Creates the middle, aqueous (watery) layer of the tear film, which maintains a smooth corneal refractive surface and mobile conjunctiva
  - Accessory glands: the glands of Krause and Wolfring in the superior fornix supplement lacrimal gland tear production

- Tear drainage:
  - "Windshield wiper" lid motion: Contraction of the orbicularis begins laterally, resulting in medial movement of tear fluid.
  - Tear lake/meniscus: Fluid accumulates in the inferior fornix near the medial canthus. The inferior punctum is normally submerged in this "lake."
  - Mechanism: Tears enter the puncta via capillary action and then drain due to the force of gravity and the canalicular pumping generated by contraction of the surrounding orbicularis.
  - Lacrimal drainage route: tear lake superior and inferior puncta superior and inferior canaliculi common canaliculus nasolacrimal sac nasolacrimal duct exit through an ostium in the nasal mucosa beneath the inferior nasal turbinate (FIG. 1A)

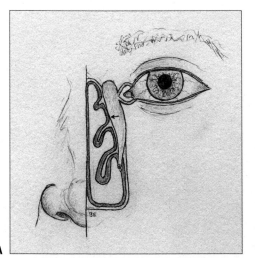

A

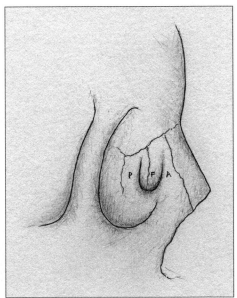

B

FIGURE 7.2.1 ◆ **(A)** The upper lacrimal drainage system consists of the superior and inferior puncta, superior and inferior canaliculi, common internal punctum, and lacrimal sac. The lower system consists of the valve of Hasner, nasolacrimal duct, and nasal mucosa exit below inferior turbinate. **(B)** The anterior and posterior lacrimal crests flank the lacrimal sac fossa, which contains the lacrimal sac.

- Nasolacrimal sac: A mucosal pouch that is located in the lacrimal fossa, a bony depression between the anterior and posterior lacrimal crests. The crests are formed by the frontal process of the maxilla and the lacrimal bone, respectively (FIG. 1A, B). The angular artery, a distal branch of the facial artery, lies just medial to the anterior lacrimal crest and is frequently encountered during surgery.

Causes of Epiphora

- Anatomic: A stricture, obstruction, foreign body, or tumor that blocks the nasolacrimal drainage system.
- Physiologic: A weak or paralyzed orbicularis that inhibits the tear-pumping mechanism; malposition of the lids and puncta (e.g., due to ectropion) can prevent tear entry into an otherwise patent drainage system.
- *Note:* Epiphora can also be seen in the absence of lacrimal drainage abnormalities. Reflex hypersecretion may occur in response to dry eye conditions or other forms of ocular surface irritation.

Classification of Obstruction
Congenital
- Due to an imperforate membrane or incomplete bony canalization in the lower drainage system
Acquired
- Idiopathic: inflammation, vascular congestion, lymphocyte infiltration, and edema develop due to an unknown cause and ultimately result in fibrosis
- Inflammatory: due to sarcoidosis, Wegener's granulomatosis, etc.
- Infectious: due to staphylococcus, streptococcus, pseudomonas, tuberculosis (TB), etc.
- Traumatic/postsurgical: can manifest after nasoethmoid fracture, sinus surgery, rhinoplasty, orbital decompression, etc.
- Malignant: due to primary lacrimal sac tumors, benign papilloma, squamous/basal cell carcinoma, lymphoma, etc.

PREOPERATIVE SCREENING

- Dye disappearance test (DDT): After topical anesthetic application, fluorescein dye is placed in the inferior fornix and the tear lake is observed with the slit lamp, using the cobalt filter. The presence of residual dye after 5 minutes suggests defective nasolacrimal drainage.
- Jones fluorescein dye test: Fluorescein is placed in the inferior fornix and the nose is examined for dye at 5 minutes. If none appears, the lacrimal sac is cannulated and irrigated with saline. Failure of dye to appear in the nose after irrigation indicates obstruction, whereas limited appearance of dye suggests stenosis.
- Lacrimal syringing: An irrigation cannula is introduced into the inferior punctum and advanced through the canaliculus. If the tip stops against bone (the floor of the lacrimal fossa), it has entered the nasolacrimal sac and the upper system is patent. If the tip stops against soft tissue, the upper system is obstructed. Saline is then infused; drainage into the nose without resistance or reflux confirms that the lower drainage system is also patent.
- Dacryocystography (DCG): This technique is occasionally used to assess patency of the nasolacrimal drainage system. Water-soluble contrast is infused prior to acquisition of digital subtraction X-ray or computed tomography (CT) scan.
- Nasal endoscopy: This technique permits observation of the nasolacrimal duct ostium.

ANESTHESIA

- A local block of the infratrochlear and anterior ethmoidal nerves is often used in conjunction with monitored anesthesia care (MAC). General anesthesia may be substituted.

PROCEDURE

SEE TABLES 7.2.1 Rapid Review of Steps and 7.2.2 Surgical Pearls, and WEB TABLES 7.2.1 to 7.2.4 for equipment and medication lists.

1. *Preoperative medication:* Nasal packing soaked with a sympathomimetic vasoconstrictor (e.g., naphazoline or cocaine) is inserted into the ipsilateral nare to reduce intraoperative bleeding (FIG. 2). Some surgeons infuse methylene blue

TABLE 7.2.1 Rapid Review of Steps
(1) Mark the incision site.
(2) Injection of local anesthetic and allow for time to work (5 minutes).
(3) Prep and drape.
(4) Incision of skin/orbicularis.
(5) Dissection to lateral nasal wall.
(6) Subperiosteal dissection to anterior lacrimal crest.
(7) Reflect lacrimal sac away from lacrimal sac fossa.
(8) Create ostium in lacrimal sac fossa.
(9) Open lacrimal sac.
(10) Create nasal mucosal flap.
(11) Pass silicone stents through ostium and secure in nose.
(12) Approximate lacrimal sac flap to nasal mucosal flap.
(13) Close skin incision in layers.

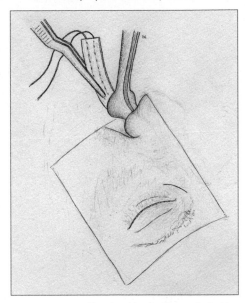

FIGURE 7.2.2 ◆ *Nasal packing:* Packing soaked with a sympathomimetic vasoconstrictor is inserted into the ipsilateral nare to reduce intraoperative bleeding.

dye into the nasolacrimal system to outline the lacrimal sac mucosa.

2. *Primary incision:* Classically, a vertical incision is made on the lateral portion of the bridge of the nose inferior to the medial canthal tendon. It is placed 10 mm medial to the canthal angle to avoid the angular vessels, which lie approximately 8 mm medial to this landmark. In prac-tice, a more lateral curvilinear incision overlying the anterior lacrimal crest provides better exposure of the fossa. The underlying angular vessels can be cauterized and cut without adverse consequences due to the presence of collateral circulation (FIGS. 3–5).

TABLE 7.2.2 Surgical Pearls

Preoperative:
- Have patient inhale decongestant solution prior to sedation or induction of general anesthesia.
- Inject anesthetic and allow for adequate time for onset.
- Consider infiltrating nasal mucosa with local anesthesia. Then pack nose with cotton pledgets soaked in additional decongestant solution.

Intraoperative:
- Hemostasis is important especially for visualization of the deep lacrimal structures.
- When removing bone, care is taken to ensure the nasal mucosa is not damaged.
- When approximating the lacrimal sac flap to the nasal mucosal flap, the suture is passed through the lacrimal flap first. Then a second bite is taken of the nasal mucosa. The nasal mucosa is very friable and easy to tear.

Postoperative:
- If monocular surgery is performed, a pressure patch can be placed on the operated side to help prevent postoperative hemorrhage.
- A nasal dressing can catch bloody nasal discharge.
- Patients should be instructed not to blow their nose for 1 week.

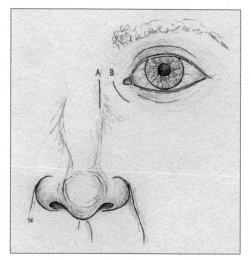

FIGURE 7.2.3 ◆ Classically, a vertical incision (A) is made on the lateral portion of the bridge of the nose inferior to the medial canthal tendon. It is placed 10 mm medial to the canthal angle to avoid the angular vessels, which lie 8 mm medial to this landmark. In practice, a more lateral curvilinear incision along the anterior lacrimal crest (B) provides better exposure of the lacrimal fossa.

3. *Lacrimal sac fossa exposure:* The orbicularis is then divided, and the dissection is carried down to the underlying periosteum, which is also incised. The periosteum is reflected laterally from the anterior lacrimal crest with a periosteal

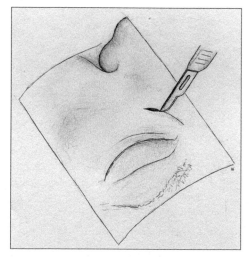

FIGURE 7.2.4 ◆ *Skin incision:* A curvilinear incision is made medial and inferior to the canthus, superficial to the anterior lacrimal crest.

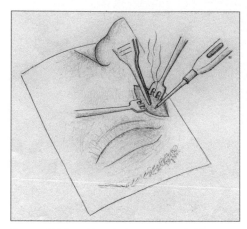

FIGURE 7.2.5 ◆ *Vessel cautery:* The underlying angular vessels are cauterized and cut. Dissection is then carried down to the periosteum overlying the anterior lacrimal crest.

elevator, revealing the sac within the lacrimal sac fossa (FIGS. 6–7). The lacrimal sac is then retracted within an envelope of periosteum to expose the fossa floor (FIG. 8).

4. *Bone removal:* To enter the nose, the floor of the lacrimal fossa is punctured at the suture line between the frontal process of maxilla and the lacrimal bone. A Kerrison rongeur is then used to remove small pieces of bone until the defect is large enough to permit the creation of a sutured fistula between the lacrimal sac mucosa and nasal mucosa (FIG. 9). In this location, the maxilla is thicker than the lacrimal bone, so natural

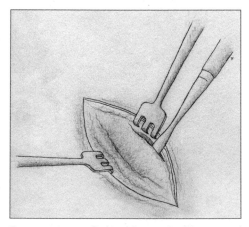

FIGURE 7.2.6 ◆ *Periosteal retraction:* The exposed periosteum is then incised and reflected laterally from the anterior lacrimal crest with a periosteal elevator.

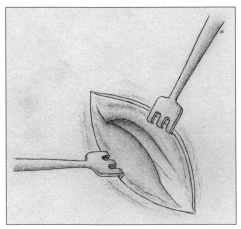

FIGURE 7.2.7 ✦ *Lacrimal fossa exposure:* Periosteal elevation reveals the lacrimal sac within its fossa; the sac is then retracted laterally within an envelope of periosteum to expose the fossa floor.

variations in suture location influence how much bone must be removed.

5. *Tract creation and stenting:* Probes connected by silicone tubing are inserted through the superior and inferior puncta into the lacrimal sac. The

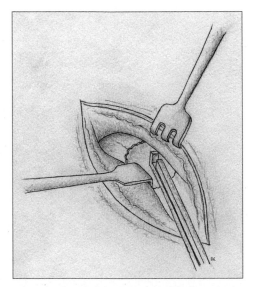

FIGURE 7.2.8 ✦ *Bony defect creation:* To enter the nose, the floor of the lacrimal fossa is punctured at the suture line. A Kerrison rongeur is then used to remove small pieces of bone until the defect is large enough to permit creation of a sutured fistula between the lacrimal sac mucosa and nasal mucosa.

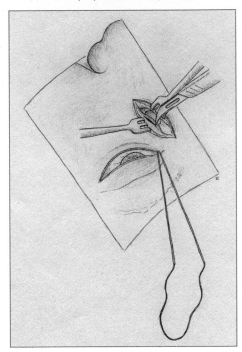

FIGURE 7.2.9 ✦ *Lacrimal sac incision:* Probes connected by silicon tubing are inserted through the superior and inferior puncta and into the lacrimal sac. The medial wall of the sac is then incised over the probe tips, creating anterior and posterior mucosal flaps.

medial wall of the sac is then incised over the probe tips, creating anterior and posterior mucosal flaps (FIG. 10). The nasal mucosa underlying the bony defect is also incised, creating anterior and posterior flaps (FIG. 11). A suction tip is then introduced into the nose and passed through the defect in the fossa floor. It is used to guide passage of the punctal probes and attached silicon tubing (FIG. 12). The mucosal flaps are then sutured posterior-to-posterior, and anterior-to-anterior to create an epithelium-lined tract (FIG. 13). Some surgeons omit posterior flap sutures, instead choosing to excise the excess mucosal tissue. The punctal probes are then detached from the silicone tubing. The free ends of the tubing are knotted together and trimmed. This knot will retract within the nare due to elastic recoil. The silicone stent is left in place for several weeks to ensure that the tract remains patent.

6. *Closure:* The periosteum and orbicularis are reapposed with interrupted sutures. The skin is then closed with a running suture.

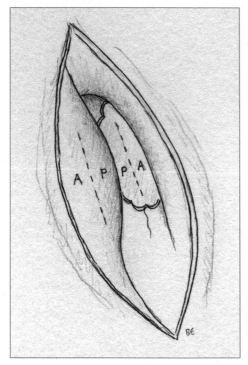

FIGURE 7.2.10 ◆ *Flaps:* The anterior and posterior flaps of the lacrimal sac are depicted on the left; those of the nasal mucosa are shown on the right through the defect in the floor of the lacrimal fossa.

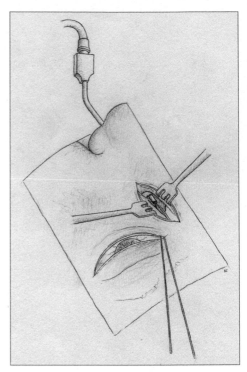

FIGURE 7.2.11 ◆ *Canalicular intubation and stenting:* A suction tip, introduced through the ipsilateral nostril and lacrimal fossa floor defect, is used as to guide the passage of the punctal probes and attached silicon tubing.

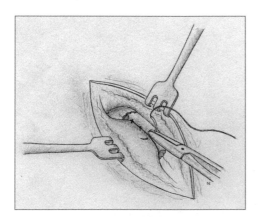

FIGURE 7.2.12 ◆ *Flap suturing:* The mucosal flaps are then sutured posterior-to-posterior, and anterior-to-anterior to create an epithelium-lined tract. Some surgeons omit suturing of the posterior flaps, instead choosing to resect the excess mucosal tissue.

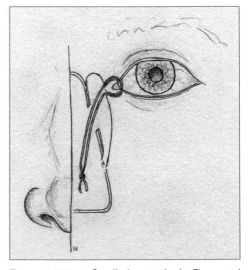

FIGURE 7.2.13 ◆ *Canalicular stent in situ:* The punctal probes are detached from the silicon tubing; the free ends are then knotted together and trimmed. This knot retracts inside the nostril due to elastic recoil. The tubing is left in place for several months to maintain tract patency.

Endoscopic surgery: A light pipe is threaded through the inferior punctum and into the lacrimal sac. The nasal mucosa is then incised around the spot of light that shines through the lacrimal fossa floor. The bone is punctured with a burrtip drill and the defect is enlarged with a Kerrison rongeur. The exposed medial wall of the lacrimal sac is incised and partially removed with scissors. Because epithelial flaps are generally not created, fistula patency must initially be maintained with an indwelling silicon stent.

COMPLICATIONS

Intraoperative

- Hemorrhage: Bleeding can be limited by cauterizing the angular veins with care, controlling systemic blood pressure, pretreating with vasoconstrictors, and using nasal packing to tamponade the mucosa.

Postoperative

- Failure to maintain patency: Administering decongestant and corticosteroid sprays can help shrink granulation tissue. Drainage system probing should be attempted prior to surgical revision.

POSTOPERATIVE CARE

- Apply topical antibiotics to the surgical wound for 1 week, and prescribe an oral antistaphylococcal antibiotic (e.g., first generation cephalosporin).

- Remove the skin suture at 5 to 7 days for optimal cosmetic results.

- Remove the silicon tubing at 6 to 12 weeks.

Further Reading

Text

Athanasiov PA, Prabhakaran VC, Mannor G, et al. Transcanalicular approach to adult lacrimal duct obstruction: a review of instruments and methods. *Ophthalmic Surg Lasers Imaging.* 2009;40(2):149–159.

Hurwitz JJ. The lacrimal drainage system. In: Yanoff M, Duker J, eds. *Ophthalmology.* 3rd ed. Philadelphia, PA: Mosby; 2009:1482–1488.

Mandeville JT, Woog JJ. Obstruction of the lacrimal drainage system. *Curr Opin Ophthalmol.* 2002;13(5): 303–309.

Wagner P, Lang GK. Lacrimal system. In: *Ophthalmology: A Pocket Textbook Atlas.* 2nd ed. New York, NY: Georg Thieme Verlag; 2007:49–66.

Watkins LM, Janfaza P, Rubin PA. The evolution of endonasal dacryocystorhinostomy. *Surv Ophthalmol.* 2003;48(1):73–84.

Primary Sources

Feretis M, Newton JR, Ram B, et al. Comparison of external and endonasal dacryocystorhinostomy. *J Laryngol Otol.* 2009;123(3):315–319.

Kansu L, Aydin E, Avci S, et al. Comparison of surgical outcomes of endonasal dacryocystorhinostomy with or without mucosal flaps. *Auris Nasus Larynx.* 2009;36(5): 555–559.

Seider N, Kaplan N, Gilboa M, et al. Effect of timing of external dacryocystorhinostomy on surgical outcome. *Ophthal Plast Reconstr Surg.* 2007;23(3):183–186.

Umapathy N, Kalra S, Skinner DW, et al. Long-term results of endonasal laser dacryocystorhinostomy. *Otolaryngol Head Neck Surg.* 2006;135(1):81–84.

7.3   ECTROPION REPAIR

- Restores an everted lower lid margin and punctum to normal positions in relation to the globe by addressing specific anatomic defects.

- Repair often entails shortening the tarsus, canthal tendons, or posterior lamella. Less commonly, the anterior lamella must be lengthened.

- Repair of the primary anatomic defect is prioritized, but it may be necessary to combine multiple techniques to achieve satisfactory results.

INDICATIONS

- Corneal breakdown due to lagophthalmos and ocular exposure.

- In the treatment of facial nerve palsy, ectropion repair is often combined with upper lid reanimation procedures such as gold weight or palpebral spring implantation.

ALTERNATIVES

Medical Therapy
- Lubrication: Artificial tears and ointments are used for mild disease.
- Bell's palsy: Ectropion is generally self-limited and administration of oral acyclovir may hasten recovery.

Surgery
- Electrocautery: Cautery spots are applied to the palpebral conjunctiva, which results in forniceal fibrosis and shortening, thus reapposing the lid to the globe. Better results are usually achieved by correcting specific anatomic defects.
- *Tarsorrhaphy:* If ectropion is associated with facial nerve palsy and "BAD syndrome" (absent **B**ell's phenomenon, **A**nesthetic corneas, and **D**ry eyes), suture tarsorrhaphy may be advisable to protect against acute corneal decompensation (see Chapter 7.8 Tarsorrhaphy).

RELEVANT PHYSIOLOGY/ANATOMY

Ectropion Overview
- The lower lid margin is everted from the globe. This leads to lagophthalmos and corneal exposure.
- Eversion of the punctum from the inferior fornix tear lake (lacus lacrimalis) inhibits nasolacrimal drainage. This causes tear fluid to run onto the cheek (epiphora).
- Poor tear drainage is exacerbated by lid laxity and loss of orbicularis tone, which eliminate the pumping mechanism (flaccid canalicular syndrome).
- If reflex tearing is inadequate to moisten the cornea, the patient will develop superficial punctate keratitis (SPK), which can progress to ulceration, superinfection, and perforation.

Ectropion Classification
- Involutional: Caused by age-related stretching of the tarsus and palpebral ligaments, and is the most common form. It generally progresses from punctal eversion to medial ectropion to generalized ectropion.

- Paralytic: Facial nerve palsy results in unilateral loss of orbicularis tone, which unmasks lid laxity. Paralysis may be temporary (e.g., Bell's palsy associated with Lyme disease, sarcoidosis, diabetes, or acquired immune deficiency syndrome [AIDS]) or permanent (e.g., trauma, surgery, or stroke affecting facial motor nucleus).
- Cicatricial: Insults such as burns, infection, and prior surgery may result in lid eversion due to scarring and contraction of the anterior lamella. This is exacerbated by coexisting horizontal laxity or lid retractor disinsertion.
- Congenital: A rare form of entropion caused by eyelid skin shortage. It is frequently associated with Down syndrome or blepharophimosis syndrome, but may also be idiopathic.
- Floppy eyelid syndrome: This is most frequently seen in overweight males with obstructive sleep apnea. Extreme lid tissue laxity is accompanied by tarsal thickening and chronic low-grade inflammation.

Lower Lid Anatomy
"Tarsoligamentous Sling" (FIG. 7.3.1)
- Formed by the inferior tarsus and canthal tendons, which keep the lid margin apposed to the

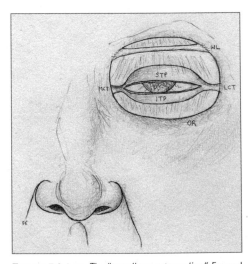

FIGURE 7.3.1 ◆ *The "tarsoligamentous sling":* Formed by the inferior tarsal plate (ITP) as well as the medial and lateral canthal tendons (MCT and LCT). It keeps the inferior lid margin and punctum apposed to the globe. Any or all parts can develop laxity, resulting in lower lid ectropion. The superior tarsal plate (STP) and Whitnall's ligament (WL) can also be visualized in the superior orbit.

globe. Any or all components can develop laxity, resulting in ectropion.

- Inferior tarsus: a dense connective tissue plate, approximately 1-mm thick and 4-mm wide in the midpupillary axis.
- Medial canthal tendon: divided into two limbs; the anterior limb anchors the medial tarsus and canthal angle to the frontal process of the maxilla (anterior lacrimal crest) while the posterior limb anchors these structures to the lacrimal bone (posterior lacrimal crest). The limbs flank the lacrimal sac, which sits in the nasolacrimal fossa.
- Lateral canthal tendon: anchors the lateral tarsus and canthal angle to Whitnall's tubercle on the inner margin of the lateral orbital rim. Other structures inserting on Whitnall's tubercle include Lockwood's ligament, the lateral check ligament, and the lateral horn of the LPS.

Lower Lid Lamellae

- Anterior lamella: consists of the lid skin and orbicularis oculi.
- Posterior lamella: consists of the inferior tarsus, capsulopalpebral fascia, and palpebral conjunctiva.
- Length imbalance between the anterior and posterior lamellae can result in lid eversion (e.g., cicatricial ectropion).

Capsulopalpebral Fascia

- Formed by the lower lid retractors, which oppose the action of the orbicularis muscle (analogous to the levator palpebrae superioris).
- Originates as an extension of the inferior rectus sheath and inserts on the inferior tarsus. This explains the depression of the lower lid in downgaze.
- Condenses to form Lockwood's ligament, which helps to support the globe within the orbit.
- Smooth muscle components receive sympathetic innervation; disruption results in "reverse ptosis."

PREOPERATIVE SCREENING

- Exam: Identify specific anatomic defect(s) and evaluate the severity of ectropion, lagophthalmos, and corneal pathology.
  - Snap test: Pull the lower lid down and away from the globe; then assess the speed of return after release (should occur spontaneously within 1 blink).

- Horizontal laxity: Pull the lid away from the globe (more than 10 mm of excursion is abnormal).
- Medial canthal tendon laxity: Pull the lid laterally and check movement of the inferior punctum (normally ≤ 1 to 2 mm).
- Lateral canthal tendon laxity: The lateral canthus should form an acute angle from 1 to 2 mm medial to orbital rim. Pull the lid medially and check movement of the angle (normally ≤ 1 to 2 mm).
- Punctal position: The inferior punctum should not be visible without manual lid eversion since it is normally submerged within the tear lake.
- Lid retractor laxity/disinsertion: Results in decreased motion of the lower lid on downgaze as well as an abnormally high resting position. Sympathetic denervation may also elevate the resting position of the lid, but should not impact motion on downgaze.
- Cicatricial changes: Observe the lower lid skin for discrete scars and check to see if tension lines form when the lid is pushed against the globe (indicates diffuse contracture).
- Orbicularis/facial nerve: Check tone during forced eye closure as well as observe for lid retraction, loss of forehead wrinkling, and mouth drop.
- Conduct a slit lamp exam with fluorescein to assess for exposure keratitis.

ANESTHESIA

- Local infiltration of anesthetic containing epinephrine to aid hemostasis

PROCEDURE

A procedure is chosen based on the anatomic defects present and the severity of disease. Although there is some overlap, these procedures can be grouped into five conceptual categories: shortening of the lateral canthal tendon, medial canthal tendon, horizontal lid, or posterior lamella, and lengthening of the anterior lamella.

1. *Lateral Canthal Tendon Shortening:*

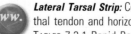 **Lateral Tarsal Strip:** Corrects lateral canthal tendon and horizontal lid laxity. (See Tables 7.3.1 Rapid Review of Steps and 7.3.2 Surgical Pearls, and Web Tables 7.3.1 to 7.3.4 for equipment and medication lists).

TABLE 7.3.1	Rapid Review of Steps

(1) Inject local anesthetic and allow for time to work (5 minutes).
(2) Prep and drape.
(3) Perform lateral canthotomy.
(4) Cantholysis of inferior crus of lateral canthal tendon.
(5) Create lateral tarsal strip.
(6) Suture lateral tarsal strip to lateral orbital rim periosteum.
(7) Reapproximate lateral commissure.
(8) Excise excess skin.
(9) Close skin incision.

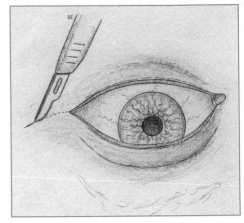

FIGURE 7.3.2 ◆ *Canthotomy skin incision:* A horizontal skin incision is made with a scalpel beginning at the lateral canthus in preparation for canthotomy and cantholysis to mobilize the lower lid.

A. *Canthotomy/Cantholysis:* A horizontal skin incision is made beginning at the lateral canthus (FIG. 7.3.2). The lateral commissure is then incised with laterally directed scissors (FIG. 7.3.3: *Canthotomy*). The inferior arm of the canthal tendon is placed on tension with forceps and transected with scissors directed toward the patient's nose (FIG. 7.3.4: *Cantholysis*). Completion of these steps result in full lower lid mobilization (FIG. 7.3.5).

B. *Orbital Rim Exposure:* The orbicularis is then divided and the periosteum overlying the lateral orbital rim is exposed with blunt dissection.

C. *Tarsal Strip Formation:* The lid margin, retractors, and anterior lamellar layers are removed with sharp dissection to expose a strip of the lateral tarsal plate (FIG. 7.3.6). The palpebral conjunctiva overlying this strip is then scraped away with a scalpel (FIG. 7.3.7).

D. *Lid Tightening:* A suture is passed through the anterior margin of the strip and then through periosteum overlying Whitnall's tubercle (FIGS. 7.3.8A,B). Tightening this suture reapposes the lid to the globe.

E. *Closure:* Passing a suture through the lateral margins of the upper and lower lids reforms the commissure (FIG. 7.3.9). Care is taken to realign the gray lines. The canthotomy incision is then closed in layers.

TABLE 7.3.2	Surgical Pearls

Preoperative:
• Warn patients that overcorrection immediately after surgery is ideal. Over the first 2 weeks, the eyelids will settle down to its normal, desired position.
• Injection of anesthetic and allow for adequate time for onset.

Intraoperative:
• Ensure that lateral canthal position is higher than medial canthal position after resuspension. Patients with relative proptosis may require a higher set lateral canthus.
• Entropion is more common in enophthalmic eyes. When placing the periosteal sutures, ensure that the suture is deep enough on the inner aspect of the orbital rim to ensure that when sutures are pulled, the eyelid reapproximates to the globe.
• Under tightening of the lateral canthal suture leads to early failure and recurrence of eyelid malposition.

Postoperative:
• Remember that at the 1-week postoperative visit, over correction is ideal in eyelid position. Therefore, reassuring a patient and holding off on revision surgery until healing is complete is important.

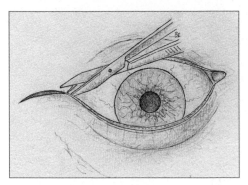

FIGURE 7.3.3 ✦ *Canthotomy:* The full thickness of the lateral commissure is incised with laterally directed scissors.

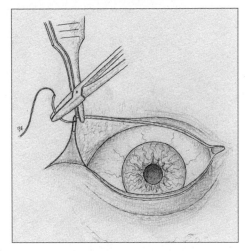

FIGURE 7.3.5 ✦ *Traction suture:* After the lid has been mobilized, a traction suture can be placed to facilitate exposure of the operative site.

2. *Medial Canthal Repairs:*
   A. *Medial Canthal Tendon Plication:* This is used for mild tendon laxity without canthal angle displacement. It is frequently combined with other horizontal shortening procedures.
     1. *Incision:* A punctal probe is placed in the inferior canaliculus to aid intraoperative identification and prevent inadvertent transection. A horizontal skin incision is then made below the medial canthus.
     2. *Plication:* After dividing the orbicularis, the tarsal insertion of the medial canthal tendon is exposed. A suture is passed from the medial tarsus to the anterior limb of the tendon, and tightened to stabilize the

canthal angle. The skin incision is then closed.
   B. *Medial Canthal Angle Resection:* Used for pronounced medial tendon laxity with angle displacement. Aggressive tendon plication alone would kink the inferior canaliculus, preventing tear drainage.
     1. *Incision:* A punctal probe is placed in the inferior canaliculus to aid intra-operative identification. A full-thickness vertical lid incision is then made medial to the inferior

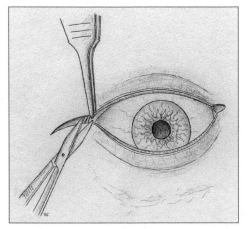

FIGURE 7.3.4 ✦ *Cantholysis:* The inferior arm of the canthal tendon is placed on tension with forceps and transected with scissors directed toward the patient's nose.

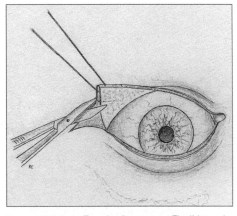

FIGURE 7.3.6 ✦ *Tarsal strip exposure:* The lid margin, capsulopalpebral fascia, and layers of the anterior lamella are removed with sharp dissection to expose a bare strip of the lateral tarsal plate.

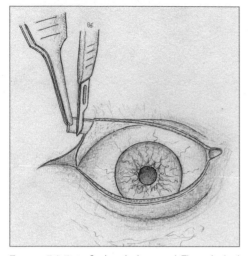

FIGURE 7.3.7 ◆ *Conjunctival removal:* The palpebral conjunctiva overlying this strip is then scraped away with a scalpel blade.

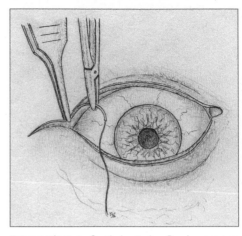

FIGURE 7.3.9 ◆ *Canthal suturing:* Passing a suture through the lateral lid margins reforms the canthal angle. Care is taken to realign the gray lines of the upper and lower lids.

punctum. The canaliculus is transected, as is the canthal tendon. The incision is then extended onto the bulbar conjunctiva.

2. *Tightening:* The posterior lacrimal crest is exposed with blunt dissection and a double-armed suture is passed through the overlying periosteum. The lid is pulled medially, and an appropriate amount is excised. The suture needles are then passed through the medial tarsus, effectively

replacing the cut posterior limb of the canthal tendon.

3. *Canalicular Fistula:* To permit tear drainage, a fistula is created between the inferior fornix and the distal canaliculus, which remains connected to the nasolacrimal duct.

4. *Closure:* The suture connecting the posterior lacrimal crest and medial tarsus is tightened and tied. The lid margin and skin are then reapproximated with sutures.

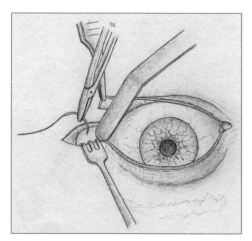

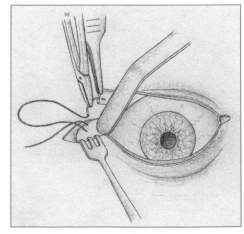

FIGURE 7.3.8 ◆ *Strip anchoring:* A nonabsorbable suture is passed through the anterior tarsal strip and the periosteum overlying Whitnall's tubercle. The globe is shielded from accidental suture penetration using a retractor. Tightening this suture reapposes the lid to the globe.

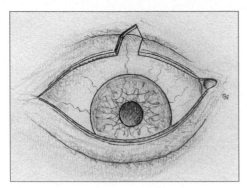

FIGURE 7.3.10 ◆ *Horizontal lid shortening:* A full thickness "pentagon" of lid tissue is removed. The incisions through the tarsus and overlying skin are made perpendicular to the lid margin and then directed to meet at an apex in the inferior fornix.

3. *Horizontal Lid Shortening:*
   A. *Full-thickness Resection:* Corrects tarsal laxity.
      1. *Incision:* Angled incisions through the tarsus would result in lid notching and tear film disruption. A full thickness "pentagon" of tissue is therefore removed (FIG. 7.3.10). The tarsus and overlying skin are transected perpendicular to the lid margin. The incisions are then angled to meet at an apex in the inferior fornix.
      2. *Closure:* The tarsal plate and lid retractors are reapproximated with partial-thickness absorbable sutures. To ensure even lid margin healing, additional sutures are passed through the gray line and lash line (FIG. 7.3.11). The tails are left long to permit easy identification and prevent corneal abrasion. Lid skin is then closed with interrupted sutures.
   B. *Lazy-T:* Corrects coexisting horizontal lid laxity and punctal eversion. Combines full-thickness lid tissue resection (see previous) with tarsoconjunctival excision (see following).

4. *Posterior Lamellar Shortening:*
   A. *Tarsoconjunctival Excision:* Localized vertical shortening of the posterior lamella corrects medial ectropion with punctal eversion.
      1. *Incision:* The lid is everted after insertion of a punctal probe to protect the inferior canaliculus. A diamond-shaped segment of tarsus and overlying conjunctiva is then removed inferior to the punctum (FIG. 7.3.12). The superior incision should

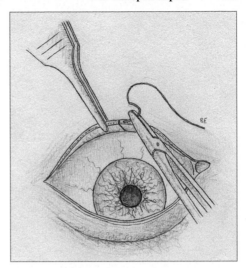

FIGURE 7.3.11 ◆ *Lid margin sutures:* To ensure lid margin alignment, sutures are passed through the gray line and lash line. The tails are left long to facilitate identification and prevent corneal abrasion. Uneven healing of the lid margin can result in tear film disruption and ocular surface damage.

be at least 2 mm below the lid margin to prevent canalicular injury during suture passage.
      2. *Closure:* Closing the defect with absorbable sutures shortens the posterior lamella, reapposing the medial lid and punctum with the

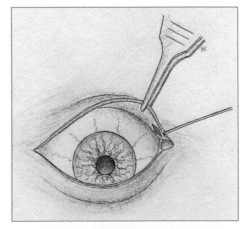

FIGURE 7.3.12 ◆ *Posterior lamellar shortening:* The lid is everted after a punctal probe is inserted to permit intraoperative identification and protection of the inferior canaliculus. A diamond-shaped segment of tarsus and overlying conjunctiva is then excised inferior to the punctum.

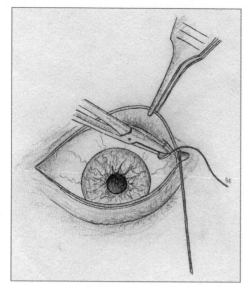

FIGURE 7.3.13 ◆ *Posterior lamellar sutures:* Closing the defect with absorbable sutures shortens the posterior lamella, reapposing the medial lid and punctum with the globe.

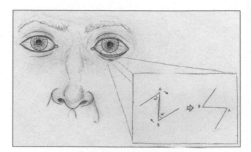

FIGURE 7.3.14 ◆ *Z plasty:* A "Z" is marked over the scar with equal length arms that intersect at 60-degree angles. It is then traced with a scalpel and the resulting flaps are undermined to permit mobilization. The flap rearrangement shown above lengthens the lid vertically while shortening it horizontally.

globe. Care is taken to bury the knots to avoid ocular surface irritation (FIG. 7.3.13).

5. *Anterior Lamellar Lengthening:*

   A. *Z Plasty:* Flap rearrangement corrects shortening due to a focal linear scar.

     1. *Incision:* A lid margin traction suture is placed through the meibomian gland orifices. A "Z" with arms that intersect at 60-degree angles is then marked over the scar and traced with a scalpel. The resulting flaps are undermined to permit mobilization (FIG. 7.3.14A).

     2. *Closure:* After scar tissue is excised, the flaps are transposed and closed with interrupted sutures (FIG. 7.3.14B). This rearrangement lengthens the lid vertically while shortening it horizontally.

NOTE: *If the scar involves the lid margin itself, full thickness excision must be performed as previously described.*

   B. *Pedicle Transposition Flap:* Excess upper lid skin is transposed to correct cicatricial lower lid ectropion. The pedicle can originate from either canthus.

     1. *Incision:* A lower lid margin traction suture is placed. The proposed upper lid flap and

lower lid incision are then marked. The flap should overlie the upper lid crease so that the defect will be well hidden after closure. The lower lid incision is made with a scalpel. Scar tissue is excised and the wound margins are undermined to permit mobilization (FIG. 7.3.15). Applying tension to the traction suture reveals the full size of the defect.

     2. *Flap Rotation:* The upper lid flap is outlined with a scalpel. The free end is then

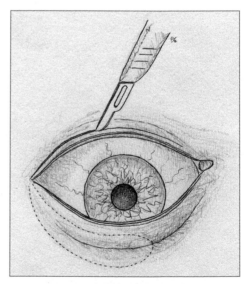

FIGURE 7.3.15 ◆ *Pedicle transposition flap:* An upper lid flap and lower lid subciliary incision are marked. The lower lid incision is made with a scalpel. Scar tissue is excised if present, and the wound margins are undermined to permit mobilization.

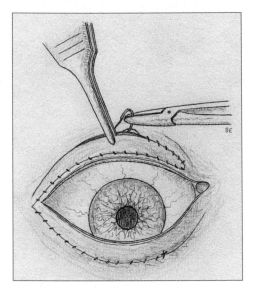

FIGURE 7.3.16 ◆ *Flap rotation and suturing:* The flap is outlined with a scalpel. The free end is undermined and rotated into lower lid defect. All skin incisions are closed with 6-0 suture.

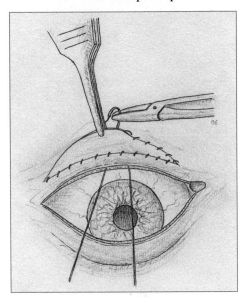

FIGURE 7.3.18 ◆ *Skin graft transfer:* After the graft is dissected from the donor bed, stab incisions are made to permit drainage, and it is sutured in place in the lower lid.

undermined and rotated into the lower lid defect (FIG. 7.3.16).

3. *Closure:* All skin incisions are closed with suture and covered with a pressure dressing for 24 hours.

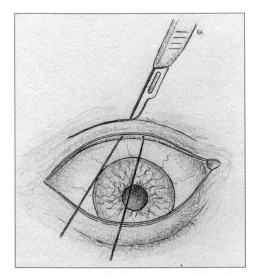

FIGURE 7.3.17 ◆ *Skin graft recipient bed preparation:* Traction sutures are placed through the lid margin, and a horizontal incision is made 2 to 3 mm below the lash line.

C. *Skin Graft:* A graft is used to correct severe ectropion due to diffuse skin shortage.

1. *Incision:* Traction sutures are placed through the lid margin, and a horizontal incision is made 2 to 3 mm below the lash line (FIG. 7.3.17). The wound margins are then undermined and scar tissue is excised. Applying tension to the traction sutures reveals the full size of the lower lid defect.

2. *Donor Site Resection:* The defect is then used to create a template for donor site resection. Postauricular, inner arm, and jugular notch skin provide good color and thickness matches.

3. *Graft Placement:* After the graft is removed from the donor bed and small stab incisions are made to permit drainage, it is sutured into place and covered with a compression dressing (FIG. 7.3.18).

NOTE: *The graft must be slightly larger than the defect to account for postoperative shrinkage.*

COMPLICATIONS

1. Undercorrection due to inadequate shortening of the tarsus or ligaments.

2. Overcorrection due to excessive lid tissue removal or ligament plication. The lid can be massaged to hasten stretching.

3. Lid notching, corneal abrasion, and trichiasis seen after full-thickness excision with angled tarsal incisions or poor realignment of the lid margin.

4. Canalicular injury can occur during medial canthal surgery. Stent the canaliculus with silicone tubing to prevent stenosis and epiphora.

5. Recurrence due to loss of suture fixation, shrinkage of grafts, etc.

POSTOPERATIVE CARE

- Apply topical antibiotic ointment to the surgical wounds.

- Prescribe an antistaphylococcal antibiotic (e.g., a first generation cephalosporin) and an oral analgesic for pain control.

- Remove the skin sutures at 5 to 7 days for optimal cosmetic results. Lid margin sutures should remain in place for 10 to 14 days to ensure adequate healing.

- Examine the ocular surface at regular intervals to ensure that defects heal after lid repair.

Further Reading

Text

Bergeron CM, Moe KS. The evaluation and treatment of lower eyelid paralysis. *Facial Plast Surg.* 2008;24(2):231–241.

Eliasoph I. Current techniques of entropion and ectropion correction. *Otolaryngol Clin North Am.* 2005;38(5):903–919.

Hintschich C. Correction of entropion and ectropion. *Dev Ophthalmol.* 2008;41:85–102.

Robinson FO, Collins JRO. Ectropion. In: Yanoff M, Duker J, eds. *Ophthalmology.* 3rd ed. Philadelphia, PA: Mosby; 2009:1412–1419.

Tasman W, Jaeger E, eds. Eyelid abnormalities: ectropion, entropion, trichiasis. *Duane's Clinical Ophthalmology.* Vol 6. Philadelphia, PA: Lippincott Williams & Wilkins; 2008:chap 73.

Vallabhanath P, Carter SR. Ectropion and entropion. *Curr Opin Ophthalmol.* 2000;11(5):345–351.

Wagner P, Lang GK. The eyelids. *Ophthalmology: A Pocket Textbook Atlas.* 2nd ed. New York, NY: Georg Thieme Verlag; 2007:chap 2.

Primary Sources

Clement CI, O'Donnell BA. Medial canthal tendon repair for moderate to severe tendon laxity. *Clin Experiment Ophthalmol.* 2004;32(2):170–174.

Della Rocca DA. The lateral tarsal strip: illustrated pearls. *Facial Plast Surg.* 2007;23(3):200–202.

Smith B. The "lazy-T" correction of ectropion of the lower punctum. *Arch Ophthalmol.* 1976;94(7):1149–1150.

Weber PJ, Popp JC, Wulc AE. Refinements of the tarsal strip procedure. *Ophthalmic Surg.* 1991;22(11):687–691.

7.4 ENTROPION REPAIR

ENTROPION REPAIR

- Restores inverted (most commonly lower) lid margin to normal position in relation to the globe by addressing specific anatomic defects.

- Repair may entail reinserting the capsulopalpebral fascia (lower lid retractor) on the tarsal plate, decreasing horizontal eyelid laxity, weakening the preseptal orbicularis muscle, removing orbital fat, or reconstructing the posterior lamella.

- Repair of the primary anatomic defect is prioritized, but it may be necessary to combine multiple techniques to achieve satisfactory results.

INDICATIONS

- Keratitis, conjunctivitis, epiphora (excessive tear production because of insufficient tear film drainage), and cosmetic reasons are all indications for surgery.

ALTERNATIVES

Medical Therapy

- Lubrication: artificial tears, ointments for mild disease

- Botulinum toxin: Effective treatment method for spastic entropion for up to 6 months per administration

- For cicatricial entropion secondary to inflammatory disease (e.g., ocular cicatricial pemphigoid), immunosuppressive agents, such as systemic corticosteroids and/or chemotherapeutics, are necessary.

Procedures

- Temporary lower lid eversion by rotating the anterior lamella and securing with tape.
- Quickert-Rathbun Sutures: Placement of several full-thickness double-arm eyelid chromic gut sutures from the inferior fornix of the lower lid, traversing obliquely through the lid, and exiting anteriorly 1 to 2 mm from the eyelid margin, which help evert the lid. Subsequent fibrosis around the sutures reinforces the everted eye position. This is a temporizing procedure as recurrence rates are high.

RELEVANT PHYSIOLOGY/ANATOMY

Lid Lamellae: (anterior vs. posterior)

- Anterior lamella: skin and orbicularis oculi
- Posterior lamella: palpebral conjunctiva and tarsus superiorly, eyelid retractors inferiorly
- Length imbalance between the anterior and posterior lamella can cause lid inversion (e.g., cicatricial entropion).

Lower Lid Retractors

- Antagonists to orbicularis
- Capsulopalpebral fascia formed by extension of inferior rectus; inserts on inferior tarsus, has sympathetic innervation

"Tarsoligamentous Sling" (Fig. 7.4.1)

- Formed by tarsus and canthal tendons; keeps lid margin apposed to globe. Any or all parts may develop laxity, resulting in ectropion.
- Inferior tarsus: dense fibrous tissue ~1 mm thick, ~4 mm high at lid center
- Medial canthal tendon: anchors medial tarsus/canthal angle to frontal bone maxillary process with anterior limb, and to posterior lacrimal crest with posterior limb
- Lateral canthal tendon: anchors lateral tarsus/canthal angle to Whitnall's tubercle at inner margin of lateral orbital rim

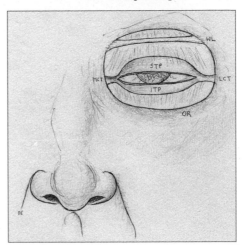

FIGURE 7.4.1 ◆ *The "tarsoligamentous sling"*: This is formed by the inferior tarsal plate (ITP) in conjunction with the medial and lateral canthal tendons (MCT and LCT), and keeps the lid margins apposed to the globe. Any or all parts may develop laxity, resulting in entropion when combined with posterior lamellar shortening or capsulopalpebral fascia disinsertion.

Entropion Overview

- Inversion of lower lid margin directs cilia toward the globe; leads to keratitis, conjunctivitis, and epiphora.
- Causal factors: horizontal lower lid laxity (generally due to weakness of lateral and/or medial canthal tendons), dehiscence/attenuation of capsulopalpebral fascia, spasticity or override of the preseptal orbicularis muscle, or vertical shortening of the posterior lamella due to inflammation or scarring

Entropion Classification

- Involutional: Most common form (aging phenomenon). Almost exclusively effects lower lid. Multiple causal factors including slowly evolving horizontal lid laxity, dehiscence of lower lid retractors, and override of the orbicularis. A lateral tarsal strip repair is generally performed. Occasionally, a combination of surgical techniques is required for adequate repair.
- Cicatricial: From scarring and contraction of the posterior lamella (palpebral conjunctiva and tarsus) secondary to an allergy, medication reaction, systemic inflammation (e.g., Steven-Johnson syndrome or ocular cicatricial pemphigoid), chemical burns, or trauma. May involve both lower and upper eyelids. Surgical management generally

involves lengthening of the posterior lamella (e.g., by grafting) and/or removal of the posterior lamellar contractures (e.g., transverse tarsotomy).

- Spastic: Due to increased muscular tone, the lower lid orbicularis shifts superiorly "overriding" the inferior tarsal border. May result from trauma, lid surgery, or inflammation. Sometimes seen in association with blepharospasm. Correction involves reversal of preseptal orbicularis override.

- Congenital: Rare. Most commonly, there is a defect in the lower lid posterior lamella leading to inverted eyelid margins.

Differential Diagnosis

- Epiblepharon: A developmental aberration in which a redundant fold of pretarsal skin and orbicularis extends beyond the lid margin pressing the eyelashes inward toward the globe.

- Distichiasis: A rare acquired or congenital condition in which the eyelashes arise from the meibomian gland openings in the posterior lamella versus the normal anterior lamella position. These lashes are directed toward the globe.

- Trichiasis: An acquired condition in which the eyelashes (arising from the normal anterior lamella) are directed posteriorly toward the globe as a result of inflammation and scarring of the lid margin. This is commonly seen in the developing world as a result of *Chlamydia trachomatis* infection (trachoma).

PREOPERATIVE SCREENING

- Exam: Identify specific anatomic defect(s); assess severity of entropion and corneal/conjunctival involvement.
  1. Horizontal lid laxity:
     a. Snap Test: pull lid down and away; assess speed of return after release (should be spontaneous with 1 blink)
     b. Pull lid from globe (>10 mm is abnormal)
  2. Medial canthal tendon laxity: pull lid laterally; check movement of inferior punctum (normally 1 to 2 mm).
  3. Lateral canthal tendon laxity: canthal angle should be acute (not rounded) and 1 to 2 mm medial to orbital rim at rest; pull lid medially and check movement of angle (normally 1 to 2 mm).
  4. Tear production: Schirmer's test: small filter paper tabs are inserted between lower lid and

globe and removed after 5 minutes. The wet area is measured in millimeters (normal ~15 mm without topical anesthesia).

  5. Corneal damage: slit lamp exam and fluorescein test to detect presence of corneal epithelial defects.
  6. Orbicularis tone: Look for blepharospasm, hemifacial spasm, or orbicularis spasm.

ANESTHESIA

- Most lid procedures are performed with local injections under monitored anesthesia care (MAC).

PROCEDURE

Choice of a procedure depends on the nature of underlying anatomic defects and severity of disease. Components of the procedures described below may be combined, either within the same operation or as parts of a staged repair. Though there is some overlap, these procedures can be grouped into four conceptual categories: correction of capsulopalpebral fascia dysfunction, correction of preseptal orbicularis override, correction of horizontal lower lid laxity, and rotation and/or reconstruction of the posterior lamella.

1. *Correction of horizontal lower lid laxity:*
   - **Lateral tarsal strip** procedure is most commonly performed for involutional entropion. This procedure is sometimes combined with retractor reattachment. (See Tables 7.4.1 Rapid Review of Steps and 7.4.2 Surgical Pearls, and Web Tables 7.4.1 to 7.4.4 for equipment and medication lists).
   - Lateral canthotomy and inferior cantholysis is first performed. After adequate lidocaine/epinephrine is given, a 1- to 1.5-cm incision is then placed at the lateral canthus extending temporally toward the orbital rim (Fig. 7.4.2). Using scissors, this incision is completed (full-thickness) (Fig. 7.4.3). The lower lid is elevated with forceps to visualize the lateral canthus tendon. Using sharp scissors with tips pointing toward the nose, the tendon is cut allowing adequate exposure of the lower lid conjunctiva (Fig. 7.4.4). If present, contractures of the posterior lamella can be lysed with sharp dissection (Fig. 7.4.5). The cantholysis allows for adequate exposure of the lateral orbital rim.
   - The anterior and posterior lamellae of the temporal eyelid are separated at the gray line.

TABLE 7.4.1 Rapid Review of Steps
(1) Inject local anesthetic and allow for time to work (5 minutes).
(2) Prep and drape.
(3) Perform lateral canthotomy.
(4) Cantholysis of inferior crus of lateral canthal tendon.
(5) Create lateral tarsal strip.
(6) Suture lateral tarsal strip to lateral orbital rim periosteum.
(7) Reapproximate lateral commissure.
(8) Excise excess skin.
(9) Close skin incision.

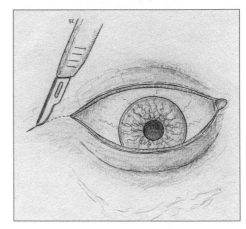

FIGURE 7.4.2 ◆ *Canthotomy skin incision:* A horizontal skin incision is made beginning at the lateral canthus in preparation for a canthotomy/cantholysis to mobilize the lower lid.

In order to isolate the tarsal strip, the palpebral conjunctiva is removed, the retractors are disinserted and the epithelium of the lid margin is excised (FIGS. 7.4.6, 7.4.7).

- Removal of excess tarsal strip: The strip is pulled gently to the lateral orbital tubercle (insertion point for lateral canthal tendon) and the excess tissue is cut with scissors. A

horizontal mattress suture is used to attach the shortened tarsus to the periosteum of the lateral orbital tubercle, reapposing the lid with the globe (FIGS. 7.4.8A, B).

- After adequate hemostasis, the lateral commissure is reformed with an interrupted resorbable suture (with careful attention to realign the gray line) (FIG. 7.4.9). The skin is closed with a simple running suture.

2. *Reattachment of Capsulopalpebral Fascia (lower lid retractor):*
   - Used to correct involutional entropion with fascia disinsertion or dehiscence. Initial approach can be transcutaneous or transconjunctival. Transcutaneous approach: a traction

TABLE 7.4.2 Surgical Pearls

Preoperative:
- Warn patients that overcorrection immediately after surgery is ideal. Over the first 2 weeks, the eyelids will settle down to its normal, desired position.
- Injection of anesthetic and allow for adequate time for onset.

Intraoperative:
- Ensure that lateral canthal position is higher than medial canthal position after resuspension. Patients with relative proptosis may require a higher set lateral canthus.
- Overtightening of the lateral canthal suture can cause the lid to pull downward, particularly on the proptotic eye. Supraplacement of the lateral canthal tendon compared to the medial canthal tendon helps prevent this.
- Undertightening of the lateral canthal suture leads to early failure and recurrence of eyelid malposition.

Postoperative:
- Remember that at the 1-week postoperative visit, overcorrection is ideal in eyelid position. Therefore, reassuring a patient and holding off on revision surgery until healing is complete is important.

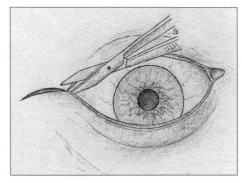

FIGURE 7.4.3 ◆ *Canthotomy:* The full thickness of the lateral commissure is then incised with laterally directed scissors.

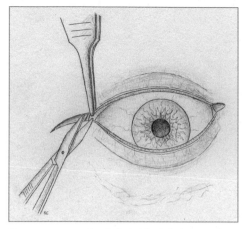

FIGURE 7.4.4 ◆ *Cantholysis:* The inferior arm of the canthal tendon is placed on tension with forceps and transected with scissors directed toward the patient's nose.

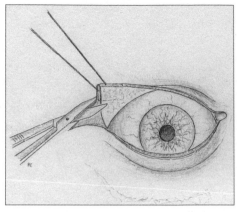

FIGURE 7.4.6 ◆ *Tarsal strip exposure:* The lid margin, capsulopalpebral fascia, and layers of the anterior lamella are removed with sharp dissection to expose a bare strip of the lateral tarsal plate.

suture is placed through the lower eyelid margin and cephalad traction is applied. A subciliary incision is placed ~4 mm inferior to the lid margin. The incision starts lateral to the punctum and continues past the lateral canthal angle.

- The orbicularis muscle is separated using scissors at the junction of the preseptal and pretarsal components.
- The inferior tarsal border and the capsulopalpebral fascia are visualized (to check for disinsertion or attenuation). The orbital septum is now penetrated and incised the full

length of the previous incisions in order to relieve tension from the lower lid retractor. The lower lid fat pads may be removed as well.

- When disinsertion is present, the fascia is advanced and sutured to the inferior tarsal border using interrupted 6-0 sutures. When the fascia is attenuated but not dehisced, it is surgically disinserted and a section is removed. The shortened capsulopalpebral fascia is then sutured to the inferior tarsal border. A running 6-0 suture can then be used to

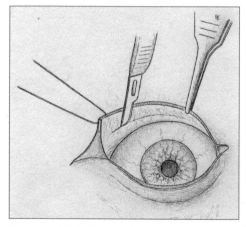

FIGURE 7.4.5 ◆ *Posterior lamellar contracture lysis:* When present, contracture are lysed with sharp dissection. This relieves the tension causing the lash line and cilia to rotate toward the globe.

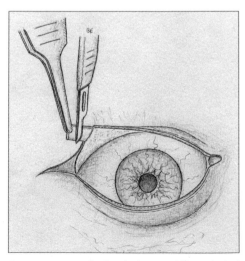

FIGURE 7.4.7 ◆ *Conjunctival removal:* The palpebral conjunctiva overlying this strip is then scraped away with a scalpel blade.

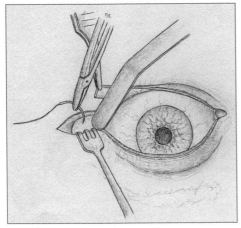 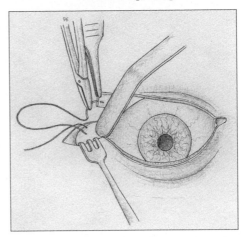

A   **B**

FIGURE 7.4.8 ◆ *Strip anchoring:* A nonabsorbable suture is passed through the anterior tarsal strip and the periosteum overlying Whitnall's tubercle. The globe is shielded from accidental suture penetration using a retractor. Tightening this suture reapposes the lid to the globe.

close the skin incision. The orbicularis muscle does not need to be reapproximated.

3. *Correction of Preseptal Orbicularis Override:*
   - Used to correct spastic entropion. A transcutaneous approach with separation of the orbicularis muscle at the preseptal and pretarsal subunits is conducted (as above). Epinephrine with lidocaine is injected into the preseptal muscle to ensure adequate anesthesia and hemostasis.
   - Following a subciliary incision, a 6- to 10-mm wide strip of preseptal orbicularis is meas-

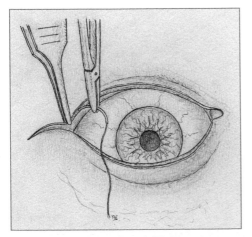

FIGURE 7.4.9 ◆ *Canthal suturing:* Passing a suture through the lateral lid margins reforms the canthal angle. Care is taken to realign the gray lines of the upper and lower lids.

ured (based on preoperative muscle override measurements) and removed (for the entire length of the muscle) using scissors.
   - After adequate hemostasis is achieved, a running 6-0 suture can be used to close the skin.

4a. *Rotation (Eversion) of the Posterior Lamella (Weis procedure):*
   - Conducted for mild-to-moderate cicatricial entropion with use of a *transverse tarsotomy* in order to free the posterior lamella contracture.
   - A traction suture is placed through the lower eyelid margin and the lid is everted over a Desmarres retractor. A horizontal incision is made 3 mm from the eyelid margin (to avoid the marginal vascular arcade) through the conjunctiva and the full thickness of the tarsus.
   - Using double-armed sutures, the eyelid is everted. The suture is first passed from anterior to posterior through the inferior tarsal plate. The suture is then passed through the superior portion of the tarsal plate, extending through the orbicularis and exiting the eyelid around the ciliary line. Mild overcorrection (ectropion) is desired immediately postoperatively to account for subsequent contraction.

4b. *Posterior Lamella Reconstruction:*
   - Conducted for severe cicatricial entropion (significant posterior lamella foreshortening) with placement of an autologous graft.

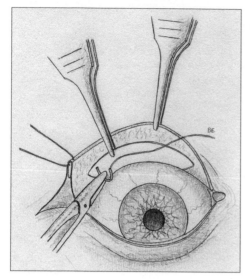

FIGURE 7.4.10 ◆ *Posterior lamellar reconstruction:* After transverse tarsotomy is performed to relieve contractures, harvested autograft (e.g., auricular cartilage) is inserted and sutured in place to lengthen the posterior lamella.

- Basic components of the graft include a semi-rigid structure that may be covered with epithelium. This includes hard palate mucosa, nasal mucoperiosteum, auricular cartilage, etc.
- A transverse tarsotomy is first performed followed by blunt dissection between the tarsus and orbicularis to relieve all traction. The posterior lamella defect is measured.
- Hard palate graft: requires local nasopalatine and greater palatine nerve blocks. Graft size is determined and mucosa and palate incised. A periosteal elevator can be used to free the graft. The palatal defect does not need to be closed.
- The slightly oversized graft (allows for postoperative contraction) is secured in the place of the posterior lamella defect by sutures along the inferior (nonmarginal) and lateral borders (FIG. 7.4.10). The rotated marginal strip (from the tarsotomy) is sutured to the anterior surface of the graft using the same suturing technique as above.

COMPLICATIONS

1. *Persistent entropion:* minimized with good preoperative planning (e.g., combined vs. single-step surgical plan).

2. *Overcorrection (ectropion):* For cicatricial entropion immediately postoperative, the patient should be overcorrected. Prolonged ectropion is likely due to excessive advancement of the capsulopalpebral fascia.

3. *Eyelid retraction:* result of excessive horizontal tightening of the tarsus or excessive advancement of the capsulopalpebral fascia.

4. *Hematoma:* inadequate hemostasis; more common with muscle manipulation.

5. *Keratopathy:* from conjunctival sutures, lagophthalmos (severe lid retraction), or posterior lamellar grafts. Uncommon complication of lower lid surgery.

6. *Symblepharon:* adhesion of eyelids to bulbar conjunctiva as a result of posterior lamella manipulation.

7. *Granuloma formation:* conjunctival granulation tissue may develop after posterior lamella surgery as a result of tissue inflammation/injury.

8. *Ptosis:* after upper eyelid posterior lamella manipulation; occurs because of injury to levator nerve fibers.

9. *Eyelash loss or eyelid necrosis:* due to damage of the vascular marginal arcade.

POSTOPERATIVE CARE

- Antistaphylococcal antibiotics (e.g., first generation cephalosporin) and oral analgesia.
- Follow up in clinic within 24 hours to screen for complications.
- Remove sutures at 5 to 7 days to prevent excessive facial scarring.

Further Reading

Text

Gigantelli JW. Entropion. In: Yanoff M, Duker J, eds. *Ophthalmology.* 3rd ed. Philadelphia, PA: Mosby; 2009: 1404–1412.

Wagner P, Lang GK. The eyelids. *Ophthalmology: A Pocket Textbook Atlas.* 2nd ed. New York: Georg Thieme Verlag; 2007:17–49.

Primary Sources

Dresner SC, Karesh JW. Transconjunctival entropion repair. *Arch Ophthlmol.* 1993;11:1144–1148.

Quickert MH, Rathbun E. Suture repair of entropion. *Arch Ophthlmol.* 1971;85:304–305.

7.5   ENUCLEATION, EVISCERATION, AND EXENTERATION

- Enucleation: Removal of the globe and a portion of the proximal optic nerve.
- Evisceration: Removal of the contents of the globe with preservation of the sclera and optic nerve.
- Exenteration: Removal of the globe and surrounding soft tissue. The extent of tissue removal depends on the presenting pathology.
- Subtotal: The periorbita and some or all of the eyelids are preserved.
- Total: The periorbita, including the entire eyelid, is removed.
- Radical: The orbital bones, paranasal sinuses, extraocular muscles, and all other soft tissues are removed.

INDICATIONS

- Enucleation: Patients with intraocular malignancies (e.g., uveal melanoma, retinoblastoma), severe trauma leading to a deformed or phthisical (atrophic) eye, or pain relief in an eye with no light perception (NLP).
- Evisceration: Pain relief in an eye with NLP, most commonly after severe infection (endophthalmitis). Procedure is preferred by some surgeons to enucleation because it allows for less disruption of the orbital tissues and a better cosmetic outcome. Contraindication includes intraocular malignancy.
- Exenteration: Patients with malignancies or fungal infections extending into the surrounding orbital tissue.

ALTERNATIVES

Intraocular Malignancy (e.g., Choroidal Melanoma): Although enucleation remains the mainstay of treatment of large intraocular tumors where vision cannot be spared, other therapies may be considered depending on tumor type, size and location, as well as on results of a metastatic workup.

- Serial observation, if suspecting small, pigmented nevus versus melanoma: For choroidal lesions, observation is generally reserved for lesions <10 mm length and <3 mm apical height without exudative retinal detachments or rapid growth. There is <5% tumor-related mortality associated with lesions of this size. Most iris lesions can be watched for growth and/or vascularization; <5% of pigmented iris lesions require intervention.
- Laser photocoagulation: For choroidal melanomas, this is reserved for lesions <3 mm thick and lesions <3 mm from the optic nerve or fovea. Tradeoff involves lower morbidity (spares direct injury to optic nerve and fovea) but requires multiple treatments and has high percentage of recurrence.
- Ionizing radiation (brachytherapy or external beam radiation): Plaque brachytherapy involves surgical placement of shielded radioisotope permitting precise targeting of lesion. If tumor is located close to the fovea or optic nerve, visual loss can be significant due to radiation exposure. External beam radiation is generally attempted for large tumors or after failed plaque therapy and involves precise external radiation targeting of tumor over a several week period.
- Local resection (iridocyclochoroidectomy): For choroidal melanoma <15 mm in diameter and <8 mm thickness, an eye wall resection may be attempted. The major advantage involves preservation of the globe. Complications include retinal detachment, cystoid macular edema (CME), vitreous hemorrhage, and incomplete resection. Tumor size positively correlates with complication rate.
- The Collaborative Ocular Melanoma Study (COMS): A multicenter, longitudinal, randomized control trial designed to systematically evaluate management of choroidal melanomas. Study groups were broken down by size.
  1. *Small Melanoma Trial (5 to 16 mm in length, 1 to 3 mm in apical height):* Evaluated the natural history of the disease. Result: Tumor growth occurred in 21% of patients at 2 years and 31% of patients at 5 years.
  2. *Medium Melanoma Trial (<16 mm in length, 2.5 to 10 mm in apical height):* Compared enucleation versus plaque radiotherapy. Result: No difference in patient survival at 5 years.

3. *Large Melanoma Trial (>16 mm in length and >2 mm in apical height, or >10 mm in apical height of any length):* Compared enucleation versus external beam radiation followed by enucleation. Result: No difference in patient survival at 5 years.

Blind Painful Eye

- Topical steroids, cycloplegics, and oral analgesics may be used to manage pain.

- Retrobulbar injection of absolute alcohol or chlor-promazine (Thorazine, GlaxoSmithKline, London, United Kingdom) can give long-term pain control.

- Custom scleral shells (made and fitted by an ocularist) may be placed directly over the disfigured eye, providing a good cosmetic result.

- If penetrating trauma occurred and the patient refuses enucleation, he or she must be counseled on the risk of developing sympathetic uveitis.

RELEVANT PATHOLOGY

Malignant Intraocular Tumors

Uveal Melanoma

- A primary malignant tumor of the uvea, which can involve the choroid (80%), ciliary body (10%), and/or iris (8%). Estimated incidence in the United States is 1,500 new cases per year.

- Choroidal melanomas are the most common primary intraocular tumor found in adults.

- Tumors may be incidentally discovered on a routine exam or may present symptomatically with blurred vision, visual field defects, floaters, light flashes, or pain.

- On funduscopic exam, choroidal lesions commonly appear gray-green or brown, occasionally with overlying orange pigment (lipofuscin). Serous retinal detachment may also be present.

- Ultrasound for evaluation of choroidal melanoma: B-scan characteristics include an internal quiet zone, choroidal evacuation, and orbital shadowing. Pathognomonic finding for melanoma is a "collar button" or mushroom shape indicating a break through Bruch's membrane. A-scan characteristics include low to medium reflectivity and spontaneous pulsations.

- Fluorescein angiography: Uveal melanoma characteristics include hot spots, leakage, and an intrinsic circulation. These findings, however, are not specific to melanoma.

- Metastasis occurs most commonly to the liver (60%), followed by subcutaneous tissue (25%) and central nervous system (CNS) (2%). Workup includes positron emission tomography/computed tomography (PET/CT) and liver function testing.

- Differential diagnosis for pigmented choroidal lesion includes malignant melanoma, nevus, congenital hypertrophy of the retinal pigment epithelium (RPE), choroidal detachment (e.g., localized suprachoroidal hemorrhage), subretinal hemorrhage from age-related macular degeneration (drusen typically present), and melanocytoma of the optic nerve.

Uveal Metastases

- The most common intraocular tumor. Metastasis to this region is common due to the highly vascular nature of the choroid and ciliary body.

- Women: The most common primary is carcinoma of the breast.

- Men: Common primary sites include lung, gastrointestinal (GI), and genitourinary (GU) malignancies.

- Lymphoma and lymphoproliferative processes can also metastasize to the uvea.

- On funduscopic exam, lesions are generally pale, nonpigmented elevations of the choroid, occasionally accompanied by serous retinal detachment.

- Ultrasound: B-scan characteristics include a solid mass with no excavation or quiet zone and no orbital shadowing. A-scan characteristics include medium-to-high reflectivity, climbing posterior spike, and no spontaneous pulsations.

- Differential diagnosis for nonpigmented choroidal lesion includes metastatic carcinoma, choroidal hemangioma (typically red or orange), choroidal osteoma, lymphoma, or posterior scleritis.

Retinoblastoma

- A malignant retinal tumor of photoreceptor origin most commonly seen in children younger than 3 years of age. May be spontaneous (generally unilateral) or inherited (generally bilateral).

- Up to 30% of cases present with bilateral retinoblastoma. A third neoplastic focus is occasionally found in the pineal gland ("trilateral retinoblastoma").

- Malignant transformation is caused by inactivation of a tumor suppressor gene (Rb). Tumor formation requires the silencing of both alleles. In the hereditable form, one allele is congenitally silenced, while the other must undergo spontaneous mutation. In the nonheritable form, both alleles must undergo spontaneous mutation.

- A tumor is most commonly detected due to presentation with leukocoria (white pupil), strabismus, or intraocular inflammation.

- Differential for leukocoria–congenital cataract, Coat's disease, primary hyperplastic vitreous (PHPV), etc.

- Funduscopic exam reveals a white, nodular mass that may be subretinal (exophytic) or extend into the vitreous (endophytic).

- Tumor may extend posteriorly into the optic nerve and brain or into the orbital tissues.

Adnexal Tumors with Orbital Spread
Basal Cell Carcinoma (BCC)

- The most common malignant eyelid tumor (85% to 95% of all epithelial eyelid malignancies), usually presenting on the lower lid. It is generally slow growing and painless. The lesion typically presents with a pearly raised lesion with overlying telangiectasias (superficial and nodular types). The lesion may ulcerate centrally (ulcerative type).

- Morphea-type (sclerosing) basal cell carcinoma present as a pale, indurated plaque. Diagnosis is difficult because the lesion lies mostly beneath the surface. Furthermore, tumor borders are indistinct, resulting in high rates of incomplete excision. In a patient with chronic, ulcerative blepharitis, rule out sclerosing BCC.

- Tumor invades locally but rarely metastasizes. Ulcerative-type BCCs are generally more infiltrative than other types.

Squamous Cell Carcinoma (SCC)

- A slow-growing, painless tumor that generally starts as a hyperkeratotic growth. Lesions frequently appear very similar to basal cell carcinoma.

- Actinic keratosis: flat, scaly, keratotic lesions occurring in sun-damaged skin. Approximately 10% of these lesions evolve into SCCs.

- These tumors spread locally and may metastasize via the lymphatic system.

Melanoma

- A slow-growing, painless tumor that is usually darkly pigmented. Amelanotic melanomas, however, do occur and are more difficult to diagnose.

- Skin melanomas are classified as: lentigo maligna melanoma, superficial spreading, and nodular.
  1. *Lentigo Maligna Melanoma:* Occurs on sun-exposed areas of the skin. Lesion begins as a tan macular lesion, gradually grows, and changes color. Growth follows a "radial growth phase" followed by a more dangerous "vertical growth phase." Prognosis is good as the tumor is generally diagnosed during the "radial growth phase."
  2. *Superficial Spreading Melanoma:* This is the most common form of cutaneous melanoma (~70%). Tumor has gradual growth with predominantly "radial growth." "Vertical growth phase" follows much later. Prognosis is good.
  3. *Nodular Melanoma:* Lesion generally is nodular with a uniform blue-black color. Amelanotic nodular lesions also occur. Growth is predominantly "vertical" and hence has the worst survival outcome.

- Prognosis is contingent on depth of tumor invasion. Original studies by Breslow and Clark have confirmed this. Breslow staging: Tumors <0.76 mm thickness have a 1% tumor-related mortality at 5 years. Patients with tumors = 1.0 mm have 20% mortality at 10 years, and tumor >4 mm have 50% tumor-related mortality at 10 years.

- Note: BCC, SCC, and melanoma are the three most common tumors requiring exenteration due to significant orbital invasion.

Severe Fungal Infection
Mucormycosis

- A rare, but often fatal, fungal infection seen in debilitated patients, particularly uncontrolled diabetics.

- Responsible species include mucor, absidia, and rhizopus. Inoculation occurs via the respiratory tract and fungi may invade small vessels of the sinus and orbit, producing significant tissue necrosis.

- Treatment includes systemic Amphotericin B, correction of ketoacidosis, and potential orbital exenteration (resection is based on the extent of invasion/tissue necrosis).

Trauma: *Please see "Open Globe"*

Sympathetic Uveitis

- A rare but severe granulomatous inflammatory response that arises in the contralateral eye after penetrating ocular trauma. It is thought to occur due to sensitization of body to uveal antigens or retinal S antigen.
- Incidence: estimates range from 0.3% to 2% depending on the study cited.
- Enucleation of the damaged eye within 2 weeks is thought to decrease this risk almost to zero.
- Evisceration does not decrease this risk.

Preoperative Assessment

- History: ocular surgery or trauma, cancer, systemic disease, constitutional symptoms (fever, fatigue, weight loss, anorexia), onset of visual symptoms (e.g., blurred vision, diplopia)
- Ocular exam: visual acuity, visual fields, slit lamp exam ("cell and flare"), lid examination, dilated funduscopic exam (for retinal/choroidal tumor)
- Computed tomography/magnetic resonance imaging (CT/MRI) of the orbits and brain: The position and extent of tumor or infectious invasion can often be determined.
- A-scan and/or B-scan ultrasound: confirms the presence of retinal/choroidal masses, particularly when the anterior optic media is opacified
- Fine needle aspiration (FNA): if suspecting intraocular tumor
- Biopsy: if suspecting extraocular tumor
- Laboratory tests: complete blood count (CBC; if infection suspected); aspartate aminotransferase/alanine aminotransferase (AST/ALT); gamma-glutamyl transpeptidase (GGT); alkaline phosphatase (melanoma most commonly metastasizes to liver); chest x-ray (CXR, if metastasis is suspected)

Anesthesia

- Retrobulbar block (with epinephrine) plus intravenous (IV) sedation is often sufficient for evisceration procedures.
- General anesthesia plus retrobulbar block (with epinephrine) is performed for enucleations and exenterations.

PROCEDURE

Enucleation: (SEE TABLES 7.5.1 Rapid Review of Steps and 7.5.2 Surgical Pearls, and WEB TABLES 7.5.1 to 7.5.4 for equipment and medication lists).

1. *Confirmation of Correct Eye:* Although posttraumatic eyes are usually easy to discern, eyes with intraocular tumors and blind eyes may be difficult to differentiate from normal eyes on gross exam. Dilated funduscopic examination to visualize the tumor and confirmation with a careful preoperative assessment is generally warranted before proceeding.

2. *Muscle Identification/Isolation:* A 360-degree perilimbal incision (peritomy) is made through the conjunctiva and Tenon's capsule. While retracting the conjunctiva and Tenon's capsule with forceps, scissors are used to bluntly dissect along the sclera between the insertion points of the four rectus muscles. Adjoining fascia is then stripped from the extraocular muscles starting at the insertion point and progressing posteriorly.

3. *Suture Placement/Disinsertion of Rectus Muscles:* A muscle hook is used to isolate and elevate each muscle from the sclera so that the suture may pass without penetrating the globe. Once the rectus muscle has been isolated, fine double-armed sutures are passed through each muscle approximately 1 mm to the scleral insertion site. (This is particularly important in retinoblastoma cases as

TABLE 7.5.1 Rapid Review of Steps
(1) Perform 360-degree conjunctival peritomy.
(2) Perform blunt dissection between all four intramuscular quandrants.
(3) Isolate each rectus muscle and place vicryl suture through muscle belly.
(4) Detach rectus muscles.
(5) Isolate and bisect oblique.
(6) Place traction sutures through muscle stumps.
(7) Palpate optic nerve with enucleation scissors and bisected.
(8) Remove globe and pack orbit for hemostasis.
(9) Place implant in intraconal space.
(10) Sew muscles to implant.
(11) Close tenons and conjunctiva in layers.
(12) Place conformer.

TABLE 7.5.2 Surgical Pearls

Preoperative:
- A long discussion with patient and family about postoperative issues including fitting of prosthesis and functioning with one eye including activities of daily living, driving, and employment is essential for the patient to start accepting the ramifications of the loss of an eye.
- A retrobulbar block with local anesthesia is important for postoperative pain management.

Intraoperative:
- Isolation and detachment of the four major recti muscles is important so that later reattachement onto an integrated, porous implant is possible to maximize postoperative motility. However, the oblique muscles are typically isolated and bisected. Attachment of the oblique muscles can cause implant motility problems.
- Closure over the implant should be meticulous and in layers—tenons in a single layer followed by conjunctiva in a second layer. This will help prevent exposure or extrusion of the implant.
- Suture tarsorrhaphy of the eyelids after the procedure can prevent postoperative hemorrhage or edema from dislodging the conformer. Some surgeons advocate pressure dressings, but these can be uncomfortable, whereas with a tarsorrhaphy in place, the patient can remove a light patch in 48 hours and shower.

Postoperative:
- The conformer must be maintained until the prosthesis is fit. During initial postoperative visits, examine the eye socket through the conformer; resist removing the conformer as it may be difficult to replace.

tumor seeding is thought to occur with globe perforation.) Locking bites are taken at both edges of the muscle to ensure suture retention (FIG. 7.5.1). The tendon is cut just distal to the suture placements, leaving the muscles suspended on the sutures. This is repeated for all four muscles. Silk

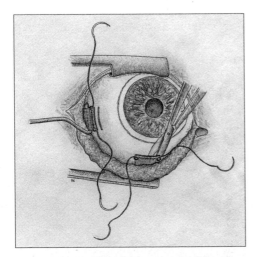

FIGURE 7.5.1 ◆ *Enucleation muscle disinsertion:* Once the rectus muscles have been isolated, fine double-armed sutures are passed through each muscle just distal to the scleral insertion. Locking bites are taken at both edges of the muscle to ensure suture retention. Each tendon is then cut just proximal to the insertion, leaving the muscles suspended on the sutures.

sutures are passed through the residual rectus muscle stumps to permit the application of upward traction when approaching the optic nerve.

4. *Cutting of Oblique Muscles:* Identification of the oblique muscles is significantly easier after disinsertion of the rectus muscles. The superior and inferior oblique are then identified, cauterized, and transected.

5. *Cutting of Optic Nerve:* This may be performed with enucleation scissors or a Foster snare.
   A. *Enucleation Scissors:* Upward traction is placed on the muscle stump sutures to permit palpation of the optic nerve with enucleation scissors. A hemostat may be placed across the optic nerve and vessels and clamped securely. Enucleation scissors are then used to transect the nerve and vessels anteriorly to the clamp. The globe is removed from the socket and sent to pathology for evaluation. The optic nerve stump is cauterized before releasing the hemostat and the globe socket is packed with sterile gauze sponges to further aid in hemostasis.
   B. *Foster Snare:* The snare is placed around the globe and advanced posteriorly while upward traction is applied to the muscle stump sutures. Care is taken to not include the rectus muscles or lid tissue within the snare. The snare is then tightly clinched, crushing the nerve while providing adequate hemostasis. After approximately 5 minutes, the snare is

further tightened to completely transect the optic nerve. After globe removal, the orbital socket is packed with sterile gauze.

6. *Placement of Orbital Implant:* An orbital implant made of a porous material (hydroxyapatite [HA] or a porous polyethylene [trade name: Medpor]) or smooth material (acrylic or silicone) is generally placed in the orbital socket. Porous implants allow for muscles to be sewn to the implant and for fibrovascular ingrowth. However, they tend to be more expensive and can have a higher risk of exposure due to their porous and rough surface. This can be avoided by wrapping with processed donor sclera, autologous fascia, or polyglactin (Vicryl) mesh. This wrapping facilitates suturing of the extraocular muscles to the implant and guards against exposure. Smooth implants are less expensive but have a higher rate of extrusion because fibrovascular tissue does not integrate with the implant. An appropriately sized implant is selected by using trial-size implants to approximate the best fit in the orbital socket (generally 20 to 22 cm in diameter).

7. *Reattachment of Rectus Muscles:* The suspended rectus muscles are then sutured to the implant at locations that correspond to their anatomic insertion points (FIG. 7.5.2). This allows for good mobility of the implant.

8. *Closure:* Tenon's capsule is then closed over the implant with several interrupted sutures followed by a running suture to close the conjunctiva. A meticulous layered closure is required in order to minimize the risk of implant exposure. A conformer is placed to maintain the conjunctival fornices followed by a topical antibiotic ointment. The eyelids may be tarsorrhaphied over top. The orbit is then pressure patched for up to 1 week.

Evisceration: The following procedure describes an evisceration with corneal removal.

1. *Confirmation of Correct Eye:* As in the enucleation procedure, an intraoperative dilated funduscopic examination is generally warranted before proceeding.

2. *Muscle Identification/Isolation:* A 360-degree peritomy is made through the conjunctiva and Tenon's capsule.

3. *Evisceration Step:* A full-thickness scleral incision is made approximately 2 mm behind the limbus. Sharp scissors are then used to cut circumferentially around the globe to remove the cornea (FIG. 7.5.3). (Note: If the goal is to preserve the cornea, the incision may stop just short of 360 degrees, leaving a scleral hinge. However, some surgeons feel leaving the cornea risks having persistent postoperative pain.) An evisceration spoon or a periosteal elevator is used to remove all of the scleral contents (FIG. 7.5.4) (retina, uvea, lens, and vitreous). Hemostasis is achieved with

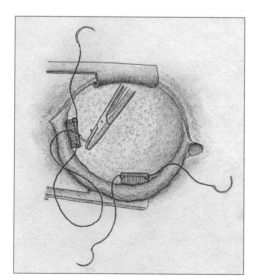

FIGURE 7.5.2 ◆ *Enucleation implant placement:* The suspended rectus muscles are then sutured to the implant at locations that correspond to their anatomic insertion points. This allows for good mobility of the implant.

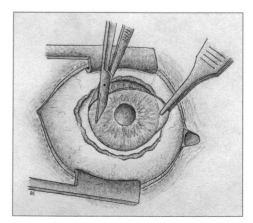

FIGURE 7.5.3 ◆ *Evisceration corneal removal:* A full-thickness scleral incision is made behind the limbus. Sharp scissors are then used to cut circumferentially around the globe to remove the cornea.

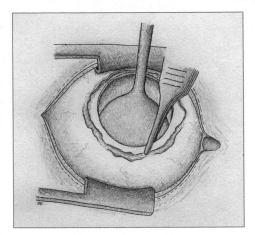

FIGURE 7.5.4 ◆ *Evisceration globe evacuation:* An evisceration spoon or a periosteal elevator is used to remove all of the scleral contents.

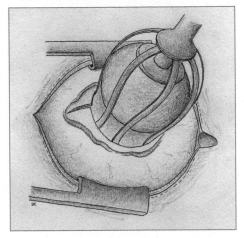

FIGURE 7.5.6 ◆ *Evisceration implant placement:* An implant is placed into the scleral cavity using a specialized inserter after windows are cut in the posterior scleral shell to permit vascular ingrowth and decrease the likelihood of extrusion.

electrocautery. Absolute alcohol-covered cotton tips are then used to remove all the remaining pigment. This is thought to denature uveal proteins to help prevent sympathetic uveitis. Finally, the intact sclera is irrigated with sterile saline.

4. *Placement of Orbital Implant:* Four scleral relaxing incisions are made in an anterior-to-posterior direction in all four intramuscular quadrants (FIG. 7.5.5). An orbital implant (porous HA or Medpor implant of generally 14 to 18 mm) is inserted into the scleral cavity (FIG. 7.5.6).

5. *Closure:* A careful layered closure significantly decreases the likelihood of implant extrusion.

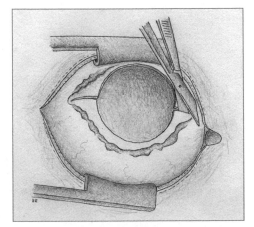

FIGURE 7.5.5 ◆ *Evisceration relaxing incisions:* Relaxing incisions are made in the sclera to permit the insertion of an appropriately sized implant.

The sclera is first closed over the implant with multiple interrupted sutures. Tenon's is then closed with interrupted sutures followed by a running suture to close the conjunctiva. A conformer is placed to maintain the conjunctival fornices followed by a topical antibiotic ointment. The eyelids may be tarsorrhaphied over top. The orbit is then pressure patched for up to 1 week.

Exenteration: This procedure varies significantly depending on the extent and nature of tissue invasion. Furthermore, the expertise of head and neck, craniofacial, and neurosurgeons may be required to achieve full debridement. The following procedure describes a total orbital exenteration with reconstruction.

1. *Approach to orbital rim:* After confirmation of the correct eye (with dilated exam and review of the preoperative assessment), an incision line is drawn around the orbital rim. Before proceeding, the lids are closed with a running suture. An incision is made over the marked line and extended down to the orbital rim (FIG. 7.5.7).

2. *Periosteal elevation and removal of the periorbita:* A circumferential incision is made in the periosteum overlying the orbital rim. Starting anteriorly, a periosteal elevator is used to bluntly dissect the periorbita away from the walls of the orbit. The large vessels traversing the orbital apex

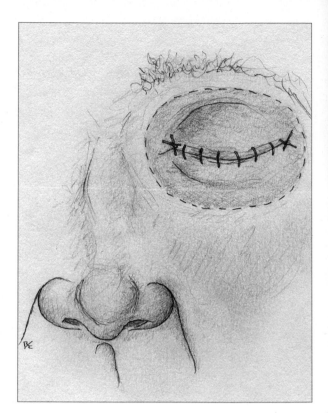

FIGURE 7.5.7 ◆ *Exenteration:* After confirmation of the correct eye, an incision line is drawn around the orbital rim. Before proceeding, the lids are closed with a running suture. An incision is then made over the marked line and extended down to the orbital rim.

are identified and cauterized prior to transection in order to maintain adequate hemostasis. Particularly along the medial orbital wall, care is taken to avoid traumatic fracture, which may result in the formation of fistulas between the orbit and sinuses. The optic nerve is identified, clamped with a hemostat, and transected with enucleation scissors. Electrocautery over the clamp may be necessary to achieve hemostasis. The periorbita and orbital contents may then be lifted out of the socket and sent to pathology. Hemostasis is achieved with meticulous cautery.

3. *Pathologic Assessment:* Before proceeding, stat frozen sections may be required to ensure that tissue invasion has not progressed beyond the orbit. If the margins are "clean" (devoid of pathologic tissue/tumor invasion), orbital reconstruction and closure may be performed.

4. *Orbital Reconstruction:* Various possibilities are available:
   A. *Granulation:* This is the simplest form of "reconstruction." The orbit is simply pressure packed with iodinated gauze for 1 week. This allows for early granulation to occur. After gauze removal, the granulation tissue must be cleaned daily. The full granulation process takes around 2 months.
   B. *Skin graft:* A split-thickness skin graft is harvested from the thigh or buttock and is sewn to the adnexal skin to cover the orbital defect. The orbit is then pressure packed over the graft with iodinated gauze for 1 week. An advantage of this procedure over simple granulation is faster wound healing.
   C. *Regional or free flap:* A frontotemporal, parietotemporal, or a microvascular free flap is used to cover the orbital defect. The orbit is then pressured packed with iodinated gauze for 1 week. This method, although time consuming and technically challenging, decreases the risk of sino-orbital fistula formation.

After appropriate healing of the socket, silicone-based prosthetics, attached to the skin or bone, are fitted to achieve adequate cosmesis.

Further Considerations for Enucleation or Evisceration

Prosthesis: Patients may be referred to an ocularist to develop a prosthesis 6 to 8 weeks after enucleation or evisceration. The prosthesis fits directly over the implant and maintains the conjunctival fornices.

Peg Placement: Used to further improve the mobility of the implant. After significant vascularization of the implant (usually 6 to 12 months postoperatively; confirmed by MRI), a titanium peg may be drilled into the implant. The peg is then coupled to a special prosthesis developed by the ocularist, providing greater mobility of the implant. Risks of peg placement include improper peg location (off center or incorrectly angled), peg fall out, discharge, pyogenic granuloma formation, prosthesis clicking, and increased risk of infection or exposure.

COMPLICATIONS

Enucleation and Evisceration

1. *Hemorrhage/hematoma:* Can generally be avoided with meticulous intraoperative hemostasis.

2. *Implant extrusion/tissue breakdown:* This complication is diminished with a combination of a meticulous closure and newer implants that permit vascular ingrowth.

3. *Socket discharge due to irritation/inflammation:* Giant papillary conjunctivitis is the most common cause of discharge.

4. Ptosis, enophthalmos, and/or superior sulcus deformity due to orbital volume loss.

5. *Socket contraction with shallow conjunctival fornices and lid deformities:* This may be due to excessive wound healing. The conformer is placed postoperatively to minimize the risk of this complication. Late socket contraction is due to chronic inflammation in the socket.

Exenteration

1. *Hemorrhage:* Largely prevented by adequate intraoperative hemostasis.

2. *Sino-orbital or naso-orbital fistula:* Patient presents with discharge, crusting, and/or wound breakdown. Fistula generally occurs if orbital walls are penetrated inadvertently or if they are purposefully resected (e.g., to achieve clear tumor margins).

3. *Cerebrospinal fluid leak:* iatrogenic injury to orbital roof

4. Osteomyelitis

5. Intracranial infection/abscess

POSTOPERATIVE CARE

General

- Apply compressive dressing for 1 week to minimize swelling/inflammation.
- Apple ice packs for 48 hours to minimize swelling/inflammation.
- Apply topical antibiotic ointment in socket for 2 to 4 weeks.
- Administer prophylactic oral antibiotics for ~5 days.
- Administer mild oral analgesia.

Enucleation/Evisceration (with corneal removal)

- Continued conformer use for first 1 to 2 months prevents shortening and scarring of the conjunctival fornices.
- Permanent eye prosthesis fitted at 6 to 8 weeks by the ocularist.
- Peg placements after vascularization (6 to 12 months) to improve implant mobility (optional).

Exenteration

- After adequate socket healing (variable time based on reconstruction method), a silicone-based prosthetic eye is fitted by the ocularist.
- For more extensive tissue removal, bone-anchored titanium plates may be placed by the surgeon followed by a prosthetic eye fitting. This allows for placement of a maxillofacial prosthesis in addition to the orbital prosthesis.

Further Reading

Text

Char DH. *Clinical Ocular Oncology.* 3rd ed. Toronto, Canada: BC Decker; 2000.

Dutton JJ. Enucleation, evisceration, and exenteration. In: Yanoff M, Duker J, eds. *Ophthalmology.* 3rd ed. Philadelphia, PA: Mosby; 2009:1478–1482.

Nunery WR, Hetzler K. Enucleation. In: Hornblass A, ed. *Oculoplastic, Orbital and Reconstructive Surgery.* Baltimore: Williams and Wilkins; 1990:1200–1220.

Sullivan, JH. Orbit. In: *Vaughan and Asbury's General Oph-thalmology*. New York, NY: Lange Medical Books/Mc-Graw-Hill; 2004:249–259.

Vaughn GL, Dortzbach RK, Gayre GS. Eyelid malignancies. In: Yanoff M, Duker J, eds. *Ophthalmology*. 3rd ed. Philadelphia, PA: Mosby; 2009:1434–1443.

Primary Sources

Christmas MD, Gordon CD, Murray TG, et al. Intraorbital implants after enucleation and their complications: a ten year review. *Arch Ophthalmology*. 1998;116(9):1199–1203.

Collaborative Ocular Melanoma Study Group. Factors predictive of growth and treatment of small choroidal melanoma. COMS report no. 5. *Arch Ophthalmol*. 1997;115(12):1537–1544.

Collaborative Ocular Melanoma Study Group. The Collaborative Ocular Melanoma Study (COMS) randomized trial of pre-enucleation radiation of large choroidal melanoma. I: Characteristics of patients enrolled and not enrolled. COMS report no. 9. *Am J Ophthalmol*. 1998;125(6):767–778.

Grossniklaus HE, McLean IW. Cutaneous melanoma of the eyelid. Clinicopathologic features. *Ophthalmology*. 1991; 98(12):1867–1873.

Lubin JR, Albert DM, Weinstein M. Sixty-five years of sympathetic ophthalmia: a clinicopathologic review of 105 cases (1913–1978). *Ophthalmology*. 1980;87(2):109–121.

Melia BM, Abramson DH, Albert DM, et al. Collaborative Ocular Melanoma Study (COMS) randomized trial of I-125 brachytherapy for medium choroidal melanoma. I. Visual acuity after 3 years. COMS report no. 16. *Ophthalmology*. 2001;108(2):348–366.

Perry AC. Integrated orbital implants. *Adv Ophthalmic Plastic Reconstructive Surgery*. 1990;8:75–81.

Vaziri M, et al. Clinicopathologic features and behavior of cutaneous eyelid melanoma. *Ophthalmology*. 2002; 109(5):901–908.

7.6   ORBITAL DECOMPRESSION

- Controlled removal of one or more orbital walls to permit decompression of the orbit and prolapse of its contents

INDICATIONS

- Most commonly performed for thyroid eye disease (Graves' ophthalmopathy, thyroid-related orbitopathy, or dysthyroid immune related ophthalmopathy) (FIG. 7.6.1)
- Considered for conditions causing severe proptosis with exposure keratitis and diplopia or com-pressive optic neuropathy that has failed medical therapy

ALTERNATIVES

Medical Therapy (for Treatment of Graves' Ophthalmopathy)
- Optimal control of thyroid status by an endocrinologist
- Exposure keratitis (initially managed by topical lubricants)
- Diplopia from muscle infiltration/restriction (initially managed by prisms that simulate changes in eye position by altering the path of incident light)
- Compressive optic neuropathy (high-dose systemic corticosteroids, immunomodulation [i.e., rituximab], and/or external beam radiotherapy to the orbit)

Surgery
- Exposure keratitis (lateral tarsorrhaphy [fusion of upper and lower lids], lengthening of lid retractors, or Botulinum toxin induced ptosis)

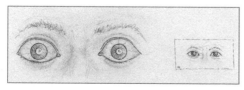

FIGURE 7.6.1 ◆ *Exophthalmos due to thyroid eye disease:* The proptotic globe causes lid retraction, significantly increasing the marginal reflex distance and resulting in superior scleral show. Normally, the upper lid margin partially covers the superior irides in primary gaze (inset).

- Diplopia (strabismus surgery after ophthalmopathy has stabilized [~6 months without change])

RELEVANT PHYSIOLOGY/ANATOMY

Graves' Ophthalmopathy (FIG. 7.6.2)

- Presumed autoimmune process (thyroid-stimulating immunoglobulin present in ~50% of cases).
- Lymphocytic infiltration of muscles (myositis) with edema and production of hyaluronic acid and other glycosaminoglycans (GAG). Muscles become progressively fibrotic and enlarged, which combined with GAG deposition, leads to proptosis.
- Proptosis and lid retraction leads to lagophthalmos, resulting in exposure keratopathy.
- Fibrosis and enlargement of muscles can lead to restriction of ocular motility and subsequent diplopia. Inferior rectus is most commonly affected.
- Significant extraocular muscle enlargement can lead to compressive optic neuropathy.
- Inflammatory infiltration and GAG deposition tends to plateau 1 to 3 years after onset.

Orbital Anatomy

Orbital Walls: seven bones total (FIG. 7.6.3)

- Superior wall (roof): frontal bone and lesser wing of the sphenoid bone (posteriorly)
- Lateral wall: zygomatic bone (strongest portion of the orbit) and greater wing of the sphenoid bone (posteriorly)
- Inferior wall (floor): maxilla, zygomatic bone (laterally), and palatine bone (posteriorly)
- Medial wall: ethmoid bone (lamina papyracea), frontal bone, maxilla, lacrimal bone (anteriorly), and body of sphenoid (posteriorly). Although the ethmoidal bones are the thinnest of the orbit, they are not the weakest due to their honeycomb configuration.

Connective Tissues of Orbit

- Periorbita: periosteum surrounding the orbit
- Orbital septal system: connective tissue that surrounds extraocular muscles, optic nerve, and orbital fat lobules in order to provide structural support. (Note: this is different from the orbital septum, which is a membranous sheet delineating the anterior boundaries of the orbit.) This connective tissue becomes densely fibrotic in

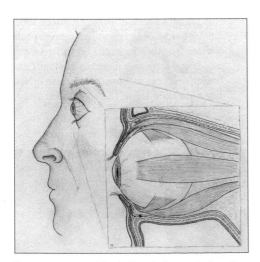

FIGURE 7.6.2 ✦ *Muscle fibrosis:* Parasagittal section of the orbit, demonstrating proptosis and lid retraction caused by extraocular muscle fibrosis and enlargement. The dashed line demonstrates the transconjunctival approach to the orbital floor, which is removed in a controlled fashion to permit the eye to recede within the orbit.

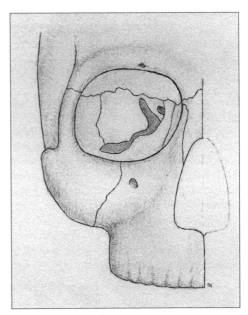

FIGURE 7.6.3 ✦ *Orbital anatomy:* The orbit is a conical structure with contributions from the frontal, lacrimal, ethmoid, zygomatic, maxillary, palatine, and sphenoid bones.

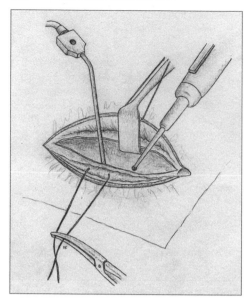

FIGURE 7.6.7 ◆ *Maxillary bone defect:* Once the orbital floor has been exposed, a burr tip drill (shown) or hemostat is used to puncture the maxillary bone medially to the infraorbital nerve. The instrument tip will enter the maxillary sinus.

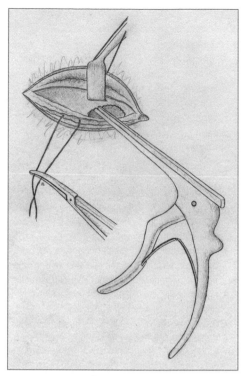

FIGURE 7.6.8 ◆ *Orbital floor removal:* A Kerrison rongeur is then used to remove the orbital floor in a controlled fashion. Care is taken to avoid injury to the infraorbital neurovascular bundle. Depending on the degrees of globe recession desired, the medial and lateral walls of the orbit may be removed as well.

the hole in the orbital floor is expanded to the posterior wall of the maxillary sinus (FIGS. 7.6.7, 7.6.8). Some surgeons will leave the inferior orbital neurovascular bundle covered by bone, whereas others will elect to unroof this structure. Bone lateral to the structure can be removed as well.

7. *Medial Wall Removal:* Continuing with the rongeur, bone removal is extended nasally from the orbital floor to the ethmoid bone. The superior margin of bone removal is the anterior and posterior ethmoidal foramen where the ethmoidal neurovascular bundles pass. Above this is the start of the cribriform plate. The transition of the orbital floor to the medial orbital wall, the inferomedial strut is often left intact so as the globe does not sublux completely into the maxillary sinus causing hypoglobus and diplopia.

8. *Blunt Dissection of Orbital Septal Tissue:* The periorbital is incised to allow the orbital fat to prolapse into the decompressed orbit. In thyroid eye disease, fibrosis of the septal tissue sometimes prevents adequate orbital prolapse. Using blunt dissection, the fibrotic septa can be separated to allow better prolapse of tissue. Care must be

taken to avoid neurovascular structures. Periorbital fat may also be removed to allow further decompression (FIGS. 7.6.9A, B).

9. *Closing of Periorbita:* The periorbita may be sutured open in order to allow adequate prolapse into the maxillary and ethmoid sinuses. Anteriorly, interrupted sutures are placed to reappose the periosteum over the orbital rim where the incision was first placed (FIG. 7.6.10).

10. *Closing of Conjunctiva* (FIGS. 7.6.11): Both traction sutures are removed and the conjunctiva is closed with a fine running suture.

COMPLICATIONS

Intraoperative

1. Optic nerve injury from retractors. Periodic monitoring of pupillary reactions is necessary.

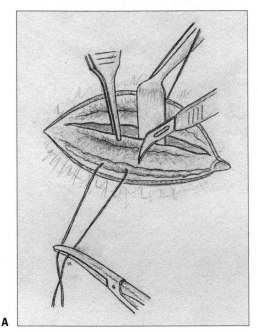

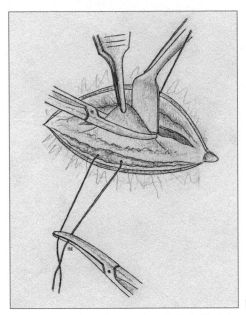

A   **B**

FIGURE 7.6.9 ◆ *Orbital fat resection:* Removal of orbital fat permits further decompression of the orbit. Periorbita is incised to permit exposure of fat, which is then cross-clamped and excised. Hemostasis is achieved with electrocautery.

2. Excessive globe pressure from retractors leading to decreased VA.

3. Overcorrection or undercorrection may require reoperation after observation and nonsurgical treatment.

Postoperative

4. Orbital hemorrhage results from inadequate cauterization and/or vessel tear on bony edge. Patient presents with proptosis, orbital pain, and decreased visual acuity.

5. *Diplopia:* The inferior oblique lies below the orbital septum and is particularly susceptible to damage. Diplopia may resolve spontaneously or

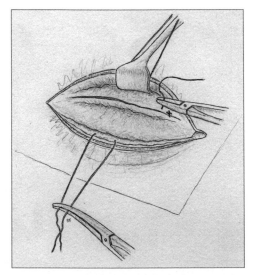

FIGURE 7.6.10 ◆ *Periosteal closure:* The orbital rim periosteum is then reapproximated with sutures.

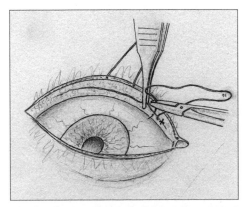

FIGURE 7.6.11 ◆ *Conjunctival closure:* The palpebral conjunctiva is reapproximated with sutures.

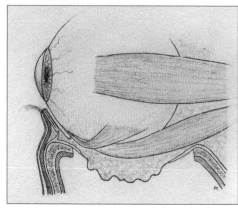

FIGURE 7.6.12 ◆ *Decompressed orbit:* Parasagittal section of the orbit demonstrating passage of the orbital soft tissues into the maxillary sinus through the bony defect created in the orbital floor. This decreases pressure on the globe, permitting it to sink back into the orbit. The globe usually comes to occupy a lower position than its fellow. Strabismus surgery may, therefore, be necessary after the decompression has stabilized.

may require subsequent strabismus surgery (FIG. 7.6.12).

6. Lower eyelid deformities (i.e., ectropion, epiblepharon) result from injury to lower lid (capsulopalpebral) fascia or scarring of orbital septum.

POSTOPERATIVE CARE

- VA and pupillary reflexes should be assessed frequently postoperatively in the first 2 hours.
- Systemic antibiotics and nasal decongestants should be given for 1 week.
- Topical antibiotic ointment plus mild analgesia should be applied to incision for 1 week.

Further Reading

Text

Dutton JJ. *Atlas of Clinical and Surgical Anatomy.* Philadelphia, PA: WB Saunders; 1994.

Dutton JJ. Orbital surgery. In: Yanoff M, Duker J, eds. *Ophthalmology.* 3rd ed. Philadelphia, PA: Mosby; 2009: 1466–1474.

Whitcher, J, Riordan-Eva P. *Vaughan and Asbury's General Ophthalmology.* New York, NY: Lange Medical Books/ McGraw-Hill; 2004.

Primary Sources

Anderson RL, Linberg JV. Transorbital approach to decompression in Graves' disease. *Arch Ophthalmol.* 1981;99(1): 120–124.

Kennerdell JS, Maroon JC. An orbital decompression for severe dysthyroid exophthalmos. *Ophthalmology.* 1982;89(5): 467–472.

Linberg JV, Anderson RL. Transorbital decompression. Indications and results. *Arch Ophthalmol.* 1981;99(1): 113–119.

7.7   PTOSIS REPAIR

- There are multiple surgical techniques for elevating a drooping upper eyelid.
- Selection depends on ptosis etiology, degree of levator palpebrae superioris function, and surgeon preference.

FRONTALIS SUSPENSION

- Elevates the upper lid to a functionally and cosmetically acceptable position by anchoring the superior tarsal plate to the frontalis muscle with a fascial or silicon sling.
- The patient must learn to elevate and depress the lid by manipulating the frontalis muscle.

Indications

- Severe ptosis with poor levator function.
- Ptosis surgery is usually elective but pediatric patients with unilateral ptosis may require urgent repair to prevent the development of amblyopia.

ANTERIOR LEVATOR APONEUROSIS ADVANCEMENT

- Elevates the upper lid by shortening the levator aponeurosis via an anterior approach.

Indications

- Moderate-to-severe ptosis with some degree of residual levator function.

- Incision location permits simultaneous blepharoplasty in patients with significant dermatochalasis or the desire for cosmetic improvement (see Chapter 7.1 Upper Lid Blepharoplasty).

FASANELLA-SERVAT PROCEDURE

- Elevates the upper lid through posterior wedge resection of tarsus, Müller's muscle, and palpebral conjunctiva.

Indications

- Effective for mild ptosis with preserved levator function.
- Cosmetically advantageous because the lid incision is hidden.

ALTERNATIVES

Medical Therapy

- Conservative management: Observe acquired ptosis for resolution.
- Ptosis crutches: Attach to eyeglasses and prop the upper lid open.
- Etiology specific: For example, proscribe acetylcholinesterase inhibitors for myasthenia gravis.

Surgery

- External tarso aponeurectomy (ETA): A full-thickness ellipse of upper lid tissue is excised and used as a lower lid graft to permit large ptosis corrections without the development of lagophthalmos.

PTOSIS BASICS

- The upper eyelid margin is abnormally low and may obstruct the visual axis.
- Depending on etiology, this finding may be unilateral or bilateral.
- It is more correctly known as blepharoptosis (*blepharo* = lid + *ptosis* = drooping). This differentiates the condition from other types of ptosis encountered in ophthalmic practice (e.g., brow ptosis).

Classification

Ptosis Severity	Measurement (mm)	Levator Function
Mild	1–2	Good
Moderate	3	Fair
Severe	4	Poor

Congenital

- Myogenic: This is the most common congenital form of ptosis. Fibrofatty tissue replaces the underdeveloped levator, impairing elevation and relaxation.
- Neurogenic: Examples include oculomotor palsy (CN III), Horner's syndrome (e.g., from brachial plexus injury during delivery), and Marcus-Gunn jaw winking syndrome (jaw movements to elicit ptosis due to CN V synkinesis).
- Aponeurotic: Involves the improper insertion of the levator aponeurosis on the anterior tarsus and lid skin; it is associated with birth trauma.
- Mechanical: The lid is depressed by mass effect from a capillary hemangioma, dermoid cyst, or neurofibroma.
- Blepharophimosis: A syndrome characterized by severe bilateral ptosis and horizontally shortened palpebral fissures.
- *Note:* 75% of cases are unilateral, and pose a high risk of amblyopia.

Acquired

- Aponeurotic/involutional: This is the most common acquired form of ptosis. Gradual stretching and dehiscence of the levator aponeurosis can result from aging, trauma, inflammation, and extended hard contact lens use.
- Neurogenic: Oculomotor palsy may result from trauma, microvascular disease, intracranial masses, and Circle of Willis aneurysms. Lesions to the sympathetic pathways, such as Pancoast tumors and internal carotid artery dissection, may cause Horner's syndrome.
- Mechanical: Weight due to scar formation, tumor, dermatochalasis, or edema can cause the eyelid to droop.
- Myotonic: An example is myasthenia gravis.

- Myogenic: An example is chronic progressive external ophthalmoplegia (CPEO).

   NOTE: *Acquired ptosis from reversible causes (trauma, inflammation) should be observed for resolution over the course of several months, whereas most congenital ptosis requires surgical intervention.*

RELEVANT ANATOMY

Facial Muscles (FIG. 7.7.1)

Sensory Innervation

- Upper lid sensation is transmitted by the supraorbital, supratrochlear, and lacrimal branches of the ophthalmic division of the trigeminal nerve (V_1).

Motor Innervation

- Pretarsal orbicularis oculi forcefully closes the eye and is supplied by the zygomatic branch of the facial nerve (CN VII).

- Frontalis muscle raises the eyebrows and wrinkles the forehead; it is supplied by the temporal branch of the facial nerve.

- Levator palpebrae superioris is the main upper lid retractor and is supplied by the core fibers of the oculomotor nerve.

- Müller's muscle is an accessory upper lid retractor supplied by sympathetic nerves from the posterior hypothalamus/superior cervical ganglion.

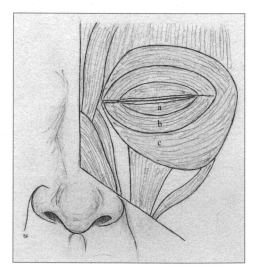

FIGURE 7.7.1 ♦ *Muscles of the upper face:* The frontalis muscle is directly superior to the orbicularis oculi, which consists of pretarsal (a), preseptal (b), and orbital (c) divisions. The upper lid retractors (not pictured) lie deep to the preseptal and pretarsal divisions.

Upper Lid Blood Supply

- The peripheral arcade travels just above the tarsus, whereas the marginal arcade runs superior to the lid margin.

- These arcades are fed by the superior medial palpebral branch of the ophthalmic artery and the superior lateral palpebral branch of the lacrimal artery.

PREOPERATIVE EVALUATION

- Rule out pseudoptosis. This may be due to ipsilateral enophthalmos (e.g., from prior orbital trauma) or contralateral proptosis (e.g., from unilateral thyroid eye disease or pseudotumor).

- Pharmacologic Müller's testing: Significant lid elevation (up to 2 mm) after topical phenylephrine administration suggests deinnervation hypersensitivity and supports use of the Fasanella-Servat procedure if ptosis is mild.

- Exam measurements: (FIG. 7.7.2)
   1. *Palpebral fissure height:* the distance between the upper and lower lid margins in primary gaze (normally 6–10 mm)
   2. *Marginal reflex distance (MRD):* the distance between the pupillary light reflex and upper lid margin in primary gaze (normally ~ 4 mm)
   3. *Levator excursion:* elevation of the upper lid margin from full downgaze to full upgaze; an indicator of levator function (normally 16–20 mm)
   4. *Upper eyelid crease:* the distance from the upper lid margin to the lid crease in downgaze (normally 8–10 mm, though frequently shorter or absent in Asians; may also be absent in congenital ptosis)

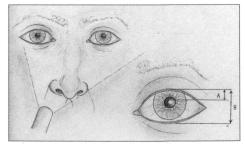

FIGURE 7.7.2 ♦ *Ptosis measurements:* Demonstration of the pupillary light reflex in primary gaze. The marginal reflex distance (MRD) is the distance between the pupillary light reflex and the upper lid margin (A). The palpebral fissure width is the distance between the upper and lower lid margins in the midpupillary axis (B).

5. *Horizontal lid laxity:* measured by ease of displacing the lid from the globe (If present, laxity can be addressed surgically at the time of ptosis repair.)

ANESTHESIA

- Local anesthesia is generally used for ptosis surgery to facilitate the intraoperative adjustment of lid height.
- Harvest of fascial autograft for frontalis suspension may require general anesthesia.

PROCEDURE

Frontalis Suspension

1. *Sling Choice:* Suspension can be achieved with harvested tensor fascia lata or a 1 mm-diameter flexible silicon rod. Autologous fascia has been the gold standard for repair because of durability, but the additional operative site increases morbidity and operating room (OR) time. Adequate harvest is generally not possible in children younger than 3 to 4 years of age. Silicon implants are easier to adjust or remove, but carry an increased risk of breakage, detachment, and extrusion.

   Fascial Harvest (omit with silicon rod): A small vertical incision is made in the lateral thigh just above the flexed knee. Dissection through subcutaneous fat reveals the underlying tensor fascia lata. Full exposure of this surgical plane permits insertion of a fascial stripper, which is used to harvest a narrow band of fascia 20 to 25 cm long. This strip is then cut to the appropriate dimensions prior to lid implantation.

2. *Primary Lid Incision:* An incision is made in the upper lid, following the contour of the natural crease, if present (FIG. 7.7.3). Dissection through the pretarsal orbicularis and subcutaneous tissue exposes the tarsal plate. The sling is then anchored to the upper tarsus using partial-thickness, nonabsorbable sutures (FIG. 7.7.4).

3. *Stab Incisions:* Three short brow incisions are made with a scalpel tip and deepened to the plane of the frontalis muscle (FIG. 7.7.3).

4. *Sling Passage:* With a silicon rod, preattached needles are used to pass the arms of the sling, first through the medial and lateral stab incisions, and then through the central incision (FIGS. 7.7.5A, B). With fascia, passage is accomplished with a curved

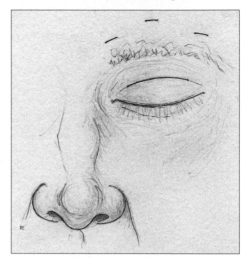

FIGURE 7.7.3 ◆ *Frontalis suspension:* An incision is made in the upper lid, following the contour of the natural crease. Three short stab incisions are made in the brow with a scalpel tip and deepened to the plane of the frontalis muscle.

Wright needle. With both methods, the arms of the sling are advanced deep to the orbital septum.

5. *Closure:* The lid crease is reconstituted by incorporating deep tissues into the skin closure. After reapproximation of the primary incision, lid height is adjusted and the free ends of the sling are joined

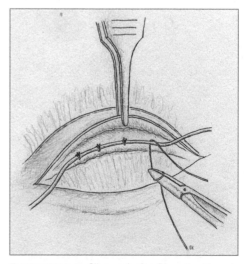

FIGURE 7.7.4 ◆ *Sling anchoring:* Dissection through the pretarsal orbicularis and subcutaneous tissue exposes the tarsal plate. The sling is then anchored to the upper tarsus using partial-thickness, nonabsorbable sutures.

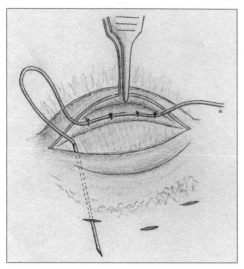

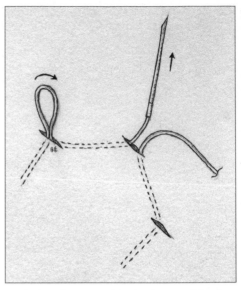

A

B

FIGURE 7.7.5.A,B ◆ *Sling passage:* With a silicon rod, preattached needles are used to pass the arms of the sling, first through the medial and lateral stab incisions, and then through the central incision.

with a silicon sleeve (silicon rod) or permanent suture (fascia). An absorbable suture can be placed around the silicon sleeve for additional security. Excess sling material is then trimmed and the free ends are tucked under the skin (FIG. 7.7.6). The brow incisions are closed in two layers.

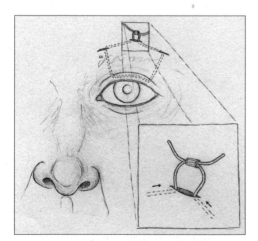

FIGURE 7.7.6 ◆ *Sling adjustment:* After the primary incision is reapproximated, lid height is adjusted, and the free ends of the sling are fastened together with a silicon sleeve (shown). Permanent suture is used in conjunction with fascia. Excess material is then trimmed and the free ends are tucked under the skin.

 Anterior Levator Aponeurosis Advancement: (SEE TABLES 7.7.1 Rapid Review of Steps and 7.7.2 Surgical Pearls, and WEB TABLES 7.7.1 to 7.7.4 for equipment and medication lists).

1. *Primary Incision:* An incision is made in the upper lid, following the contour of the natural crease (FIG. 7.7.7). The preseptal orbicularis is then divided parallel to its fibers, and the orbital septum is incised. The fat pads are retracted

TABLE 7.7.1 Rapid Review of Steps
(1) Inject anesthetic and allow time to work (5 minutes).
(2) Prep and drape.
(3) Incise lid crease.
(4) Excise excess skin (optional).
(5) Debulk orbital fat pads (optional).
(6) Dissect to anterior surface of tarsus.
(7) Dissect levator aponeurosis off tarsus and underlying Müller's muscle.
(8) Pass sutures through tarsus.
(9) Pass sutures through levator aponeurosis.
(10) Sit patient up and check eyelid contour.
(11) Adjust suture position to adjust eyelid height.
(12) Secure suture and close skin incision.

TABLE 7.7.2 Surgical Pearls

Preoperative:
- Determining whether skin and orbital fat removal should be performed at the same time as ptosis repair is important for surgical planning. Also, in cases of unilateral ptosis, deciding whether to operate on the obviously ptotic eyelid alone or bilaterally is important.

Intraoperative:
- Overcorrecting to account for epinephrine's action on Müller's muscle is important to get a good postoperative result.

Postoperative:
- Slight asymmetry at the 1-week postoperative period often resolves with improvement of edema. However, significant asymmetry should be revised in the early postoperative period (2 weeks).

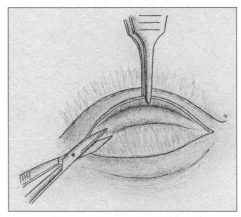

FIGURE 7.7.8 ◆ *Levator disinsertion:* After exposure of the anterior tarsus, the levator aponeurosis is disinserted with sharp dissection.

after dissection from the underlying levator aponeurosis, or removed to produce a change in lid contour.

2. *Aponeurosis Disinsertion:* After exposure of anterior tarsus with blunt dissection, the levator aponeurosis is sharply disinserted (FIG. 7.7.8). The freed aponeurosis is then reflected superiorly and separated from the underlying Müller's muscle.

3. *Aponeurosis Advancement:* The cut levator is advanced onto the tarsus in accordance with the degree of ptosis. A double-armed suture is passed through a partial thickness of the tarsus in the midpupillary axis, and then through the overlapping aponeurosis (FIGS. 7.7.9, 7.7.10). This suture is initially fastened with a slipknot to permit adjustment of the lid height, which is evaluated with the patient in an upright position (FIG. 7.7.11). After a

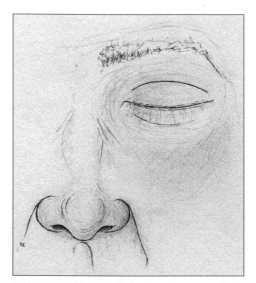

FIGURE 7.7.7 ◆ *Anterior levator advancement incision:* An incision is made in the upper lid, following the contour of the natural crease.

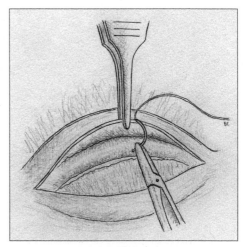

FIGURE 7.7.9 ◆ *Tarsal suture:* A double-armed suture is passed through a partial thickness of the superior tarsus in the midpupillary axis.

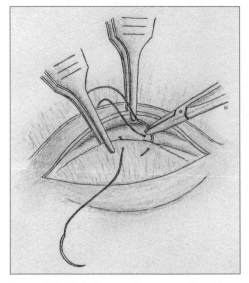

FIGURE 7.7.10 ✦ *Levator advancement:* The cut levator is then advanced onto the tarsus in accordance with the degree of ptosis, and both arms of the suture are passed through the overlapping aponeurosis.

satisfactory height is achieved, the suture is permanently knotted and excess levator is resected.

4. *Closure:* Redundant orbicularis is removed to prevent a thickened lid contour. The lid crease is then reformed by incorporating bites of levator into the skin closure.

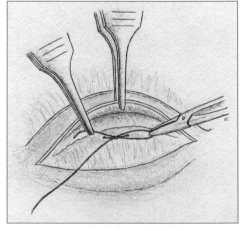

FIGURE 7.7.11 ✦ *Lid height adjustment:* This suture is initially secured with a slipknot to permit adjustment of the lid height, which is evaluated with the patient in an upright position. After satisfactory lid height is achieved, the suture is permanently knotted and excess levator is excised.

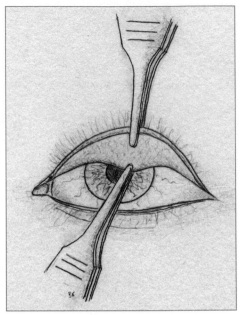

FIGURE 7.7.12 ✦ *Fasanella-Servat:* The upper lid margin is grasped with forceps and the eyelid is everted. This exposes the posterior surface of the tarsal plate beneath a layer of adherent palpebral conjunctiva. The conjunctiva is then grasped with a second pair of forceps at the superior tarsal margin, and traction is applied to elevate the posterior lid tissue.

Fasanella-Servat Procedure

1. *Posterior Exposure:* The upper lid margin is grasped with forceps and the eyelid is everted. This exposes the posterior surface of the tarsal plate beneath a layer of adherent palpebral conjunctiva (FIG. 7.7.12). The conjunctiva is grasped at the superior tarsal margin with a second pair of forceps, and traction is applied to elevate posterior lid tissue. Two hemostats are then placed across the elevated tissue in opposite directions.

2. *Suture Placement:* A suture is passed though the full eyelid thickness, beginning from the medial lid crease skin. It is then run behind the hemostats using a continuous horizontal mattress stitch (FIG. 7.7.13). Upon completion, it is again passed through the full-lid thickness, exiting at the lateral lid crease. The two free ends of the suture are then tied together (FIG. 7.7.14).

3. *Tissue Resection:* The hemostats are removed and the tissue that they crushed is excised. Initial hemostat placement is therefore critical to determining the degree of correction.

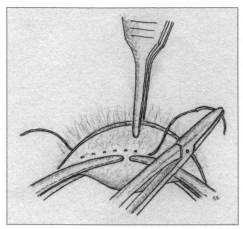

FIGURE 7.7.13 ◆ *Suture placement:* Two hemostats are placed across the elevated tissue in opposite directions. A suture is passed from the medial lid crease skin through the full thickness of the eyelid. It is then run behind the hemostats with a continuous mattress stitch.

COMPLICATIONS

General
1. *Undercorrection:* A second surgery may be necessary if the desired elevation of the lid margin is not achieved.

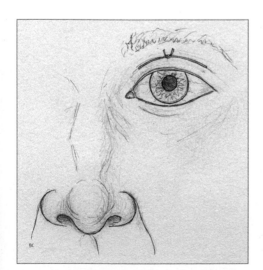

FIGURE 7.7.14 ◆ *Lid suture in situ:* Upon completion, the suture is again passed through the full-lid thickness, exiting the skin in the lateral lid crease. The two ends are then tied together.

2. *Overcorrection:* This can contribute to exposure keratitis, which is initially treated with lubricants and/or punctal plug insertion. Eyelid massage and closure exercises can help lower the lid. In extreme cases, reoperation may be necessary to avoid progression to corneal ulceration and superinfection.
3. *Contralateral ptosis:* significant elevation of the operated lid may unmask ptosis in the other due to Hering's law. (The innervation of corresponding extraocular muscles is linked.)

Operation Specific
1. Frontalis suspension failure is more common in patients with poor sight since visual field improvements reinforce proper lid manipulation with the frontalis.
2. Uneven levator aponeurosis advancement can produce an abnormal lid contour.
3. Excessive Müller's resection or aponeurosis advancement may cause prolapse of the superior conjunctival fornix due to tension on the suspensory ligaments.

POSTOPERATIVE CARE

- Apply antibiotic ointment to the lid wound.
- Prescribe mild oral analgesics.
- Apply ice packs for the first 48 hours to decrease lid edema and ecchymosis.
- Limit activity if fascia lata has been harvested.
- Remove skin sutures at the 1-week visit for optimal cosmetic results.
- In general, observe the patient until edema resolves and lid position stabilizes before reoperating.
- If necessary due to progressive ocular surface defects, revision within the first week will cause little additional bleeding or edema.

Further Reading
Text

Baroody M, Holds JB, Vick VL. Advances in the diagnosis and treatment of ptosis. *Curr Opin Ophthalmol.* 2005; 16(6):351–355.

Cetinkaya A, Brannan PA. Ptosis repair options and algorithm. *Curr Opin Ophthalmol.* 2008;19(5):428–434.

Custer PL. Blepharoptosis. In: Yanoff M, Duker J, eds. *Ophthalmology.* 3rd ed. Philadelphia, PA: Mosby; 2009: 1397–1404.

Wagner P, Lang GK. The eyelids. In: *Ophthalmology: A Pocket Textbook Atlas.* 2nd ed. New York, NY: Georg Thieme Verlag; 2007:17–49.

Primary Sources

DeMartelaere SL, Blaydon SM, Cruz AA, et al. Broad fascia fixation enhances frontalis suspension. *Ophthal Plast Reconstr Surg.* 2007;23(4):279–284.

Gündisch O, Vega A, Pfeiffer MJ, et al. The significance of intraoperative measurements in acquired ptosis surgery. *Orbit.* 2008;27(1):13–18.

Karsloglu S, Serin D, Ziylan S. Simple alternative to the Wright needle in frontalis sling surgery. *Ophthal Plast Reconstr Surg.* 2007;23(3):231–232.

Morris CL, Buckley EG, Enyedi LB, et al. Safety and efficacy of silicone rod frontalis suspension surgery for childhood ptosis repair. *J Pediatr Ophthalmol Strabismus.* 2008;45(5):280–288, 289–290.

Patel SM, Linberg JV, Sivak-Callcott JA, et al. Modified tarsal resection operation for congenital ptosis with fair levator function. *Ophthal Plast Reconstr Surg.* 2008; 24(1):1–6.

7.8   TARSORRHAPHY

TARSORRHAPHY

- Closure or lateral fusion of the eyelids reduces corneal exposure, helping to heal or preventing the development of ocular surface defects.
  - Temporary closure is usually done to promote rapid healing.
  - By contrast, permanent closure is usually partial and lateral to maintain useful vision while preventing corneal decompensation.

INDICATIONS

- Lagophthalmos with exposure keratitis or ulceration (e.g., from facial nerve palsy)
- Neurotrophic keratitis or ulceration (e.g., from herpes simplex virus [HSV] infection)
- Persistent epithelial defects associated with prior corneal surgery (e.g., penetrating keratoplasty)
- Poor response to alternative treatments: lateral tarsorrhaphy is often avoided due to cosmetic concerns, but may be necessary to protect the ocular surface in cases of "BAD syndrome," a combination of absent **B**ell's phenomenon, **a**nesthetic corneas, and **d**ry eyes.

ALTERNATIVES

Medical Therapy

- Lubrication: Preservative-free artificial tears are used during the day, and higher viscosity ointments are applied at night. Products containing preservative should be limited due to the risk of corneal toxicity and contact dermatitis.
- Oral antivirals (e.g., acyclovir, valacyclovir): Administration may accelerate recovery from virally mediated Bell's palsy.
- Punctal occlusion: Plug insertion or punctal closure with electrocautery decreases aqueous drainage through the nasolacrimal system, augmenting the tear lake and moistening the cornea.
- Pressure patches or bandage contact lenses: These facilitate healing by protecting the cornea from exposure, but may increase the risk of infection.
- Cyanoacrylate glue: The application of this glue permits short-term ocular closure akin to suture tarsorrhaphy, but the effective duration is highly variable and use precludes interval examination of the eye.
- Botulinum toxin injection: The injection induces severe ptosis by paralyzing the levator palpebrae superioris. It protects the cornea for weeks to months, but significantly obstructs the visual axis.

Surgery

- Lid weight or palpebral spring (see Chapter 7.9 Upper Lid Reanimation): This restores lid closure in cases of facial nerve palsy by reducing lagophthalmos and ocular exposure.
- Amniotic membrane graft: A "biologic contact lens" is created with preserved membrane to facilitate healing of the corneal epithelium.

The membrane can also be layered to fill deep refractory ulcers, reducing the risk of perforation.

- Conjunctival flaps: A bulbar conjunctival flap is mobilized and rotated to cover corneal defects, promoting epithelial healing.
- Levator recession: A spacer graft is inserted to lengthen the levator aponeurosis, eliminating upper lid retraction and reducing corneal exposure.

RELEVANT ANATOMY/PATHOPHYSIOLOGY

Lid Anatomy (Fig. 7.8.1)

The lid consists of two principle layers, or lamella.

Anterior Lamella

- Skin: This includes the thinnest skin in the body with scant underlying connective tissue for maximum mobility.
- Orbicularis oculi: The primary lid closer is innervated by the temporal and zygomatic branches of the facial nerve (CN VII). Fibers exit at the lid margin to form the *gray line*, an important external landmark for differentiating the anterior and posterior lamellae.

Posterior Lamella

- Tarsus: This is a stiff connective tissue plate containing the meibomian glands. It stabilizes the lid and permits insertion of the lid retractors.
- Lid retractors:
  - Upper lid:
    - Levator palpebrae superioris: The main upper lid retractor is innervated by the oculomotor

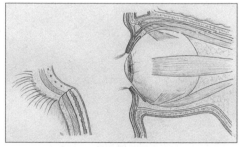

FIGURE 7.8.1 ◆ *Lid anatomy:* The anterior lid lamella consists of skin and orbicularis; the posterior lamella consists of tarsus, lid retractors, and palpebral conjunctiva. The gray line is formed by the orbicularis fibers (muscle of Riolan) and delineates the lamellae at the lid margin. The meibomian gland orifices can be seen posterior to the gray line and are important landmarks for temporary suture tarsorrhaphy.

nerve (CN III). It inserts on the tarsus and upper lid skin.
  - Müller's muscle: This muscle is an underlying, accessory retractor that is innervated by sympathetic fibers. It inserts on the superior tarsal margin.
- Lower lid:
  - Capsulopalpebral fascia: This is an extension of the inferior rectus muscle sheath that inserts on the inferior tarsal margin and depresses the lower lid in downgaze.
- Palpebral conjunctiva: This is a moist mucus membrane tightly adherent to the posterior tarsal surfaces. It glides smoothly over the bulbar conjunctiva during eye movements.

Facial Nerve Palsy/Exposure Keratitis

- When the facial nerve is damaged, lid retractors are unopposed by the paralyzed orbicularis. This leads to lagophthalmos and excessive drying from corneal exposure.
- Superficial punctate keratitis (SPK): With exposure, epithelial defects develop over the inferior one-half to one-third of the cornea. If unchecked, this can progress to corneal erosion, superinfection, and perforation.
- Lesions to the facial nerve and nucleus may be temporary or permanent:
  - Temporary: Bell's palsy may be associated with Lyme disease, sarcoid, human immunodeficiency virus (HIV), and other conditions. Acyclovir PO (by mouth) may hasten recovery.
  - Permanent: Causes include surgery to the parotid gland or cerebellopontine angle (e.g., for acoustic neuroma), stroke affecting facial motor nucleus, and trauma to the facial nerve.

Neuroparalytic Keratitis

- Damage to branches of the ophthalmic division of the trigeminal nerve (CN V_1) can lead to decreased corneal sensitivity.
- When the blink rate drops below the threshold necessary to maintain a healthy corneal surface, SPK develops. This can progress to ulceration, superinfection, and corneal perforation.
- Contributing factors may include HSV keratitis, trigeminal nerve surgery, and laser-assisted in situ keratomileusis (LASIK) procedures (nerve fibers are cut during corneal flap elevation).

PREOPERATIVE ASSESSMENT

- Slit lamp exam: Apply fluorescein dye to the cornea to evaluate for keratitis and persistent epithelial defects. Rose Bengal dye will show devitalized cells that have not yet been shed.

- Lid margin exam: Observe carefully for irregularities, such as notching and trichiasis, that can perpetuate corneal epithelium defects.

- Tear film evaluation: Confirm adequacy of the tear film by conducting the Schirmer's test and assessing tear breakup time. Low values are often indicative of dry eye conditions that may require additional treatment.

- Corneal sensation: Test reflex closure of the lids with a sterile cotton applicator tip. Poor closure suggests the presence of a neurotrophic cornea.

- Tarsorrhaphy selection: The need for temporary versus permanent tarsorrhaphy is determined by gauging the acuity of corneal decompensation and the likelihood of eventual recovery.

ANESTHESIA

- The upper and lower lids are infiltrated with lidocaine plus epinephrine to aid hemostasis.

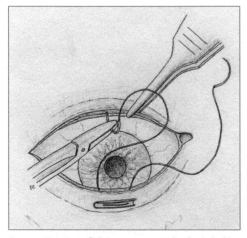

FIGURE 7.8.2 ◆ *Bolster suture tarsorrhaphy:* A double-armed suture is passed through a bolster and then through the upper lid. Both needles are then passed through the tarsus so that they exit the lid margin through the meibomian gland orifices. They are next passed through the lower lid meibomian orifices and tarsus.

PROCEDURE

There are a wide variety of techniques for performing tarsorrhaphy. The following outline examples of common variations that may be encountered.

Temporary Suture Tarsorrhaphy

Tarsorrhaphy with bolsters

- *Bolster Selection:* Bolsters are used to protect the skin from suture tension and can be made from various materials. Common examples include the foam from suture packaging or pieces of plastic tubing (e.g., intravenous [IV] catheter) that have been sectioned lengthwise.

- *Suture Passage:* A double-armed suture is passed through a bolster and then through the upper lid skin, 3 to 4 mm above the lid margin. Both needles are passed through the tarsus so that they exit the lid margin through the meibomian gland orifices. They are then passed through the lower lid meibomian orifices and tarsus to exit the skin 2 to 3 mm below the lid margin (FIG. 7.8.2). Both needles are passed through a second bolster.

- *Tarsorrhaphy Closure:* In a standard bolster tarsorrhaphy, the suture ends are then secured with a knot (FIG. 7.8.3). In the drawstring technique described at the University of Iowa, the needles are instead passed through a third bolster and the suture ends are tied with slack. This bolster can then be slid to open or close the tarsorrhaphy, permitting interval evaluation of the ocular surface (FIG. 7.8.4).

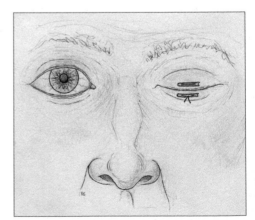

FIGURE 7.8.3 ◆ *Tarsorrhaphy in situ:* The left palpebral fissure is shown closed by a standard bolster tarsorrhaphy.

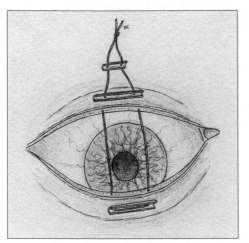

FIGURE 7.8.4 ♦ *Drawstring tarsorrhaphy:* In the drawstring technique, the needles are passed through a third bolster. The suture ends are then tied, leaving slack that permits the bolster to be slid up or down to close or open the tarsorrhaphy.

Tarsorrhaphy without bolsters

- *Suture Passage:* Bolsters are not required since the sutures do not penetrate the lid skin in this technique. A thicker, typically 4-0, suture is passed in and out of the upper lid margin through the meibomian gland orifices, firmly anchoring the tarsus.

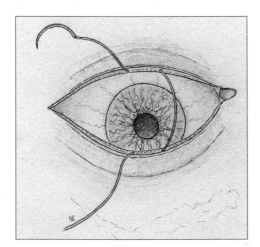

FIGURE 7.8.5 ♦ *Bolster-free suture tarsorrhaphy:* A 4-0 suture is passed through the upper lid meibomian gland orifices and tarsus. After exiting the upper lid margin, the suture is passed through the lower lid margin and the free ends are fastened.

TABLE 7.8.1 Rapid Review of Steps
(1) Inject anesthetic and allow time to work (5 minutes).
(2) Prep and drape.
(3) Excise lid marginal tissue of both upper and lower eyelid.
(4) Separate anterior from posterior lamella of both eyelids.
(5) Approximate tarsus of both eyelids.
(6) Close the skin.

- *Tarsorrhaphy Closure:* After exiting the upper lid, the suture is passed through corresponding points in the lower lid margin and the free ends are secured (FIG. 7.8.5). Suture tails are cut long to permit easy identification.

LATERAL TARSORRHAPHY

 SEE TABLES 7.8.1 Rapid Review of Steps and 7.8.2 Surgical Pearls, and WEB TABLES 7.8.1 to 7.8.4 for equipment and medication lists.

The goal is to close the lateral palpebral fissure sufficiently to prevent ocular surface decompensation. Some techniques minimize the alteration of lid anatomy whereas others entail mobilization of skin or tarsal flaps. A common procedure with minimal lid modification follows.

- *Lid Margin Preparation:* A fine blade is used to separate a lateral section of the upper lid into

TABLE 7.8.2 Surgical Pearls
Preoperative:
• Determining the amount and location of eyelid closure is important.
Intraoperative:
• Multilayered closure is essential for long-lasting results—tarsus to tarsus, orbicularis to orbicularis, skin to skin. If reversing of the tarsorrhaphy is anticipated, lashes should be left intact; if tarsorrhaphy is to be long-standing, excise lashes will hide the tarsorrhaphy.
Postoperative:
• With deep closure, skin sutures may be removed within 1 week.

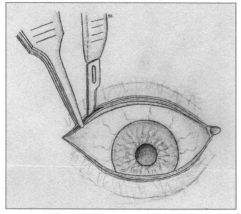

FIGURE 7.8.6 ◆ *Lateral tarsorrhaphy:* A fine blade is used to separate the lateral lids into anterior and posterior lamellae. This is achieved by incising the lid margins at the gray line.

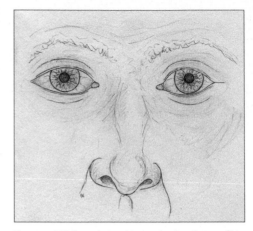

FIGURE 7.8.8 ◆ *Lateral tarsorrhaphy closure:* Skin and orbicularis of the anterior lamella are then closed with interrupted sutures. Postoperatively, the left palpebral fissure is visibly shorter.

anterior and posterior lamellae (FIG. 7.8.6). This is achieved by incising the lid margin at the gray line. The process then repeated for the corresponding lower lid. Palpebral conjunctiva adjacent to the upper and lower lid margins is removed with scissors to create raw tarsal surfaces that can heal together.

- *Suture Passage:* The exposed tarsal plates are then approximated with partial thickness mattress sutures over the desired length (FIG. 7.8.7). The skin and orbicularis are closed with interrupted sutures. The lateral lashes are preserved in case it becomes possible to reverse the tarsorrhaphy at a later date (FIG. 7.8.8).

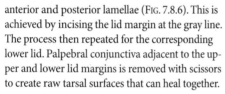

FIGURE 7.8.7 ◆ *Tarsal approximation:* The exposed tarsal plates are then approximated with partial thickness mattress sutures over the desired length.

COMPLICATIONS

1. Lid margin deformity and trichiasis may occur after reversal of long-term tarsorrhaphy. The risk increases with the degree of anatomic alteration.

2. *Dehiscence:* The risk is greater with temporary closure since the lid margin is not altered to create raw edges that heal together; durability depends on suture strength alone.

3. *Stretching:* Tissue laxity tends to increase over time, reducing tarsorrhaphy effectiveness.

4. Visual field limitation occurs when a lateral tarsorrhaphy is long enough to obstruct the pupillary axis.

5. Corneal irritation may be caused by exposed tarsal sutures.

POSTOPERATIVE CARE

- Administer topical antibiotic ointment.

- Prescribe mild oral analgesics.

- With permanent tarsorrhaphy, remove skin sutures at 2 weeks to permit adequate healing.

- Evaluate ocular surface health at regular intervals.

Further Reading

Text

Bergeron CM, Moe KS. The evaluation and treatment of lower eyelid paralysis. *Facial Plast Surg.* 2008;24(2):231–241.

Lang GK. Cornea. In: *Ophthalmology: A Pocket Textbook Atlas,* 2nd ed. New York, NY: Georg Thieme Verlag; 2007:115–160.

Pfister RR. Clinical measures to promote corneal epithelial healing. *Acta Ophthalmol Suppl.* 1992;(202):73–83.

Seiff SR, Chang J. Management of ophthalmic complications of facial nerve palsy. *Otolaryngol Clin North Am.* 1992;25(3):669–690.

Tuli SS, Schultz GS, Downer DM. Science and strategy for preventing and managing corneal ulceration. *Ocul Surf.* 2007;5(1):23–39.

Primary Sources

Cosar CB, Cohen EJ, Rapuano CJ, et al. Tarsorrhaphy: clinical experience from a cornea practice. *Cornea.* 2001;20(8):787–791.

Kitchens J, Kinder J, Oetting T. The drawstring temporary tarsorrhaphy technique. *Arch Ophthalmol.* 2002;120(2):187–190.

McInnes AW, Burroughs JR, Anderson RL, et al. Temporary suture tarsorrhaphy. *Am J Ophthalmol.* 2006;142(2):344–346.

7.9 UPPER LID REANIMATION

UPPER LID REANIMATION

- Prevents corneal breakdown in patients with facial nerve paralysis by increasing upper lid excursion with blinking and by enabling lid closure during sleep.
- Lid weight implantation is the most common strategy, but palpebral springs and temporalis muscle transfer are also used.

INDICATION

- Patients with lagophthalmos from facial nerve palsy who have failed conservative management are candidates. Reanimation techniques are generally preferred to long-term tarsorrhaphy because they more closely approximate the function and appearance of normal lid movement.

ALTERNATIVES

Medical Therapy

- Artificial tears and/or a moisture chamber can help limit daytime drying of the ocular surface.
- High viscosity gels and patching can protect the eye at night when vision is not required. Taping the lids shut is generally more difficult for patients and is less effective.
- A patient can be trained to manually close the affected eye when symptoms become pronounced (e.g., burning, foreign body sensation).
- Lower lid ectropion and retraction contribute to corneal drying and can be temporarily managed with horizontal taping.
- Botulinum toxin—induced ptosis can protect the cornea for several weeks per injection, but obstructs the visual axis during daytime hours.

Surgery

- Upper lid reanimation is often combined with procedures to address paralytic ectropion (see Chapter 7.3 Ectropion Repair). In older patients, involutional changes to the tarsus and canthal tendons are frequently unmasked by loss of orbicularis tone.
- Suture tarsorrhaphy (see Chapter 7.8 Tarsorrhaphy): The palpebral fissure is temporarily closed with sutures passed through the upper and lower lid margins. This is generally used for short-term management of acute corneal decompensation.
- Lateral tarsorrhaphy (see Chapter 7.8 Tarsorrhaphy): The lateral lid is sewn shut to reduce the exposed corneal surface area and to facilitate lid closure, often at the expense of partial visual axis obstruction.

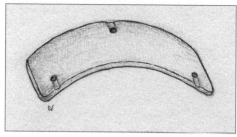
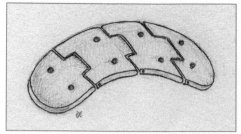

A   **B**

FIGURE 7.9.1 ✦ *Lid weights:* Weights are made of dense, inert metals and come in a various sizes. Gold weights are generally rigid plates **(A)**, while some platinum weights have articulating links to permit conformation to the patient's lid curvature **(B)**. Platinum weights can be implanted in patients with gold allergy.

REANIMATION OVERVIEW

Lid Loading

- A gold or platinum weight is sutured to the tarsus in the midpupillary axis, enabling lid closure by opposing the active levator palpebrae superioris (LPS) with the force of gravity.
  - Gold weight: A rigid plate that is curved to fit the eyelid and has holes for sutures (FIG. 7.9.1A). While gold is inert, some patients develop allergic lid inflammation and must have the weight removed.
  - Platinum weight: some models are made with articulating links to accommodate a range of lid curvatures (FIG. 7.9.1B). Platinum weights can be implanted in patients with a gold allergy.

- Weight range: Lid weights range from 0.6 to 2.8 grams to accommodate varying LPS strengths. The 1-gram model is used most frequently.
  - Advantages: Implantation is simple and easy to reverse. Weights contain no fatigable moving parts.
  - Disadvantages: Weights do not function when a patient is supine. He or she must therefore sleep with additional pillows or use eye patches. Lid closure is significantly slower than a natural blink.

Palpebral Spring

- Tension generated by a handcrafted stainless steel spring opposes the active LPS (FIG. 7.9.2).
- The lower arm is secured to the tarsus, the fulcrum loop to the lateral orbital rim periosteum, and the upper arm to the superior orbital rim (FIG. 7.9.3).

- Advantages: Since springs are not gravity dependent, they work in all positions. They also permit the eyelid to snap shut, providing a more natural blink. Springs are particularly effective with "BAD syndrome" (poor **B**ell's phenomenon, corneal **a**nesthesia, and **d**ry eyes).
- Disadvantages: Implantation is technically challenging and outcomes are more dependent on surgeon experience. Springs are fatigable; they can break, and tension may diminish with time.

Temporalis Transfer

- Thin flaps of muscle and fascia, mobilized from the ipsilateral temporalis, are tunneled into the upper and lower lids to restore motility in cases of permanent facial nerve paralysis.

- Advantages: Reliable lid closure has been demonstrated in small patient cohorts. No foreign bodies are implanted.

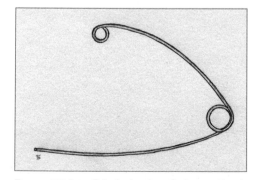

FIGURE 7.9.2 ✦ *Palpebral springs:* Springs are handmade by the surgeon from resilient stainless steel wire. The central loop serves as a fulcrum, whereas the upper and lower arms exert tension on surrounding tissues. This tension opposes the action of the lid retractors.

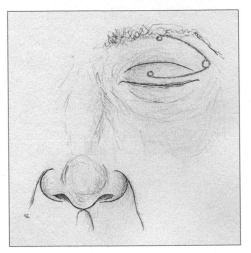

FIGURE 7.9.3 ◆ *Palpebral spring in situ:* The outline of a palpebral spring can be seen in the upper lid. Once implanted, the lower arm is secured to the tarsus, the fulcrum loop to the lateral orbital rim, and the upper arm to the superior orbital rim.

- Disadvantages: This is a very challenging procedure with significant interoperator variability in outcomes.

RELEVANT PHYSIOLOGY/ANATOMY

Upper Lid Anatomy (FIG. 7.9.4)
Anterior Lamella
- Skin is thin with scant underlying connective tissue for maximum mobility.
- Orbicularis oculi is the primary lid closer, innervated by the temporal and zygomatic branches of

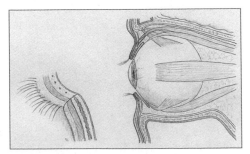

FIGURE 7.9.4 ◆ *Layers of the lid:* The anterior lid lamella consists of the skin and orbicularis; the posterior lamella consists of the tarsus, lid retractors, and palpebral conjunctiva.

the facial nerve (CN VII). It has orbital, preseptal, and pretarsal divisions.

Posterior Lamella
- Superior tarsus is a stiff connective tissue plate that contains the meibomian glands. It keeps the lid closely apposed to the globe and provides points of insertion for the lid retractors.

- Lid retractors:
  - The levator palpebrae superioris (LPS) is the main upper lid retractor, innervated by the oculomotor nerve (CN III). It originates on the lesser wing of the sphenoid bone and inserts on the tarsal plate and upper lid skin (after interdigitating with the overlying orbicularis fibers).
  - Müller's muscle is an accessory retractor innervated by sympathetic fibers. It originates on the inferior surface of the LPS and inserts on the superior tarsal margin.

- Palpebral conjunctiva is a moist mucus membrane that articulates with the bulbar conjunctiva during eye movement and is firmly adherent to the posterior tarsus.

Tear Film
The tear film protects against corneal desiccation and consists of three layers:

1. The outer layer includes oil from the meibomian glands, as well as the glands of Moll and Zeiss, which stabilizes the outer surface of tear film, preventing rapid evaporation.

2. The middle includes watery secretions from the lacrimal gland, and accessory glands of Krause and Wolfring make the greatest contribution to tear volume.

3. The inner layer includes mucin from conjunctival goblet cells, which stabilizes the inner surface of the tear film on the corneal epithelium.

Eye Closure
- The lids act as "windshield wipers" to distribute the tear film across the cornea during blinking. With orbicularis contraction, the palpebral fissure narrows laterally to medially, moving tears toward the puncta for nasolacrimal drainage.

- Upper lid movement dominates this process and is more affected by facial nerve palsy (lower lid excursion during eye closure is only 1 to 2 mm).

- Adequate closure during sleep is extremely important because it prevents evaporation of the protective tear film.
- Bells phenomenon: The globe rotates upward when the lids are closed. This provides additional protection to the corneal surface.

Facial Nerve Palsy

- Lid retractors are unopposed by the paralyzed orbicularis. This leads to lagophthalmos and excessive drying from corneal exposure (FIG. 7.9.5).
- Superficial punctate keratitis (SPK) develops over the inferior one-half to one-third of the cornea and can progress to erosion, superinfection, and perforation.
- Lesions to the facial nerve and nucleus may be temporary or permanent.
  - Temporary: Bell's palsy may be associated with Lyme disease, sarcoid, human immunodeficiency virus (HIV), and other conditions. PO acyclovir may hasten recovery.
  - Permanent: Causes include surgery to the parotid gland or cerebellopontine angle (e.g., for acoustic neuroma), stroke affecting facial motor nucleus, and trauma to the facial nerve.

Preoperative Assessment

- Slit lamp exam: Assess corneal pathology with fluorescein dye.
- Lower lid exam: Check for horizontal laxity, punctal eversion, and frank ectropion.

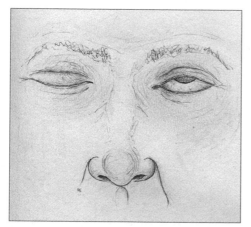

FIGURE 7.9.5 ◆ *Left CN VII palsy:* In facial nerve palsy, the lid retractors are unopposed by the paralyzed orbicularis. The eye, therefore, cannot be closed, leading to lagophthalmos and excessive drying from corneal exposure.

- Rule out BAD syndrome: Check corneal sensation and tear breakup time, and perform the Schirmer's test to quantify tear fluid production.
- Lid weight selection: Choose the weight that maximizes closure during passive blinking without causing significant ptosis in primary gaze. The optimum weight depends on LPS strength. Sizing kits with trial implants are available to aid selection. Alternatively, weights can be taped to the external lid and then resterilized prior to implantation.
- Spring adjustment: Palpebral springs are molded to the patient's lid contour in the clinic and sterilized prior to implantation. Tension is adjusted intraoperatively to ensure proper lid closure. Often, more than one spring is made to guarantee proper fit.

Anesthesia

- Local infiltration or regional blocks are usually adequate for lid surgery. General anesthesia may be advisable for more elaborate procedures, such as temporalis muscle transfer.

PROCEDURE

Lid Weight: (SEE TABLES 7.9.1 Rapid Review of Steps and 7.9.2 Surgical Pearls, and WEB TABLES 7.9.1 to 7.9.4 for equipment and medication lists).

1. *Incision/Dissection:* An incision is made in the upper lid crease (FIG. 7.9.6), and fibers of the underlying orbicularis are divided. A pocket is then dissected anterior to the tarsus to permit weight placement (FIG. 7.9.7).
2. *Plate Fixation:* The weight is fixed to the anterior tarsus with partial-thickness sutures to decrease the risk of extrusion (FIG. 7.9.8). It is centered above the point of maximum lagophthalmos, which usually corresponds to the midpupillary axis.

TABLE 7.9.1 Rapid Review of Steps
(1) Injection of anesthetic and allow time to work (5 minutes).
(2) Prep and drape.
(3) Incise lid crease.
(4) Dissect anterior surface of tarsus.
(5) Secure gold weight to tarsus.
(6) Close incision in layers.

TABLE 7.9.2 Surgical Pearls

Preoperative:

- Determining the appropriate gold weight size is important. Too heavy causes ptosis, too light leaves residual lagophthalmos. Trial weights can be stuck onto the outside of the eyelid or patients can try weights at home.

Intraoperative:

- Positioning of the gold weight is important. Some surgeons like to place the weight more medial or higher in the eyelid, so it is less noticeable. However, in these locations, the weight has less mechanical advantage and, therefore, needs to be upsized in size.
- Securing the gold weight to the tarsus with a permanent suture prevents late postoperative migration. Layered closure of the incision also prevents extrusions or exposures. Some surgeons like to wrap the gold weight with a dermal or fascial graft.

Postoperative:

- Motility of the eyelid and eyelid position improves as swelling goes down. Therefore, patients must be counseled that initial results may be less than desired, but may improve with time.

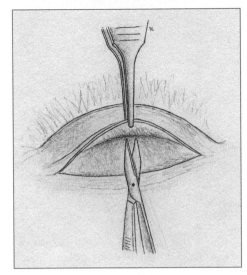

FIGURE 7.9.7 ◆ *Lid dissection:* A pocked is dissected in the soft tissue anterior to the tarsus to permit lid weight placement.

3. *Closure:* The incision is then closed in layers. Incorporation of the levator aponeurosis in the skin closure reforms the lid crease (FIG. 7.9.9).

Palpebral Spring

1. *Incision/Dissection:* After insertion of a scleral shell to protect the globe, an incision is made along the lateral two-thirds of the lid crease. Dissection in the tissue plane between the orbicularis and

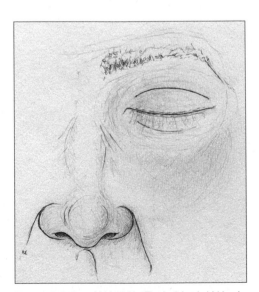

FIGURE 7.9.6 ◆ *Lid incision:* The incision is hidden in the upper lid crease, which is generally 8 to 10 mm above the lash line in the midpupillary axis (although it is often lower or absent in Asians).

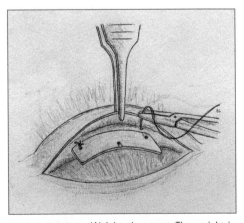

FIGURE 7.9.8 ◆ *Weight placement:* The weight is fixed to the anterior tarsal surface with partial thickness sutures to decrease the risk of extrusion. It is centered above the point of maximum lagophthalmos, which usually corresponds to the midpupillary axis.

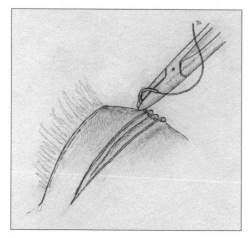

FIGURE 7.9.9 ◆ *Lid crease formation:* Incorporation of the levator aponeurosis in the skin closure reforms the lid crease. The inelastic orbital septum is not included, as this can contribute to postoperative lid retraction.

orbital septum is used to expose the superior and lateral orbital rim.

2. *Spring Placement:* A spinal needle with stylet is then passed between the orbicularis and tarsus, approximately 5 mm above the lid margin. This serves to guide subsequent spring placement. After the stylet is removed, the lower arm of the spring is passed through the lumen of the needle (FIG. 7.9.10). The needle is then removed, leaving the spring in place.

3. *Spring Attachment/Adjustment:* The spring fulcrum (central loop) is secured to lateral orbital rim periosteum with a nonabsorbable 4-0 suture (FIG. 7.9.11). The end of the lower spring arm is bent into a loop just medial to the midpupillary axis. It is then secured to the tarsus with sutures and/or a Dacron patch that permits soft tissue ingrowth. The upper arm is tucked under the superior orbital rim and tension is checked with the patient in both supine and upright positions. After spring tension is adjusted to match levator

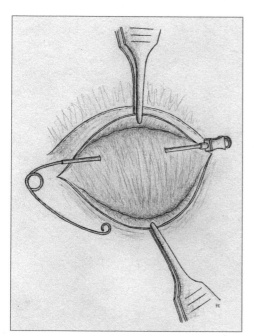

FIGURE 7.9.10 ◆ *Spring insertion:* A spinal needle and stylet are passed anterior to the tarsus, approximately 5 mm above the lid margin. After the stylet is removed, the lower arm of the spring is passed through the lumen of the needle. The needle is then removed, leaving the spring in place.

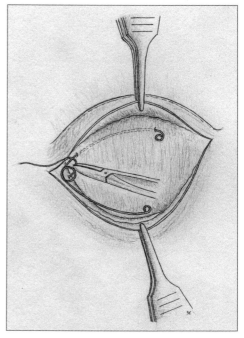

FIGURE 7.9.11 ◆ *Spring suturing:* The fulcrum of the spring (the central loop) is sutured to the lateral orbital rim periosteum. The end of the lower spring arm is bent into a loop just medial to the midpupillary axis. It is then secured to the tarsus with sutures and/or a Dacron patch that permits soft tissue ingrowth. The upper arm is then tucked under the superior orbital rim and sutured to periosteum.

strength, the upper arm is secured to the periosteum with a nonabsorbable 4-0 suture.

4. *Closure:* The lid incision is then closed in layers. Incorporation of the levator aponeurosis into the skin closure reforms the lid crease.

Additional Considerations

A strong levator makes lid weight implantation more challenging since larger weights are harder to conceal and more likely to cause complications. Use of a spring with greater tension, however, yields a more rapid and natural blink. In palpebral spring procedures, levator strength is therefore frequently augmented ("enhanced") by passing a suture through the tarsus and LPS body prior to spring placement.

Complications

Lid Weight

1. *Migration, extrusion, or infection:* The risk decreases with careful suturing of the weight to the tarsus.

2. *Overcorrection/pseudoptosis:* When a normal eye is opened, the orbicularis is turned off and does not oppose the LPS. An implanted weight, however, always opposes the LPS and can cause significant ptosis if it is too heavy.

3. *Cosmetic problems:* The weight may bulge visibly or shine through the skin in bright light conditions.

4. *Astigmatism:* A heavy weight that is placed too low in the lid will exert a distorting pressure on the superior cornea.

5. *Undercorrection:* This occurs when the implanted weight is too light to counterbalance the power of the LPS.

6. *Gold allergy:* Though inert, gold occasionally elicits a chronic inflammatory response, resulting in lid edema and erythema. This can be treated with corticosteroids or explantation. Platinum weights can be substituted following explantation.

Palpebral Spring

1. *Migration, extrusion, or infection:* The incidence is higher due to the dynamic nature of the implant.

2. *Spring fatigue and/or breakage:* Spring tension often decreases with time, whereas the risk of breakage increases.

3. *Lid function recovery:* Implants should be removed if orbicularis strength returns, but springs often develop a connective tissue capsule that renders lid dissection more difficult.

Postoperative Care

- Apply topical antibiotics to the lid crease wound.
- Prescribe oral antibiotics and mild oral analgesics.
- Apply ice packs for the first 48 hours to reduce lid swelling, then apply heat.
- Even though springs are ferromagnetic, most patients can safely undergo MRI after connective tissue encapsulation has occurred.

Further Reading

Text

Bergeron CM, Moe KS. The evaluation and treatment of upper eyelid paralysis. *Facial Plast Surg.* 2008;24(2): 220–230.

Lang GK. Cornea. In: *Ophthalmology: A Pocket Textbook Atlas.* 2nd ed. New York, NY: Georg Thieme Verlag; 2007: 115–160.

Tate JR, Tollefson TT. Advances in facial reanimation. *Curr Opin Otolaryngol Head Neck Surg.* 2006;14(4): 242–248.

Wagner P, Lang GK. Lacrimal system. In: *Ophthalmology: A Pocket Textbook Atlas.* 2nd ed. New York, NY: Georg Thieme Verlag; 2007:49–66.

Primary Sources

Avni-Zauberman N, Rosen N, Ben Simon GJ. Induced corneal astigmatism by palpebral spring for the treatment of lagophthalmos. *Cornea.* 2008;27(7):840–842.

Levine RE, Shapiro JP. Reanimation of the paralyzed eyelid with the enhanced palpebral spring or the gold weight: modern replacements for tarsorrhaphy. *Facial Plast Surg.* 2000;16(4):325–336.

Miyamoto S, Takushima A, Okazaki M, et al. Retrospective outcome analysis of temporalis muscle transfer for the treatment of paralytic lagophthalmos. *J Plast Reconstr Aesthet Surg.* 2008:16 [Epub ahead of print].

CHAPTER 8

Retina

Ron Adelman, John J. Huang, and James E. Kempton

8.1 INTRAVITREAL INJECTIONS

- A fine needle is inserted into the vitreous through the pars plana to deliver intraocular medication (FIG. 8.1.1).

INDICATIONS

- Intravitreal injections are an increasingly common therapeutic tool for addressing various retinal pathologies. Examples include:
  - Antivascular endothelial growth factor (VEGF) agents for neovascular ("wet") age-related macular degeneration (AMD) or proliferative diabetic retinopathy (PDR)
  - Corticosteroids for cystoid macular edema (CME) due to diabetes, central retinal vein occlusion (CRVO), or branch retinal vein occlusion (BRVO)
  - Antimicrobials for bacterial or fungal endophthalmitis
  - Antivirals for retinal necrosis in immunocompromised patients

CONTRAINDICATIONS

- Active blepharitis: This increases the risk of inoculating the vitreous with bacteria and should be treated with lid scrubs and topical antibiotics prior to injection.

ALTERNATIVES

Medical Therapy

- Macular degeneration: Nutritional supplements (antioxidants plus zinc) and smoking cessation have been shown to slow the progression from nonexudative ("dry") macular degeneration to the "wet" neovascular form.[1]

Lasers/Surgery

- Macular degeneration: Prior to the development of anti-VEGF agents, various laser treatments were commonly used for AMD. These include:
  1. Laser photocoagulation: Laser spots are applied to areas of choroidal neovascularization (CNV). This technique is only effective with well-demarcated CNV. It also has high rates of recurrence, and results in laser-induced scotoma when burns are placed near the macula.
  2. Photodynamic therapy (PDT): A photosensitizing agent (verteporfin) is administered intravenously. The retina is then exposed to a low-energy 689 nm laser for 83 seconds, which activates the agent and results in neovascular closure. Patients must be cautioned to avoid direct sunlight for several days following each treatment because of the risk of photosensitivity reactions.

- Bacterial endophthalmitis: Pars plana vitrectomy permits physical removal of intraocular organisms and inflammatory mediators, as well as direct administration of antibiotics. Sufficient vitreous specimens are easily obtained. In post-cataract extraction patients with visual acuity that is better than light perception upon presentation, however, needle biopsy with intravitreal antibiotic injection produces equivalent outcomes.[2]

RELEVANT PATHOPHYSIOLOGY

Age-Related Macular Degeneration (AMD)

- AMD is the leading cause of irreversible vision loss in the elderly.

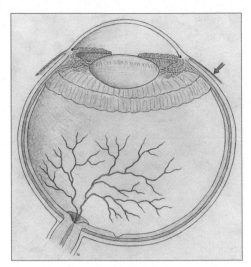

FIGURE 8.1.1 ◆ A fine needle is inserted into the vitreous through the pars plana to deliver intraocular medications (arrow). This prevents damage to the highly vascular ciliary body anteriorly and the sensory retina posteriorly.

- Progressive deterioration of the macula results in central vision loss.
- It occurs in two forms:
  1. *Nonexudative ("dry"):* Subacute degeneration of the macula characterized by retinal pigment epithelium atrophy and the accumulation of subretinal deposits, or drusen. This condition may progress to "wet" AMD.
  2. *Neovascular ("wet"):* Development of choroidal neovascularization (CNV) leads to fluid extravasation and serous detachment of the retinal pigment epithelium due to breaks in Bruch's membrane. This produces severely blurred central vision and metamorphopsia.

Anti-VEGF Agents

- VEGF-A: Vascular endothelial growth factor-A stimulates choroidal/retinal neovascularization and increases vessel permeability.
- Three anti-VEGF agents have been approved by the Food and Drug Administration (FDA).
  1. *Bevacizumab (Avastin):* Bevacizumab was FDA approved in 2004 for intravenous treatment of metastatic colon cancer, and used off-label for intravitreal injections. It contains a full-length monoclonal antibody that inhibits all active VEGF-A isoforms.
  2. *Ranibizumab (Lucentis):* Ranibizumab was FDA approved in 2006 for exudative AMD. It

contains a monoclonal antibody–binding fragment that inhibits all active VEGF-A isoforms. Lucentis costs significantly more per dose than Avastin and trials comparing efficacy are currently underway.
  3. *Pegaptanib sodium (Macugen):* Pegaptanib sodium was FDA approved in 2004 for classic exudative AMD. It contains an RNA oligonucleotide (aptamer) linked to polyethylene glycol that specifically binds to and inhibits VEGF 165. It has been superseded by the development of Lucentis and Avastin.

- Monthly injections are required in many patients, but it is possible to vary the frequency of administration based on macular ocular coherence tomography (OCT) findings.

Cystoid Macular Edema (CME)

- Cytokine release from activated inflammatory cells is thought to trigger breakdown of the blood-retinal barrier, leading to accumulation of fluid in the outer plexiform layer of the macula.
- This distorts central vision and produces cystic spaces visible on OCT.
- It occurs in a various disorders, inducing diabetes, central retinal vein occlusion (CRVO), and branch retinal vein occlusion (BRVO).
- It is also a potential complication of cataract extraction and other intraocular surgery.
- Initial treatment is with topical steroids or nonsteroidal anti-inflammatory drugs (NSAIDS). If this fails, sub-Tenon's or intravitreal steroid injections (e.g., triamcinolone) may be given.

Infectious Endophthalmitis

- Infection of intraocular compartments and adjacent layers can result from direct inoculation (e.g., open globe injury, intraocular surgery) or hematogenous spread.
- Potential signs and symptoms include ocular pain, decreased visual acuity, conjunctival injection, chemosis, hypopyon, and the presence of anterior chamber "cell and flare" on slit lamp examination.
- If endophthalmitis is suspected, specimens of the aqueous and/or vitreous should be obtained for culture and sensitivity using needle biopsy or vitrectomy.
- Most antibiotics have limited ability to penetrate the vitreous if administered topically, systemically,

or as a sub-Tenon's injection. Intravitreal injection is therefore the best strategy for achieving therapeutic drug levels. Direct contact with intraocular tissues, however, increases the risk of retinal toxicity.

- Bacterial endophthalmitis: Onset is usually acute. Empiric treatment must be instituted pending culture results. Vancomycin is generally used for gram-positive coverage, whereas amikacin (an aminoglycoside) or ceftazidime (a third generation cephalosporin) is added for gram-negative coverage. Antibiotic coverage is narrowed and focused once an etiologic agent has been identified.

- Fungal endophthalmitis: Progression is usually more indolent. Amphotericin B was the traditional therapy of choice, but azole antifungals are less toxic to the retina and have gained popularity.

- The addition of intravitreal corticosteroids helps to reduce inflammation, but does not appear to influence long-term visual outcomes.

PREOPERATIVE ASSESSMENT

- Slit lamp exam: Check the anterior chamber for "cell and flare" as well as for hypopyon, which layers in the inferior angle.

- Dilated fundus exam: Assess for posterior segment pathology, including neovascularization, CRVO, BRVO, macular drusen, or vitreous stranding and cells.

- Macular OCT: Examine images for evidence of drusen or cystoid edema.

- Fluorescein/indocyanine green angiography: Assess for dye diffusion patterns suggestive of retinal or choroidal neovascularization. Normal retinal vessels retain fluorescein dye, but it leaks from neovascular beds, which have increased permeability. Fluorescein diffusely enhances the choroidal circulation because its fenestrated capillaries are permeable to the dye. Indocyanine green, however, is normally retained and leakage helps to pinpoint areas of occult choroidal neovascularization.

ANESTHESIA

- Topical anesthetic drops are applied to the inferior fornix.

- The injection site can be further anesthetized with subconjunctival infiltration (e.g., lidocaine) or with an application of topical anesthetic jelly.

PROCEDURE

1. *Preparation:* Topical antibiotic drops may be administered for several days preceding the injection. The lids, lashes, and ocular surface are carefully painted with Betadine prior to lid speculum insertion.

2. *Injection:* A 0.5 inch 27- to 30-gauge needle is passed through the pars plana to avoid damage to the highly vascular ciliary body anteriorly and the sensory retina posteriorly. It should be inserted 3.5 to 4 mm from the limbus in a phakic eye, or 3 mm from the limbus in a pseudophakic or aphakic eye (FIG. 8.1.2). The inferotemporal quadrant is selected most frequently due to ease of access. The globe can be stabilized with a cotton-tipped applicator during injection. The needle, directed toward the center of the globe, is steadily advanced over 1 second to a depth of half the needle length. As the needle is withdrawn, this applicator is used to tamponade the injection site, preventing leakage (FIG. 8.1.3).

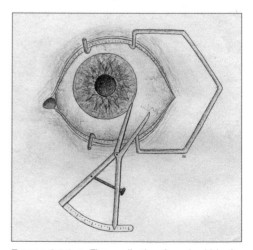

FIGURE 8.1.2 ◆ The needle therefore should be inserted 3.5 to 4 mm from the corneal limbus in a phakic eye, or 3 mm from the limbus in a pseudophakic eye. This distance can be measured with calipers.

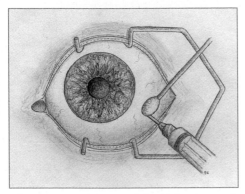

FIGURE 8.1.3 ◆ As the needle is withdrawn, an applicator is used to tamponade the injection site, preventing leakage.

COMPLICATIONS

1. *Sudden decreased visual acuity:* This most commonly occurs as a result of a transient increase in intraocular pressure (IOP) with rapid and spontaneous resolution. If symptoms do not resolve in 1 minute, however, an anterior chamber paracentesis should be performed.

2. *Floaters:* These are due to injected medication or air bubbles in the visual axis and should resolve rapidly.

3. *Secondary cataract or glaucoma:* These are frequent complications of intravitreal steroids. Careful monitoring is warranted while receiving such injections.

4. *Endophthalmitis:* Infection is very rare with proper adherence to sterile technique.

5. *Vitreous hemorrhage:* This is also a rare complication with appropriate needle insertion.

POSTOPERATIVE CARE

- After injection, view the fundus with an indirect ophthalmoscope to rule out complications.
- It is not necessary to check the IOP with applanation tonometry if the optic nerve appears well-perfused following injection.
- Instruct the patient to apply topical antibiotic drops for several days after the injection.

- Counsel the patient to report severe ocular discomfort or reduction in visual acuity, but reassure him or her that transient blurring or dark patches in the visual fields (bubbles) are to be anticipated.

Further Reading

Text

Andreoli CM, Miller JW. Anti-vascular endothelial growth factor therapy for ocular neovascular disease. *Curr Opin Ophthalmol.* 2007;18(6):502–508.

Fu A, Bui A, Rae R, et al. Cystoid muscular edema. In: Yanoff M, Duker J, eds. *Ophthalmology.* 3rd ed. Philadelphia, PA: Mosby; 2009:696–701.

Lang GK. Vitreous body. In: *Ophthalmology: A Pocket Textbook Atlas.* 2nd ed. New York, NY: Georg Thieme Verlag; 2007:285–304.

Read RW. Endophthalmitis. In: Yanoff M, Duker J, eds. *Ophthalmology.* 3rd ed. Philadelphia, PA: Mosby; 2009: 815–819.

Rosenfeld PJ, Martidis A, Tennant MTS. Age-related mucular degeneration. In: Yanoff M, Duker J, eds. *Ophthalmology.* 3rd ed. Philadelphia, PA: Mosby; 2009:558–673.

Primary Sources

Age-Related Eye Disease Study Research Group. A randomized, placebo-controlled, clinical trial of high-dose supplementation with vitamins C and E, beta carotene, and zinc for age-related macular degeneration and vision loss: AREDS report no. 8. *Arch Ophthalmol.* 2001; 119(10):1417–1436.

Arevalo JF, Fromow-Guerra J, Sanchez, et al.; Pan-American Collaborative Retina Study Group. Primary intravitreal bevacizumab for subfoveal choroidal neovascularization in age-related macular degeneration: results of the Pan-American Collaborative Retina Study Group at 12 months follow-up. *Retina.* 2008;28(10):1387–1394.

Brown DM, Kaiser PK, Michels M, et al.; ANCHOR Study Group. Ranibizumab versus verteporfin for neovascular age-related macular degeneration. *N Engl J Med.* 2006;355(14):1432–1444.

Endophthalmitis Vitrectomy Study Group. Results of the Endophthalmitis Vitrectomy Study. A randomized trial of immediate vitrectomy and of intravenous antibiotics for the treatment of postoperative bacterial endophthalmitis. *Arch Ophthalmol.* 1995;13(12): 1479–1496.

Ferrara N, Damico L, Shams N, et al. Development of ranibizumab, an anti-vascular endothelial growth factor antigen binding fragment, as therapy for neovascular age-related macular degeneration. *Retina.* 2006;26(8): 859–870.

Rosenfeld PJ, Brown DM, Heier JS, et al.; MARINA Study Group. Ranibizumab for neovascular age-related macular degeneration. *N Engl J Med*. 2006;355(14):1419–1431.

VEGF Inhibition Study in Ocular Neovascularization (V.I.S.I.O.N.) Clinical Trial Group; Chakravarthy U,

Adamis AP, Cunningham ET Jr, Goldbaum M, Guyer DR, Katz B, Patel M. Year 2 efficacy results of 2 randomized controlled clinical trials of pegaptanib for neovascular age-related macular degeneration. *Ophthalmology*. 2006;113(9):1508.e1–25.

8.2   PARS PLANA VITRECTOMY (PPV)

Small instruments, inserted through the pars plana, are used to cut and remove vitreous, peel membranes, and laser photocoagulate providing treatment to various posterior segment pathologies.

INDICATIONS

Common indications include (but are not limited to):

- Proliferative diabetic retinopathy (PDR)
- Proliferative vitreoretinopathy (PVR)
- Retinal detachment with or without breaks
- Macular hole
- Macular pucker (epiretinal membrane)
- Persistent or recurring vitreous hemorrhage
- Vitreoretinal traction
- Complications of anterior segment surgery (e.g., dislocated lens, choroidal hemorrhage)
- Infection (e.g., endophthalmitis, viral retinitis) and inflammatory conditions (e.g., sarcoidosis, Behçet's syndrome)
- Persistent macular edema
- Subretinal hemorrhage
- Trauma and intraocular foreign bodies (IOFB)
- Retinopathy of prematurity
- Choroidal neovascularization (CNV)
- Tumors (e.g., lymphoma, diagnostic vitrectomy)

RELEVANT PHYSIOLOGY/ANATOMY

Vitreous
- 98% water; hyaluronic acid and collagen fibrils account for gel-like consistency.

- The outer cortex adheres to the internal-limiting membrane (ILM) of the retina.
- The outer membrane (the hyaloid membrane) adheres firmly to the ora serrata (vitreous base), posterior lens capsule, pars plana epithelium, optic nerve head, blood vessels, and perifoveal region.
- With aging, the vitreous body contracts and can pull away from the ILM leading to a posterior vitreous detachment (PVD).

Posterior Hyaloid Face
After the vitreous cortex detaches from the ILM, this thin layer remains adherent to the ILM in the macular region, providing a persistent source of retinal traction.

Retina
Nine layers (from inside to outside)

1. *Internal limiting membrane:* glial cell fibers separate from vitreous
2. *Nerve fiber layer:* from third-order neurons, converge on optic disc
3. *Ganglion cell layer:* third-order neurons
4. *Inner plexiform layer:* synapses of second and third-order neurons
5. *Inner nuclear layer:* second-order neurons, bipolar cells (horizontal and amacrine cells)
6. *Outer plexiform layer:* synapses of first and second-order neurons
7. *Outer nuclear layer:* first-order neurons, nuclei of rods and cones
8. *Outer limiting membrane:* separates rod and cone nuclei from photoreceptive elements
9. Rod and cone photoreceptors

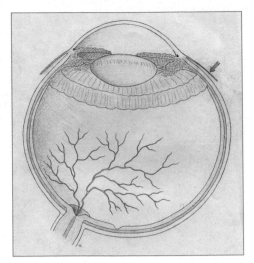

FIGURE 8.2.1 ◆ *Pars plana:* Instrument placement through the pars plana (arrow) permits the surgeon to access posterior segment pathology with the fewest potential complications.

- Retinal pigment epithelium (RPE)
- Subretinal space: lies between photoreceptors and RPE
- Bruch's membrane: choroid basement membrane (Note: CNV is thought to arise via breaks in Bruch's membrane.)

Pars Plana (FIG. 8.2.1)

- Entrance site (sclerostomy) is approximately 3.5 mm (pseudophakic eyes) to 4 mm (phakic eyes) posterior to the limbus.
- Sclerostomy allows entrance into the posterior segment without damaging the retina (anterior to the ora serrata) or causing hemorrhage (posterior to the highly vascularized pars plicata).

RELEVANT PATHOPHYSIOLOGY

Retinal Detachment: Three types

- Rhegmatogenous: Full-thickness break (e.g., hole or tear) in the sensory retina with extravasation of vitreous fluid into the subretinal space; usually preceded by a PVD.
- Tractional: Fibrovascular tissue (e.g., vitreal, epiretinal, or subretinal membranes) leads to tractional forces that separate the sensory retina from the RPE.

- Serous/Hemorrhagic: Fluid accumulates in the subretinal space without traction or retinal breakage; seen with degenerative, infectious, and inflammatory diseases.

Vitreous Hemorrhage

- Causes include PDR, branch or central retinal vein occlusion, retinal tears or detachment, or trauma.
- Mechanism generally involves vitreoretinal traction leading to rupture of small vessels.

Epiretinal Membranes

- Membranes are composed of glial cells, fibroblasts, RPE cells, and inflammatory cells; they become adherent to the retina.
- PVR: Scar tissue formation is commonly seen after retinal detachment. RPE and glial cells enter the vitreous cavity after a retinal tear, and despite adequate repair, these cells can proliferate on the retinal surface leading to retinal traction upon membrane contraction.
- When tractional forces from epiretinal membranes cause wrinkling of the retinal surface overlying the macula, this is referred to as *macular pucker*.

Macular Hole

- A macular hole involves a partial or full-thickness break in the sensory region overlying the macula. Although the exact etiology remains unknown, it is believed that vitreoretinal traction over the macula is responsible for creating these holes.
- Staging (determines treatment outcomes):
  - Stage 1: Loss of normal foveal depression; presence of yellow ring or pigmentary spot
  - Stage 2: Full-thickness hole with diameter <400 microns
  - Stage 3: Full-thickness hole with diameter >400 microns
  - Stage 4: Full-thickness hole with diameter >400 microns plus posterior hyaloid detachment
- Watzke-Allen Test: Classic clinical test used to differentiate macular holes from pseudoholes/epiretinal membranes. A narrow beam of light is placed over the macula. If the patient describes a break in the line, this is a positive test for a macular hole. This test is not always reliable, and optical coherence tomography (OCT) is often used to confirm the diagnosis.

ALTERNATIVE TREATMENTS FOR COMMON PATHOLOGIES

Diabetic Vitreous Hemorrhage

- Observation followed by laser therapy: A large percentage of diabetic bleeds clear spontaneously.
- Laser photocoagulation: This is done when any part of the retina is visible after initial hemorrhage. If hemorrhage is excessive, this is not a viable option.
- Intravitreal bevacizumab (Avastin) or ranibizumab (Lucentis)
- Anterior retinal cryotherapy (ARC): This is done if portions of the retina are visible; it is infrequently performed compared to laser photocoagulation.

The Diabetic Retinopathy Vitrectomy Study (DRVS) suggests early vitrectomy for vitreous hemorrhage; although recently, many retinal specialists are trying bevacizumab first.

Retinal Break/Detachment

- Laser/cryotherapy: Creates adhesions between the retinal pigment epithelium (RPE) and sensory retina.
- Pneumatic retinopexy: Air or gas is injected into the vitreous to keep the retina in place in conjunction with laser treatment or cryotherapy to create anchoring adhesions.
- Scleral buckle: External compression of the globe over the site of a retinal break reapposes the retina with the RPE; it is often coupled with laser or cryotherapy.

Significant Vitreoretinal Traction or Preretinal Membranes

- Close observation followed by surgical intervention (e.g., PPV and/or membrane removal)

Macular Hole

Observation: About half of stage 1 holes resolve spontaneously along with a smaller percentage of stage 2 holes.

PREOPERATIVE SCREENING

Screening involves complete history and physical (H&P), which is very important in diabetic/hypertensive patients; VA measurement and pupillary function; visual fields; and Amsler grid test for metamorphopsia (indicates macular involvement).

- Anterior segment assessment: Observe carefully for iris neovascularization as this may require panretinal photocoagulation (PRP) prior to vitrectomy.
- Lens assessment (phakia vs. pseudophakia vs. aphakia): In pseudophakic eyes, the type of intraocular lens (IOL) may influence the operative strategy (e.g., intravitreal silicone oil may adhere to a hydrophobic lens).
- Indirect biomicroscopy: Used to assess relationship and characteristics of the vitreous and retina; it is important to determine if PVD is present. If so, the extent of the posterior hyaloid surface is noted. The location of retinal breaks and the severity of membrane proliferation should also be noted.
- Ultrasound: Essential for eyes with opaque vitreous (e.g., hemorrhage). Can identify retinal detachments, membranes, intraocular foreign bodies (IOFBs), choroidal detachments, subretinal fluid, and tumor location.
- Electroretinography (ERG): ERG can be used to evaluate the functionality of the retina.
- Imaging: For trauma cases, CT scans are very helpful for localizing IOFBs and assessing bony damage. A magnetic resonance imaging (MRI) is contraindicated as metallic IOFBs may shift during scanning.

TABLE 8.2.1 Rapid Review of Steps
(1) Conjunctival exposure (in 20-gauge vitrectomy).
(2) Place infusion cannula inferotemporally and confirm the proper location with a light pipe.
(3) Place superonasal and supertemporal trocar or sclerotomies.
(4) Place vitrectomy viewing system (BIOM or handheld lens system).
(5) Insert light pipe and vitrector.
(6) Perform core vitrectomy with induction of a PVD (posterior vitreous detachment).
(7) Apply membrane peel, endolaser, or injection of gas as needed.
(8) Inspect peripheral retina with scleral indentation.
(9) Remove the trocars and, lastly, the infusion cannula.
(10) Suture the sclerotomies or leaking trocar wounds.

ANESTHESIA

Local anesthesia (e.g., retrobulbar, peribulbar, or sub-Tenon's block) is most commonly administered. Infrequently, topical anesthesia is sufficient.

General anesthesia is only considered in patients who cannot tolerate local anesthesia or who present with recent open globe.

Nitrous oxide is contraindicated in patients who are receiving intraocular gas.

PROCEDURE

The following narrative describes the introductory steps in a PPV with the intention to clear opacified

media and relieve vitreoretinal traction. Various case-dependent surgical techniques are discussed under "Further Surgical Considerations."

 See Tables 8.2.1 Rapid Review and 8.2.2 Surgical Pearls, and Web Tables 8.2.1 to 8.2.4 for review of suggested instrumentation and supplies.

General Vitrectomy Techniques:

1. *Microscope and Lens Setup:* After the operating microscope is adjusted, the surgeon must choose an appropriate lens to visualize the posterior segment. If an assistant is present, a handheld lens can be used (Fig. 8.2.2). If no assistant is present, a lens can be sutured to the sclera (e.g., Landers lens) or a noncontact system (e.g., BIOM, Oculus,

---

TABLE 8.2.2 Surgical Pearls

Preoperative:
- Communicate with the patient that the postoperative course is variable and that it may take a few weeks (rarely 1 to 2 months) to return to baseline vision.
- Based on the indication of the vitreo-retinal surgery, the patient may need to maintain a facedown position for 1 to 4 weeks.
- Include in the consent the increased risk of retinal detachment in all patients undergoing vitrectomy.

Intraoperative:
- The infusion cannula and the trocar/sclerotomies are placed 3 mm posterior to the limbus in pseudophakic/aphakic patients, and 4 mm in phakic patients. Before the infusion cannula is opened, the intraocular placement should be confirmed with a light pipe.
- Trocars are inserted by displacing the conjunctiva with a cotton-tipped applicator and creating a biplanar incision into the eye.
- Avoid rapid movement of the vitrector and the light pipe inside the eye. This minimizes vitreous traction, decreasing the risk of an iatrogenic peripheral retinal tear.
- Posterior vitreous detachment can be induced with suction of the vitrector probe or the extrusion cannula. Posterior vitreous detachment helps to ensure the vitreous in the posterior pole is removed.
- Peripheral retina in the location of the trocars/sclerotomies should be thoroughly inspected with scleral indentation at the end of the surgery.
- Consider preplacing sutures in the flaps to facilitate closure of the scleral flap.
- If the trocars/sclerotomies are created too far posterior, the retina can be torn, leading to retina detachment. Anterior placement of the trocars/sclerotomies in phakic patients can lead to damage to the lens capsule.
- Vitrectomies in phakic patients should not cross the midline to avoid contact of the vitrector or light pipe to the posterior lens capsule. In general, the core vitrectomy should be performed with the vitrector setting on low suction and a high-cut rate to reduce the amount of vitreous traction.

Postoperative:
- Carefully check for wound leaks. The peripheral retina should be carefully examined. Low postoperative intraocular pressure is usually due to a leaking trocar site.
- Communicate with the patient that they should not bend, strain, or lift heavy objects until cleared by the primary surgeon.
- Monitor for excessive postoperative inflammation. Consider oral or periocular depot steroids to control excessive inflammation.

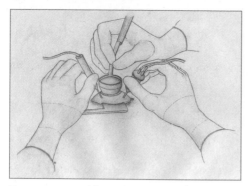

FIGURE 8.2.2 ◆ *Vitrectomy instruments:* The surgical field, demonstrating the use of a planoconcave lens (in conjunction with the operating microscope) to view intraocular structures during PPV.

Washington) can be used. For evaluation of the peripheral retina, scleral depression is combined with the use of a prismatic or wide-field viewing lens with an inverter on the microscope. A binocular indirect ophthalmoscopy may also be used.

2. *Vitrectomy Instruments:* There are two basic types of vitrectors used to cut and remove vitreous. A guillotine cutter is a blunt instrument in which a small piece of vitreous is aspirated through a side port and cut by an inner blade moving up and down. A rotary cutter is a blunt instrument in which the inner blade rotates inside the outer probe. The aspiration port is closer to the tip allowing for closer cutting to the retina. Of note, the higher the cutting speed, the less traction on the vitreous and retina (i.e., decreased risk of iatrogenic retinal tear).

The surgeon may also decide between a sutureless 23-, 25-, or 27-gauge vitrector versus a 20-gauge vitrector. Use of the 20-gauge vitrectomy instrument necessitates opening the conjunctiva and subsequent suturing to the sclera. The 23-gauge to 27-gauge vitrector ports are placed transconjunctivally and do not require suturing to the sclera.

3. *Description of sutureless (23-gauge to 27-gauge) vitrector port:* The insertion system consists of a sharp blade (trocar) surrounded by a sleeve through which the vitrector and other instruments will be inserted. Trocars are most commonly placed in the inferotemporal, superonasal, and supertemporal regions, through which the infusion cannula, fiberoptic light, and vitrector will be placed (FIG. 8.2.3).

4. *Caliper measurement:* Calipers are used to measure the desired distance from the limbus to the sclerostomy sites (4 mm in the phakic eye; 3 to 3.5 mm in the pseudophakic or aphakic eye). These measurements ensure penetration of the pars plana, rather than the pars plicata or sensory retina.

5. *Insertion of sutureless trocar:* Using fine forceps, the conjunctiva overlying the location for trocar placement is pulled toward the limbus. After confirming the caliper measurement, the trocar is inserted in a biplanar fashion through the sclera. First, the trocar penetrates half of the sclera in an oblique fashion, followed by a perpendicular penetration in which the trocar is aimed toward the center of the globe (FIG. 8.2.4). The sleeve is held by forceps while the trocar is removed (FIG. 8.2.5). The sleeve does not need to be sutured to the sclera and the vitrector or alternate instruments may now be inserted through the sleeve.

Two components of this procedure allow for a self-sealing closure. First, by pulling the conjunctiva toward the limbus, the penetration site through the conjunctiva and sclera are not directly overlapping. Second, the biplanar incision through the sclera creates a self-sealing wound. Of note, due to the small port diameter, uniplanar sclerostomies for 25-gauge and 27-gauge vitrector systems may be performed with self-sealing

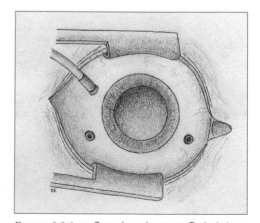

FIGURE 8.2.3 ◆ *Sutureless vitrectomy:* Typical placement of ports for 23-, 25-, and 27-gauge vitrectomy. The infusion cannula clips into one port, while the remaining two are used for the light pipe and vitrector (or other instruments).

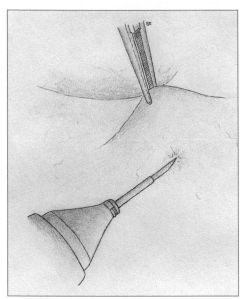

FIGURE 8.2.4 ◆ *Trocar insertion:* Using fine forceps, conjunctiva overlying the pars plana is pulled toward the limbus. A trocar with an overlying port/sleeve is then used to pierce the sclera; it is first directed obliquely (shown), and then toward the center of the globe. This creates a tunnel that will seal without sutures when the port is removed.

results. However, for 23-guage vitrectomy systems, the biplanar approach is essential for producing a sutureless incision.

NOTE: *Steps 6 through 9 describe the approach for placement of ports for a 20-guage vitrectomy.*

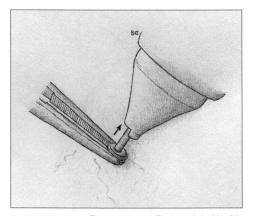

FIGURE 8.2.5 ◆ *Trocar removal:* The port is held with forceps while the trocar is removed. It does not need to be sutured to the sclera and is ready for connection of the infusion cannula or passage of instruments.

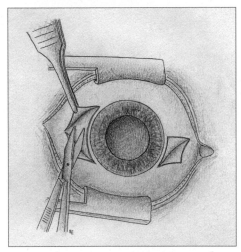

FIGURE 8.2.6 ◆ *Scleral exposure:* Creation of conjunctival flaps permits access to the underlying sclera, which must be penetrated during pars plana access.

6. *Superficial incisions:* Conjunctival/Tenon's capsule flaps are raised to expose the inferotemporal, superonasal, and supertemporal regions overlying the future sclerotomies (FIG. 8.2.6). Partial-thickness scleral sutures are then placed in the inferotemporal quadrant, permitting the infusion cannula to be secured once it is inserted (FIG. 8.2.7). Calipers are then used to measure the desired distance from the limbus to the sclerostomy sites (4 mm in the phakic eye; 3

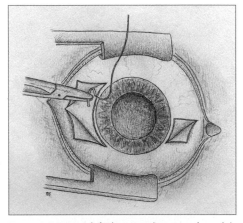

FIGURE 8.2.7 ◆ *Infusion cannula suture:* A partial-thickness scleral suture is placed to secure the infusion cannula; instruments placed through other sclerostomies must remain mobile and are not secured externally.

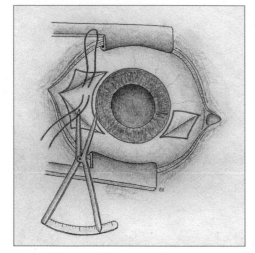

FIGURE 8.2.8 ✦ *Measurement:* Castroviejo calipers are used to measure the distance from the limbus to the site of the sclerostomy incisions (4 mm in the phakic eye versus 3 to 3.5 mm in the pseudophakic or aphakic eye).

to 3.5 mm in the pseudophakic or aphakic eye) (FIG. 8.2.8).

7. *Inferotemporal entry incision:* The inferotemporal sclerostomy is made using a microvitreoretinal (MVR) blade, which should be angled toward the optic nerve or the center of the globe in order to avoid hitting the lens (FIG. 8.2.9). The sclera and pars plana are penetrated before entering the vitreous. In retinal detachment cases,

the MVR blade angle will be relatively flatter to avoid injury to the retina.

8. *Placement of infusion cannula:* An infusion cannula is placed through the inferotemporal incision and secured with the preplaced sutures. Infusion is automated to maintain intraocular pressure (IOP) while cutting and removing vitreous. Balanced salt solution (BSS) has been shown to be the least toxic infusion agent. For diabetic patients, dextrose may be added to the solution in order to avoid osmotic shifts and lens opacification.

9. *Superior entry incisions:* Sclerostomy incisions are then made in the superonasal and supertemporal quadrants to allow for placement of the fiberoptic light and vitrector (FIG. 8.2.10).

10. *Removal of vitreous:* Starting in the center of the eye, the vitrector is used to cut and remove the vitreous while the infusion cannula maintains IOP (FIG. 8.2.11). The vitrector is then repositioned to perform vitreous shaving for peripheral vitreous removal.

11. *Removal of posterior hyaloid membrane:* If PVD is present, the posterior hyaloid membrane is often removed to prevent continued vitreoretinal traction. The membrane can be lifted with suction and excised with the vitrector.

12. *Case-dependent surgical techniques:* After the vitreous is removed and vitreoretinal traction is relieved, a specific retinal pathology can be addressed. For adjunctive laser photocoagulation, insertion of perfluorocarbons or silicone oil, pars plana lensectomy, removal of preretinal membranes, and repair of macular hole,

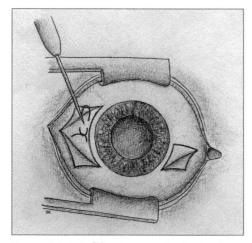

FIGURE 8.2.9 ✦ *Sclerostomy creation:* A microvitreoretinal (MVR) blade is use to make the first sclerostomy incision in the inferotemporal quadrant; the infusion cannula will be placed here.

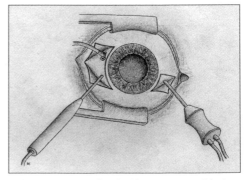

FIGURE 8.2.10 ✦ *Surgical instrument positioning:* Clockwise from upper left; the infusion cannula, vitrector, and fiber optic light.

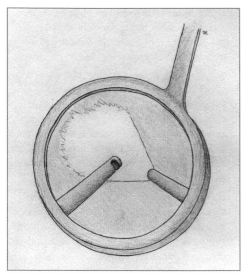

FIGURE 8.2.11 ◆ *Vitrectomy:* Vitrectomy probe (left) and fiber optic light (left) viewed through the planoconcave lens. The wide-angle lens and oblique lighting permit visualization of vitreous strands during removal.

please see the "Further Surgical Considerations" section.

13. *Peripheral retinal examination:* Prior to instrument removal and closure, the peripheral retina, using scleral depression or a wide-angled lens, is carefully inspected for retinal breaks or detachments.

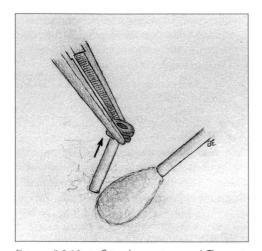

FIGURE 8.2.12 ◆ *Sutureless port removal:* The ports are slowly removed with fine forceps. Using a cotton-tipped applicator, pressure is held over the incision sites for 10 to 20 seconds

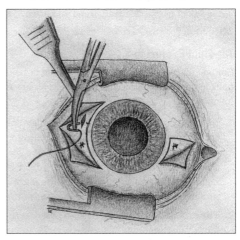

FIGURE 8.2.13 ◆ *Scleral suturing:* The sclerostomy incisions are closed with sutures to prevent leakage of silicon oil (SO) or other intraocular fluids. The conjunctival flaps are then reapproximated.

14a. *Removal of instruments for 23-gauge to 27-gauge vitrector systems:* All instruments are removed from the ports. With fine forceps, the ports are slowly removed. Using a cotton-tipped applicator, pressure is held over the incision sites for 10 to 20 seconds (FIG. 8.2.12). No sutures are generally required.

14b. *Removal of instruments for 20-gauge vitrector systems and closure:* The sutures used to secure the infusion cannula are cut and all instruments are removed. The sclerostomy incisions are closed with a 7-0 polyglactin or similar suture (FIG. 8.2.13). IOP is then measured prior to superficial closure. BSS can be injected or removed to achieve adequate IOP. The conjunctival incisions are closed with 8-0 polyglactin or plain gut suture.

15. *Subconjunctival steroid and antibiotic injections:* Care must be taken to avoid infiltration of the rectus muscles.

FURTHER SURGICAL CONSIDERATIONS

Laser Photocoagulation

- Retinal tears: Laser photocoagulation is applied around the tear using an endolaser probe or indirect ophthalmoscope; this promotes readhesion to the RPE.
- PDR: Laser burns are scattered in the retinal periphery (panretinal photocoagulation) to reduce

hole) in order to maximize the tamponading effect for up to 2 weeks.

Topical antibiotic drops (e.g., moxifloxacin) are applied for 1 week, topical steroid drops (e.g., prednisolone) are applied for 1 month, and/or dilating drops (e.g., atropine or scopolamine) are applied for 2 to 4 weeks to prevent posterior synechiae formation.

Follow up in clinic the next day to screen for complications (e.g., increase in IOP).

Avoid heavy lifting or the Valsalva maneuver.

Patients cannot fly while inert gas bubble is present (gas expands at higher altitudes).

Further Reading

Text

Engelbert M, Chang S. Vitrectomy. In: Yanoff M, Duker J, eds. *Ophthalmology*. 3rd ed. Philadelphia, PA: Mosby; 2009: 530–533.

Gass JD. *Stereoscopic Atlas of Macular Diseases: Diagnosis and Treatment*. St. Louis, MO: Mosby; 1997:904–909.

Whitcher J, Riordan-Eva P. *Vaughan and Asbury's General Ophthalmology*. New York: Lange Medical Books/Mc-Graw-Hill; 2004

Primary Sources

Blankenship GW, Machemer R. Long-term diabetic vitrectomy results: report of 10 year follow-up. *Ophthalmology.* 1985;92(4):503–506.

Blankenship GW. Preoperative prognostic factors in diabetic pars plana vitrectomy. *Ophthalmol.* 1982;89(11): 1246–1249.

Borne MJ, Tasman W, Regillo C, et al. Outcomes of vitrectomy for retained lens fragments. *Ophthalmology.* 1996; 103(6):971–976.

Chang S. Perfluorocarbon liquids in vitreoretinal surgery. *Int Ophthalmol Clin.* 1992;32(2):153–163.

Davis MD. Vitreous contraction in proliferative diabetic retinopathy. *Arch Ophthalmol.* 1965;74(6):741–751.

de Bustros S, Thompson JT, Michels RG, et al. Vitrectomy for progressive proliferative diabetic retinopathy. *Arch Ophthalmol.* 1987;105(2):196–199.

Diabetic Retinopathy Vitrectomy Study Research Group. Early vitrectomy for severe proliferative diabetic retinopathy in eyes with useful vision: clinical application of results of a randomized trial, Diabetic Retinopathy Vitrectomy Study Report 4. *Ophthalmology.* 1988; 95(10):1321–1334.

Diabetic Retinopathy Vitrectomy Study Research Group. Early vitrectomy for severe vitreous hemorrhage in diabetic retinopathy. Two-year results of a randomized trial. Diabetic Retinopathy Vitrectomy Study Report 2. *Arch Ophthalmol.* 1985;103(11):1644–1652.

Federman J, Schubert HD. Complications associated with the use of silicone oil in 150 eyes after retina-vitreous surgery. *Ophthalmology.* 1988;95(7):870–876.

Flynn HW Jr, Chew EY, Simons BD, et al., 3rd ed. Pars plana vitrectomy in the early treatment diabetic retinopathy study, ETDRS report no. 17. *Ophthalmol.* 1992;99(9):1351–1357.

Lucke KH, Foerster MH, Laqua H. Long-term results of vitrectomy and silicone oil in 500 cases of complicated retinal detachments. *Am J Ophthalmol.* 1987;104(6): 624–633.

Pastor JC. Proliferative vitreoretinopathy: an overview. *Surv Ophthalmol.* 1998;43(1):3–18.

Rice TA, De Bustros S, Michels RG, et al. Prognostic factors in vitrectomy for epiretinal membranes of the macula. *Ophthalmology.* 1986;93(5):602–610.

Ryan E, Gilbert HD. Results of surgical treatment of recent-onset full thickness idiopathic holes. *Arch Ophthalmol.* 1994;12(12):1545–1553.

Silicone Study. Vitrectomy with silicone oil or perfluoropropane gas in eyes with severe proliferative vitreoretinopathy: results of a randomized clinical trial. *Arch Ophthalmol.* 110(6):780–792.

8.3 RETINAL LASER PHOTOCOAGULATION

- Involves the use of a thermal laser to burn small portions of the retina to destroy diseased tissue or produce chorio-retinal adhesions.

- Therapeutic goals achieved by scar formation include destruction of abnormal choroidal neovascular vessels in age-related macular degeneration (AMD), sealing leaky blood vessels in diabetic macular edema, panretinal photocoagulation to remove ischemic retina in proliferative diabetic retinopathy, and forming chorioretinal adhesions for patients with retinal tear and detachment (to reappose the sensory retina to the retinal pigment epithelium [RPE] in a detachment).

INDICATIONS

- Proliferative diabetic retinopathy (PDR) with high-risk characteristics:
  1. Neovascularization of the disc (NVD) and vitreous hemorrhage
  2. NVD greater than one-fourth of the disc area
  3. Neovascularization elsewhere (NVE) greater than one-half disc area plus preretinal hemorrhage or vitreous hemorrhage (panretinal photocoagulation [PRP] administered)
- Macular edema: Focal or diffuse forms treated by focal (local application) or grid (application in ordered rows and columns) photocoagulation, respectively
- Retinal breaks: Two to three rows of laser burns around the retinal break to form chorioretinal adhesions and reduce the risk of retinal detachment
- Retinal vein occlusions:
  1. Branch retinal vein occlusion (BRVO): Grid laser photocoagulation used for the treatment of macular edema due to BRVO; sectoral photocoagulation to the area of ischemic retina (affected by the BRVO) used to reduce the risk of retinal neovascularization by preventing the release of angiogenic factors
  2. Central retinal vein occlusion (CRVO): For CRVO with significant ischemia, there is a high risk of developing the following:
     a. Rubeosis iridis (neovascularization of the iris), which can lead to neovascular glaucoma
     b. Peripheral retinal neovascularization leading to vitreous hemorrhage (Laser photocoagulation at the first sign of iris and retinal neovascularization significantly decreases the risk of this complication.)
- Extrafoveal choroidal neovascularization: from AMD or ocular histoplasmosis (Subfoveal lesions are not treated by laser therapy due to the collateral damage to the retina tissue responsible for the central vision.)
- Retinopathy of prematurity: Scatter photocoagulation in the peripheral area of nonperfused retina prevents neovascularization complications.
- Sickle cell retinopathy: Scatter photocoagulation of ischemic areas decreases neovascularization risk.
- Retinal vascular abnormalities (e.g., AV connections, Coats' disease [retinal telangiectasias], and

arterial aneurysms): Focal photocoagulation of abnormalities prevents leakage and exudative complications.
- Central serous chorioretinopathy (CSCR): only used for recurrent or persistent situations; resolution is commonly spontaneous
- Small tumors: benign (e.g., retinal and choroidal hemangioma) and malignant (e.g., retinoblastoma and choroidal melanoma); goal of photocoagulation is to achieve vascular coagulation and tumor ischemia

ALTERNATIVES

Proliferative Diabetic Retinopathy (High Risk)
- Retinal cryotherapy: useful if hemorrhage is present
- Pars plana vitrectomy (PPV): treatment for significant vitreous hemorrhage (can be used in conjunction with endolaser)
- Intravitreal injection of anti-vascular endothelial growth factor (anti-VEGF) agents such as bevacizumab (Avastin) or ranibizumab (Lucentis)

Macular Edema
- Observation: spontaneous clearance
- Topical corticosteroids and nonsteroidal anti-inflammatory drugs (NSAIDs) for the treatment of postsurgical macular edema
- Periocular or intravitreal steroids (e.g., triamcinolone)
- Intravitreal anti-VEGF agents (e.g., bevacizumab [Avastin])

Retinal Breaks
- Retinal cryotherapy: use of liquid nitrogen cooled probe to create chorioretinal adhesions
- Pneumatic retinopexy: likely treatment if progression to retinal detachment is expected
- Scleral buckle: treatment of rhegmatogenous retinal detachments

RELEVANT PHYSIOLOGY/ANATOMY

Retinal Anatomy (Fig. 8.3.1)
Retinal Pigments
- Melanin: found in RPE and choroid; absorbs all wavelengths of light

Conformational changes in the rod and cone photopigments transduce light into electrical signals that are transmitted to the occipital cortex.

The macula is located ~15° temporal and slightly inferior to the optic disc. It includes the fovea centralis, which contains only cones and is responsible for acute central vision.

- Vascular supply: The central retinal artery supplies the inner retinal layers (via the internal carotid and ophthalmic arteries); diffusion from the choroidal circulation supplies the outer retinal layers. Prolonged macular detachment therefore deprives this region of a key source of nutrition and can have catastrophic visual consequences.

- Sensory supply: No sensory nerves (aside from the optic nerve) innervate the retina, so pathology is generally painless.

Retinal Anatomy

The posterior segment has two fundamental divisions:

1. *Sensory retina:* neural tissue posterior to the ora serrata

2. *Pars plana/pars plicata:* anterior to the ora serrata

There are nine integral layers plus two closely related layers:

1. *Internal limiting membrane:* composed of glial cell fibers adjacent to the posterior hyaloid face of the vitreous

2. *Nerve fiber layer:* ganglion cell axons converge on the disc, forming the optic nerve

3. *Ganglion cell layer:* consists of the third order ganglion cell neurons

4. *Inner plexiform layer:* made up of the synapses between the second and third order neurons

5. *Inner nuclear layer:* consists of the second order bipolar cell neurons (horizontal and amacrine cells)

6. *Outer plexiform layer:* made up of the synapses between the first and second order neurons

7. *Outer nuclear layer:* consists of the first order rod and cone nuclei

8. *Outer limiting membrane:* a porous layer separating the nuclei of the rods and cones from their photoreceptive elements

9. *Rod and cone photoreceptors*

Closely related layers include the following:

1. *Retinal pigment epithelium:* A pigmented cell layer that helps to nourish the retina, and firmly adheres to Bruch's membrane.

2. *Bruch's membrane:* The basement membrane of the choroid.

Anatomy also includes the subretinal space, which is a potential space that can fill with fluid when the retina detaches from the underlying retinal pigment epithelium.

Relationship to Other Globe Layers (FIG. 8.4.1)
Retinal Detachment
- Separation of the sensory retina from the underlying RPE

Potential symptoms include flashing lights (photopsia), increasing floaters, perception of a falling curtain or rising wall, "black rain" (due to vessel avulsion with intravitreal bleeding), peripheral visual field loss, decreased visual acuity, and metamorphopsia (due to macular involvement).

Retinal detachment can also be asymptomatic; high-risk patients should be examined annually.

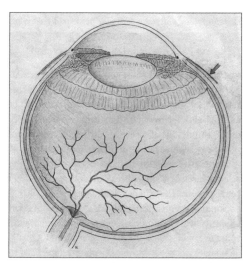

FIGURE 8.4.1 ✦ *Retinal anatomy:* The retina has two distinct parts, which merge at the ora serrata (os). These are the pars optica, or photoreceptive retina, and the pars ceca, or secretory epithelium, which covers the ciliary body and iris. The photoreceptive retina is separated from the underlying choroid and sclera by the retinal pigment epithelium and Bruch's membrane.

Three major categories (can overlap)

- Rhegmatogenous: The most common form of detachment. A full thickness break allows liquified vitreous to enter the subretinal space, elevating the retina. Frequency increases with age, posterior vitreous detachment, existing breaks, high myopia, aphakia, pseudophakia, neodymium-doped yttrium aluminum garnet (Nd:YAG) capsulotomy, lattice degeneration, and trauma. Visual prognosis is usually good with prompt treatment.

- Tractional: Detachment occurs when fibrovascular tissue exerts enough traction to exceed the force of adhesion between the retina and RPE.

- Serous/hemorrhagic: Nonvitreal fluid accumulates in the subretinal space, elevating the retina (e.g., choroidal effusion or hemorrhage, malignant effusion, or exudate from breakdown of the blood–retinal barrier).

PREOPERATIVE WORKUP

Conduct a dilated fundus exam with a slit lamp and 3-mirror lens as well as with an indirect ophthalmoscope, using scleral depression to view the periphery. Areas of detached retina will appear opaque and edematous. The bright red choroidal circulation may be seen through breaks in the retina. Identify coexisting retinal pathology and determine the number and location of detachments or breaks as this is critical to selecting an appropriate treatment.

Carefully examine of the fellow eye since up to 20% of detachments are bilateral. If there is significant refractive opacity (e.g., a mature cataract), perform B-scan ultrasound to visualize the posterior segment of the eye. If there is significant vitreous opacity (e.g., hemorrhage), vitrectomy may be performed.

In evaluating the fundus, rule out conditions that can resemble retinal detachment. These include choroidal detachment and retinoschisis, an abnormal but usually benign split within the retina, most often in the outer plexiform layer. Degenerative retinoschisis, the most common form, affects approximately 7% of the population and generally does not require treatment.

ANESTHESIA

Retrobulbar or peribulbar anesthesia is sufficient for most patients. Adjunctive infiltration or sub-Tenon's

TABLE **8.4.1** Rapid Review of Steps

(1) Provide 360° of conjunctival exposure.
(2) Dissect subconjunctivally (limbus or fornix-based approach) with blunt curved Wescott scissors.
(3) Isolate all four rectus muscles with muscles hooks.
(4) Loop 2-0 silk suture for each rectus muscle.
(5) Identify and mark the retinal tear/break with indirect ophthalmoscopy.
(6) Administer cryotherapy of the retinal tear/break.
(7) Select the proper scleral buckle element.
(8) Suture the scleral buckle element.
(9) View scleral buckle location and height with indirect ophthalmoscopy.
(10) Close incisions with Tenon's plus conjunctival closure.

injection of a local anesthetic can help reduce postoperative pain.

PROCEDURE

 SEE TABLES 8.4.1 Rapid Review and 8.4.2 Surgical Pearls, and WEB TABLES 8.4.1 to 8.4.4 for review of suggested instrumentation and supplies.

1. *Peritomy:* The initial conjunctival incision is placed at the limbus or several millimeters behind it if an obstruction is present (e.g., a filtering bleb from a prior trabeculectomy). A full 360° peritomy (circular incision around the limbus) is created. Conjunctival relaxing incisions are used to decreases the risk of tears during subsequent manipulation (FIG. 8.4.2).

2. *Muscle Isolation:* After Tenon's capsule is opened, the scleral insertions of the rectus muscles are identified and captured with muscle hooks. The rectus muscles are dissected free of connective tissue. Sutures can then be passed behind the muscles to facilitate manipulation in subsequent steps (FIG. 8.4.3).

3. *Scleral Exposure:* While Tenon's and conjunctiva are retracted, scissor tips are gently spread between the rectus muscles to lyse connections to the underlying sclera (FIG. 8.4.4). The bare sclera is then inspected to identify areas where sutures cannot safely be placed during the bucking procedure. Examples include vortex veins, regions of

TABLE 8.4.2 Surgical Pearls

Preoperative:
- Communicate with the patient that the postoperative course is variable and that it may take a few weeks (rarely 1 to 2 months) to return to baseline vision. There may be postoperative positioning needed.
- Communicate that the resolution of the subretinal fluid after surgery may take weeks.
- Include in the consent the need for additional surgery.

Intraoperative:
- Ensure proper exposure of the sclera in all four quadrants. Assess the sclera for any area of thinning to reduce the risk of perforation duration suturing of scleral buckle. Assess intraocular pressure as the scleral buckle is sutured into place. This is more commonly seen in patients with high scleral buckles.
- Consider intraoperative and postoperative corticosteroids to reduce swelling and pain.
- Place the 5-0 nylon sutures 1 mm on each side of the scleral buckle to produce imbrication.
- Ensure careful manipulation of the rectus muscle and minimize the size of the scleral buckle element to reduce the risk of postoperative ocular motility restriction.
- In patients with large bullous retinal detachments, the subretinal fluid can be drained through the sclera. Additional measures may include the injection of intraocular expandable gas such as SF6 or C3F8 with postoperative positioning.

Postoperative:
- Carefully check for intraocular pressure (IOP). Evaluate the location of the retinal tear and positioning of the scleral buckle. Ideal location of the retinal tear should be at the anterior edge or the height of the scleral buckle.
- Communicate with the patient that they should not bend, strain, or lift heavy objects until cleared by the primary surgeon.
- An encircling scleral buckle is associated with increase risk of choroidal detachment.
- An encircling scleral buckle increases the risk of anterior segment ischemia in patients with sickle cell disease.
- Monitor for excessive postoperative inflammation. Consider oral or periocular depot corticosteroids to control excessive inflammation.

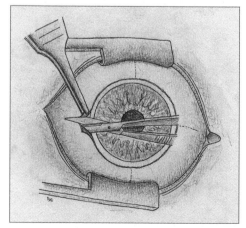

FIGURE 8.4.2 ◆ *Peritomy:* The initial conjunctival incision is generally placed at the limbus. A full 360° peritomy is made if an encircling band is to be placed. Conjunctival relaxing incisions are used to decreases the risk of tears during subsequent manipulation.

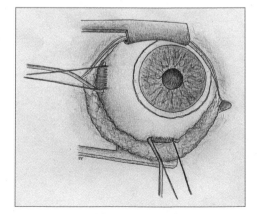

FIGURE 8.4.3 ◆ *Muscle isolation:* The scleral insertions of the rectus muscles are identified and isolated with muscle hooks. The muscles are dissected free of connective tissue; sutures can then be passed to facilitate their manipulation during buckle placement.

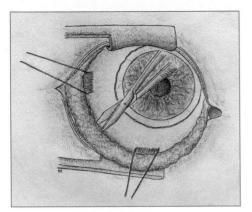

FIGURE 8.4.4 ◆ *Scleral exposure:* While Tenon's and conjunctiva are retracted, scissor tips are gently spread between the rectus muscles to lyse connections to the sclera.

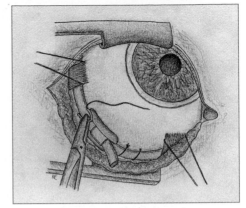

FIGURE 8.4.5 ◆ *Buckle placement:* If circumferential buckling is required, a silicone band is inserted beneath the rectus muscles. Silicon inserts of various sizes and shapes can be attached to this band to create regions of focal indentation. Mattress sutures are then placed to prevent migration of the band when it is tightened.

thinning, and staphylomas (protrusions of uveal tissue through the sclera). Rarely, one or more rectus muscles must be disinserted to adequately expose the sclera overlying the retinal break(s).

4. *Marking of Retinal Breaks:* Accurate buckle positioning is essential to a good surgical outcome. It is therefore necessary to identify and mark the surface projections of all retinal breaks. This is accomplished by using a probe to focally indent and mark the sclera while the underlying retina is visualized by indirect ophthalmoscopy.

5. *Chorioretinal Adhesion:* These various techniques use thermal energy to create adhesions that anchor the retina to underlying layers of the globe in the vicinity of the break(s). Cryopexy and diathermy are applied externally through the sclera. Laser photocoagulation is applied via an indirect ophthalmoscope. Cryopexy freezes tissue with localized delivery of liquid-phase nitrous oxide, diathermy generates heat from high frequency electrical current, and laser photocoagulation transduces focused light into heat. Cryopexy is the most commonly used.

6a. *Buckle Placement:* A silicone implant is secured to the sclera overlying the retinal break with partial thickness, nonabsorbable mattress sutures. These sutures should be passed at a depth between one-half and two-thirds of the scleral thickness. Since scleral perforation can cause serious complications, the globe should be stabilized during suture placement by grasping a rectus muscle insertion with forceps. If circumferential buckling is

required, a silicone band is placed beneath the rectus muscles. Silicon implants of various sizes and shapes can then be attached to this band to create regions of focal indentation. Mattress sutures are placed to prevent migration of the band with tightening (FIG. 8.4.5).

6b. *Internal Buckle Placement:* The buckle is placed between layers of sclera after the creation of a partial thickness flap or tunnel (FIG. 8.4.6). The sclera is then sutured closed over the implant. This technique is rarely used.

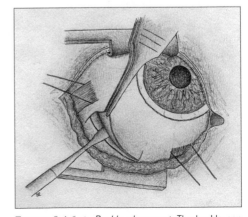

FIGURE 8.4.6 ◆ *Buckle placement:* The buckle can also be placed between layers of sclera after creation of a partial thickness flap or tunnel. This technique is rarely used.

7. *Subretinal Fluid Drainage:* Not all surgeons routinely include this step. In theory, it improves outcomes by permitting closer apposition of the retina with the underlying RPE and by moderating the rise in intraocular pressure (IOP) during buckle tightening. A fine-gauge needle is inserted through the sclera and choroid and into the subretinal space. Care is taken to avoid vortex veins and major choroidal vessels. Fluid is aspirated just prior to tightening the buckle, which helps to tamponade the drainage site. Skipping this step eliminates potential complications of transchoroidal drainage (e.g., retinal incarceration and choroidal hemorrhage). Without drainage, however, it may be necessary to administer IOP-lowering medications prior to buckle tightening.

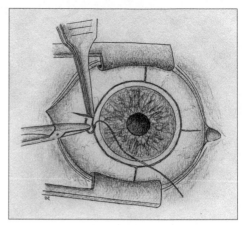

FIGURE 8.4.8 ✦ *Closure:* The conjunctival relaxing and peritomy incisions are then reapproximated with fine sutures.

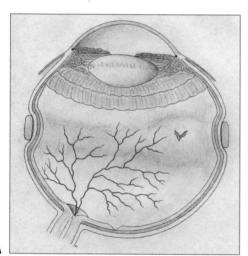

A

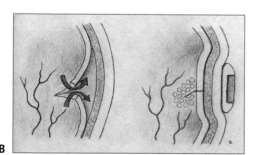

B

FIGURE 8.4.7 ✦ *Buckle tightening:* (**A**) When the mattress sutures are tightened, the silicon insert focally indents the globe. This reapposes the retinal break with the underlying RPE. (**B**) Liquified vitreous can no longer pass behind the retina to expand the detachment.

8. *Buckle Tightening:* When the mattress sutures are tightened, the silicone implant focally indents the globe. This reapposes the area of detached retina with the RPE. If a circumferential band is used, it is tightened and then secured with a silicone sleeve, suture, or clip (FIG. 8.4.7A, B). The buckle is not definitively fastened until indirect ophthalmoscopy has been used to confirm that the optic nerve remains well perfused and that the retinal breaks have been closed appropriately.

9. *Closure:* After irrigation with antibiotics and local anesthetic, Tenon's capsule is identified and closed. The conjunctival relaxing and peritomy incisions are then reapproximated with fine sutures (FIG. 8.4.8). This reduces tension on the conjunctiva and covers the buckle in two layers, reducing the risk of implant erosion.

COMPLICATIONS

Intraoperative

- Corneal clouding: Epithelial edema resulting from the increase in IOP triggered by scleral indentation. This may be treated with epithelial debridement if severe.

- Scleral perforation: If a scleral suture is placed too deep, blood, pigment, or subretinal fluid may leak from the suture tract. The retina should be carefully examined with indirect ophthalmoscopy to determine the depth of needle penetration and to check for associated breaks or hemorrhage.

- Complications of subretinal fluid drainage:
  - Retinal incarceration: The retina will appear dimpled over the drainage site and is at an increased risk of breaking.
  - Choroidal/subretinal hemorrhage: Blood will appear at the drainage site.

Postoperative

- Failure to reattach the retina: This is often seen when the break is not successfully closed or if significant retinal traction remains after buckling (e.g., from severe PVR). Incidence is decreased with appropriate patient selection.
- Infection/extrusion: The buckle is made of inert materials but can become infected. Infections are managed with antibiotics and/or implant removal (retinal detachment may subsequently recur).
- Anterior segment ischemia: This occurs due to disruption of the blood supply. The risk is increased with use of tight encircling bands, especially if one or more rectus muscles were disinserted for better exposure.
- Macular edema and submacular fluid: Accumulation of edema fluid beneath the macula is relatively common postoperatively and the impact on visual acuity is variable. Treated with corticosteroids and nonsteroidal anti-inflammatory drugs (NSAIDs).
- Glaucoma: This is often due to secondary angle closure from buckling, though other mechanisms are possible. It can be controlled with IOP-lowering mediations or laser therapy.
- Choroidal detachment: Serous or serosanguineous fluid sometimes accumulates in the suprachoroidal space as a consequence of vortex vein obstruction. This tends to be self-limited, but surgical drainage may be necessary if the detachment is severe and persistent.
- Macular pucker: A preretinal membrane forms from RPE and glial cells that have migrated through breaks in the retina. This may cause significant postoperative deficits in vision; treatment is possible with vitrectomy.

- Refractive error changes: Large segmental buckles may induce irregular astigmatism because they asymmetrically indent the globe. Encircling buckles can cause a myopic shift because they tend to elongate the globe.
- Diplopia: This is common in the first few weeks, but generally transient.

POSTOPERATIVE CARE

- Administer topical antibiotics for 1 week.
- Apply topical steroids and dilating eye drops for 1 month to limit inflammation.
- Prescribe oral analgesics for postoperative pain.
- Carefully screen for postoperative complications during clinic follow-up.
- Educate the patient to recognize the signs of new retinal detachments.

Further Reading

Text

Lang GE, Lang GK. Retina. In: *Ophthalmology: A Pocket Textbook Atlas*. 2nd ed. New York: Georg Thieme Verlag; 2007:305–372.

Schwartz SG, Flynn HW. Primary retinal detachment: scleral buckle or pars plana vitrectomy? *Curr Opin Ophthalmol*. 2006;17(3):245–250.

Sodhi A, Leung LS, Do DV, et al. Recent trends in the management of rhegmatogenous retinal detachment. *Surv Ophthalmol*. 2008;53(1):50–67.

Williams GA. Scleral buckling surgery. In: Yanoff M, Duker J, eds. *Ophthalmology*. 3rd ed. Philadelphia, PA: Mosby; 2009:530–533.

Primary Sources

Brazitikos PD, Androudi S, Christen WG, et al. Primary pars plana vitrectomy versus scleral buckle surgery for the treatment of pseudophakic retinal detachment: a randomized clinical trial. *Retina*. 2005;25(8):957–964.

Covert DJ, Wirostko WJ, Han DP, et al. Risk factors for scleral buckle removal: a matched, case-control study. *Am J Ophthalmol*. 2008;146(3):434–439.

Gopal L, D'Souza CM, Bhende M, et al. Scleral buckling: implant versus explant. *Retina*. 2003;23(5):636–640.

Mahdizadeh M, Masoumpour M, Ashraf H. Anatomical retinal reattachment after scleral buckling with and without retinopexy: a pilot study. *Acta Ophthalmol*. 2008;86(3):297–301.

CHAPTER 9

Trauma

C. Robert Bernardino and John J. Huang

9.1 CANTHOTOMY/CANTHOLYSIS

- These procedures involve transection of the inferior limb of the lateral canthal tendon to relieve excess pressure within the orbit and globe.

INDICATIONS

- Severe or progressive retrobulbar (orbital) hemorrhage causing orbital compartment syndrome with risk of permanent blindness.
  - Retrobulbar hemorrhage must be ruled out in all cases of blunt facial trauma.
  - It may also arise following orbital surgery, aggressive blepharoplasty, endoscopic sinus surgery, or traumatic retrobulbar injection.
  - Canthotomy/cantholysis is also used to expose the lateral orbital wall or during entropion/ectropion repair.

ALTERNATIVES

Medical Therapy

- Small orbital bleeds may be self-limited and resolve without adverse consequences. If there is no evidence of optic neuropathy, intraocular pressure (IOP) can be controlled with mannitol and carbonic anhydrase inhibitors.
- Due to the potential for devastating visual consequences, however, the threshold for surgical decompression should be very low.

RELEVANT PHYSIOLOGY/ANATOMY

Orbital Compartment Syndrome

- The orbital contents, including the optic nerve and globe, are contained within a dense fascial sheath anteriorly defined by the orbital septum and bony cone with a fixed volume.
- Anterior movement of the globe is limited by the fibrous tarsal plates, which are anchored to the orbital rim by the medial and lateral canthal tendons.
- Small increases in orbital volume can be offset by globe proptosis and orbital fat prolapse; larger increases very rapidly elevate the orbital and intraocular pressures.
- As the orbital pressure approaches the systolic pressure of the central retinal artery and optic nerve feeder vessels, perfusion of the nerve and retina are compromised, resulting in ischemia. Increases in pressure can also cause damage via direct compression of the optic nerve.

Lateral Canthus

- An acute angle formed by convergence of the superior and inferior lid margins near the lateral orbital rim.
- The lateral canthal tendon anchors the canthal angle to Whitnall's tubercle on the inner margin of the lateral orbital rim. It consists of a superior limb emanating from the superior tarsus and an inferior limb from the inferior tarsus.
- Lateral division of the canthus (canthotomy) separates the superior and inferior lid margins, but leaves the limbs of the canthal tendon intact. Only transection of the inferior limb (cantholysis) produces significant orbital decompression.

PREOPERATIVE SCREENING

- Gross exam: Check the suspected eye for proptosis, decreased extraocular motility, tight and edematous lids, chemosis, and conjunctival hemorrhage. Also assess the integrity of the orbital rim to rule out associated fractures.

- Pupillary exam: Carefully observe for a relative afferent pupillary defect, which suggests the presence of unilateral optic neuropathy.
- Tonometry: Increased orbital pressure is usually transmitted to the globe; IOP should fall with appropriate decompression.
- Vision: Check visual acuity and color vision.
- Fundus exam: Observe for papilledema, central retinal artery pulsations, and choroidal folds. Venous pulsations may be seen in normal eyes, but arterial pulsations suggest increased IOP with compromised perfusion. Choroidal folds indicate external compression of globe.
- Retrobulbar hemorrhage is a clinical diagnosis and use of imaging or other ancillary tests must not delay intervention. The following modalities may be useful in equivocal cases or may have been ordered prior to consultation:
  - CT scan: Orbital images rarely reveal focal collections of blood; look for diffuse infiltration of the orbital fat accompanied by globe proptosis. Generally speaking, more than half of the globe should be posterior to a line drawn between the medial and lateral orbital rim on axial slices. The optic nerve makes a gentle "S" curve through orbit; if straight ("on stretch"), there has been a significant increase in orbital volume. In severe cases, the taut optic nerve will deform ("tent") the posterior globe.
  - Bedside ultrasound: This is less time consuming than a CT scan, but requires a skilled operator.

ANESTHESIA

- After cleaning, the skin surrounding the lateral canthus is infiltrated with 1% to 2% lidocaine containing epinephrine to aid hemostasis. The needle is directed laterally to avoid inadvertent penetration of the globe.
- *Note:* with significant lid swelling, the tissue edema and accompanying acidosis may decrease the efficacy of local anesthetic.

PROCEDURE

1. *Premedication:* Pharmacologic reduction of the IOP is often used in conjunction with surgical

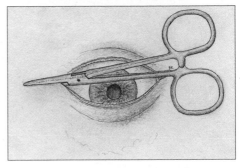

FIGURE 9.1.1 ◆ *Cross Clamping:* A hemostat can be placed across the full thickness of the lateral canthus to aid hemostasis and improve subsequent visualization.

decompression of the orbit. Mannitol and carbonic anhydrase inhibitors are typically used. Corticosteroids may be administered if a traumatic component to the observed optic neuropathy is suspected. Medications to control pain, agitation, and emesis are given on a case-by-case basis.

2. *Cross Clamping:* Place a straight clamp or hemostat across the full thickness of the lateral canthus (FIG. 9.1.1). Focal tissue compression for up to a minute aids hemostasis and improves visualization during subsequent steps of the procedure.

3. *Canthotomy:* After removing the hemostat, the crushed tissue is incised with laterally directed scissors (FIG. 9.1.2).

4. *Cantholysis:* The inferior limb of the canthal tendon is placed on tension with toothed forceps

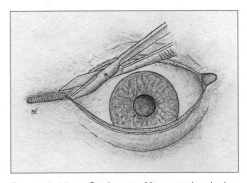

FIGURE 9.1.2 ◆ *Canthotomy:* After removing the hemostat, the crushed tissue is incised with laterally directed scissors. This provides access to the inferior limb of the canthal tendon, but does not release a significant amount of orbital pressure.

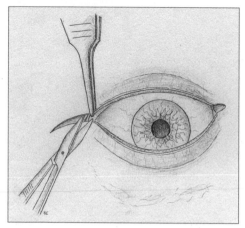

FIGURE 9.1.3 ◆ *Cantholysis:* The inferior limb of the canthal tendon is placed on tension with toothed forceps lifted toward the ceiling and transected with scissors pointed toward the patient's nose. When the inferior limb of the canthal tendon has been successfully cut, the lower lid should pull away from globe completely.

and transected with scissors pointed toward the patient's nose (FIG. 9.1.3). Visualization is often poor due to bleeding and tissue edema, so the procedure may need to be done by feel. When the inferior limb of the canthal tendon has been successfully cut, the lower lid should pull away from globe completely. Large quantities of blood may not extravasate after decompression, but exploration of the globe should be avoided due to the risk of traumatic damage.

COMPLICATIONS

1. *Bleeding:* This is anticipated but usually resolves without cauterization of the cut vessels. If persist-

ent, hemostasis can usually be achieved by applying pressure over the lateral orbital rim.

2. *Incomplete decompression:* It is essential to complete the cantholysis as inadequate decompression can result in irreversible optic neuropathy and blindness.

POSTOPERATIVE CARE

• Recheck the IOP and visual acuity after decompression to confirm improvement.

• Periodically apply ice packs to reduce lid edema.

• The lower lid may spontaneously heal without the need for additional surgery. If canthoplasty is required for cosmetic reasons, it may be completed within 1 to 2 weeks.

Further Reading

Text

Goodall KL, Brahma A, Bates A, et al. Lateral canthotomy and inferior cantholysis: an effective method of urgent orbital decompression for sight threatening acute retrobulbar haemorrhage. *Injury.* 1999;30(7):485–490.

Lima V, Burt B, Leibovitch I, et al. Orbital compartment syndrome: the ophthalmic surgical emergency. *Surv Ophthalmol.* 2009;54(4):441–449.

Vassallo S, Hartstein M, Howard D, et al. Traumatic retrobulbar hemorrhage: emergent decompression by lateral canthotomy and cantholysis. *J Emerg Med.* 2002;22(3):251–256.

Wagner P, Lang GK. The eyelids. In: *Ophthalmology: A Pocket Textbook Atlas.* 2nd ed. New York, NY: Georg Thieme Verlag; 2007:17–49.

Primary Sources

Yung CW, Moorthy RS, Lindley D, et al. Efficacy of lateral canthotomy and cantholysis in orbital hemorrhage. *Ophthal Plast Reconstr Surg.* 1994;10(2):137–141.

9.2 LID AND CANALICULAR LACERATION REPAIR

• Surgical repair of damage to the eyelids and/or lacrimal drainage system:
  • Simple suture approximation of the affected layers is generally adequate, but significant tissue loss may require use of flaps or grafts.

• Canalicular lacerations should be suspected with injury to the medial lid and require stenting of the drainage system to preserve patency.

INDICATIONS

- Traumatic damage to the lids, including lacerations, deep abrasions, tissue avulsion, puncture wounds, and blunt trauma.
- Patient stabilization takes precedence over lid repair.
- Cases requiring special management include:
  - Lid margin injuries: Particular care is required because improper repair may lead to serious ocular surface defects.
  - Canalicular injuries: Careful repair of the lacrimal drainage system is critical to preventing chronic epiphora and associated complications.

ALTERNATIVES

Conservative Management

- Some superficial injuries can be adequately treated with lid taping.
- Some puncture wounds can be permitted to heal by granulation if underlying structures have not been damaged.

RELEVANT PHYSIOLOGY/ANATOMY

Lid Anatomy (See Fig. 9.2.1A, B)

Lacrimal Drainage System Anatomy (See Fig. 9.2.2)

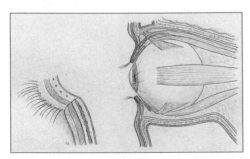

Figure 9.2.1 ◆ *Lid and lid margin anatomy:* The anterior lid lamella consists of skin and orbicularis; the posterior lamella consists of tarsus, lid retractors, and palpebral conjunctiva. The gray line is formed by the orbicularis fibers and delineates the lamellae at the lid margin. The meibomian gland orifices can be seen posterior to the gray line as can the mucocutaneous line, which marks the border between the tarsal plate and adherent palpebral conjunctiva.

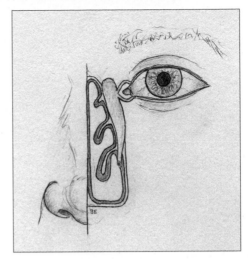

Figure 9.2.2 ◆ *Lacrimal drainage system anatomy:* The upper lacrimal drainage system consists of the superior and inferior puncta, superior and inferior canaliculi, common internal punctum, and lacrimal sac. The lower system consists of the valve of Hasner, nasolacrimal duct, and nasal mucosa exit below inferior turbinate.

PREOPERATIVE ASSESSMENT

- Obtain a complete history, including timing and mechanism of injury, immunization status of patient and if animal bite involved (e.g., tetanus, rabies), and anticoagulant use.
- Document injuries with photographs and/or illustrations that include measurements of all defects.
- Retrobulbar hemorrhage must be ruled out due to the risk of permanent vision loss. Signs and symptoms include severe pain, reduced ocular motility and visual acuity, as well as increased intraocular pressure (IOP), edema, proptosis, and ecchymosis. If suspicion is high, perform a lateral canthotomy and cantholysis to decompress the orbit and prevent compressive optic neuropathy (see Chapter 9.1 Canthotomy/Cantholysis).
- Clarify the depth of the injury and the anatomical structures involved with a detailed external and slit lamp exam. Devote special attention to examining the lid margin and lacrimal drainage system and to assessing tissue loss.
- Palpate the facial and orbital bones for crepitus, step-offs, and instability. Computed tomography (CT) images of the face and orbits should be

obtained if the exam or mechanism of injury suggests fracture.

- Check medial and lateral canthal tendon integrity to rule out traumatic dehiscence. This is accomplished by pulling the lid laterally and medially while observing movement of the puncta and lateral canthal angle, respectively (normally ≤1 to 2 mm).

- Rule out traumatic injury of the levator aponeurosis by assessing levator excursion (the difference in lid position between downgaze and upgaze). Normal excursion ranges from 16 to 20 mm; lower values suggest potential damage.

- Obtain baseline measurements with a Hertel's exophthalmometer because enophthalmos is a common long-term consequence of trauma. Conversely, retrobulbar hemorrhage can produce proptosis. Anticipated normal values differ slightly based on race and gender. A difference between the eyes greater than 2 to 3 mm suggests a unilateral or asymmetric process.

- Assess visual acuity and check for an afferent pupillary defect (APD), which suggests unilateral or asymmetric damage to the retina or optic nerve.

- Probe and irrigate the canalicular system to assess integrity if there is any suspicion of injury. Saline should freely drain through the ipsilateral nare. Punctal reflux or wound site leakage is abnormal and should prompt further investigation.

ANESTHESIA

- Local infiltration of lidocaine with epinephrine can be used for most repairs. Adding hyaluronidase facilitates anesthetic distribution and decreases tissue distortion.

- Regional blocks that target branches of the trigeminal nerve produce less tissue swelling than local injections. Infraorbital, supraorbital, supratrochlear, and infratrochlear blocks are commonly used when repairing injuries to the ocular adnexa.

- General anesthesia may be required for young children and patients with complex defects or bony involvement.

- Topical anesthesia must be applied to the nasal mucosa prior to passing a silicon stent during canalicular laceration repair.

PROCEDURE

1. *Repair Timing:* If the patient can be stabilized, lid repairs are ideally conducted between 12 and 24 hours of injury. This permits reduction of tissue edema, which is particularly important for identifying the cut ends of a lacerated canaliculus. If repair is delayed, the wounds should be covered with saline-moistened dressings to prevent tissue desiccation. It is also prudent to place a protective eye shield to prevent further damage.

2. *Medications:* It may be necessary to update the patient's tetanus immunization. Antibiotic prophylaxis is particularly important in cases of human or animal bites.

3. *General Principles:*
   - Prior to repair, it is important to irrigate the wound and remove embedded debris. Any devitalized tissue should be débrided.
   - An operative plan is then developed that addresses each damaged structure.
   - Penetration of the orbital septum can lead to fat prolapse and levator aponeurosis injury. If present, this is addressed with suture repair of the levator and overlying orbicularis. The orbital septum itself should not be closed due to the potential for postoperative lid retraction.
   - Even without septal involvement, defects in the orbicularis should be reapproximated to avoid the development of lid contour irregularities.
   - Skin can be closed with a running stitch, but interrupted sutures are preferred if the wound margins are irregular. Skin edges should be slightly everted during repair.

4. *Lid Margin Repair:* Careful approximation is essential to prevent lid notching and other defects that may damage the ocular surface.
   - *Tarsal Reconstruction:* Irregular tarsal lacerations should be trimmed to produce even surfaces (FIG. 9.2.1). A temporary suture can then be passed through the meibomian gland orifices on either side of the defect. Applying tension to this suture ensures even apposition of the cut tarsal edges (FIG. 9.2.2). Interrupted partial-thickness sutures are then placed to reapproximate the tarsus (FIG. 9.2.3).
   - *Lid Margin Reconstruction:* The lid margin is realigned by passing fine silk sutures through the gray line and posterior lash line. A third

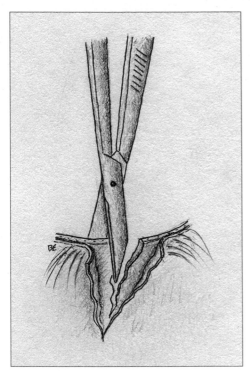

FIGURE 9.2.3 ✦ Irregular tarsal lacerations can be trimmed to produce even surfaces that can be closely approximated.

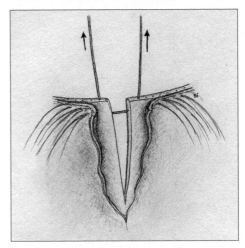

FIGURE 9.2.4 ✦ A temporary suture can then be passed through the meibomian gland orifices on either side of the defect. Applying tension to this suture ensures even apposition of the cut tarsal edges.

is only 1 to 1.5 mm in diameter, however, and the distal end may be hard to identify if there is significant tissue swelling. In difficult cases, dilute fluorescein or another distinctive liquid can be injected into the opposite canaliculus

suture through the mucocutaneous margin offers additional stability (FIG. 9.2.4). Sutures should enter and exit the lid margin 2 mm from the laceration and travel 2 mm deep within the lid tissue (FIG. 9.2.5). After they are tied, the tails are left long and tied away from the globe for easy identification and to guard against corneal abrasion.

- *Superficial Closure:* The orbicularis and skin are closed independently with interrupted sutures (FIG. 9.2.6). To prevent corneal irritation, the lid margin suture tails can be incorporated into the knots of the skin sutures (FIG. 9.2.7).

5. *Canalicular Laceration:* Repair entails identification of the cut canalicular ends, stenting of the lacrimal system, and suture repair.
   - *Canalicular Identification:* Several methods exist for identifying the cut canalicular ends. The simplest entails inserting a punctal probe. As it is advanced, the probe should exit the proximal cut end of the canaliculus, and point to the distal cut end (FIG. 9.2.8). The canaliculus

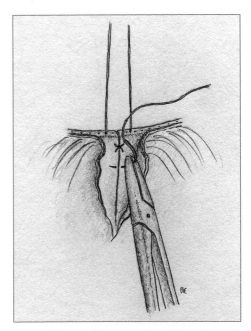

FIGURE 9.2.5 ✦ *Tarsal sutures:* Interrupted partial-thickness sutures are then placed to reapproximate the tarsus.

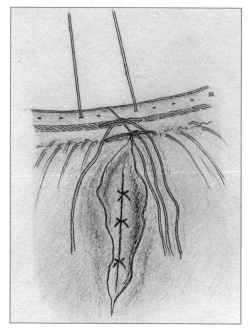

FIGURE 9.2.6 ✦ *Lid margin sutures:* The margin is re-aligned by passing fine silk sutures through the gray line and posterior eyelash line. A third suture can be placed through the mucocutaneous margin for additional stability.

to facilitate identification (FIG. 9.2.9A). Alternatively, the surgical site can be flooded with saline. Air injected into the opposite canaliculus will then produce bubbles at the distal cut end (FIG. 9.2.9B).

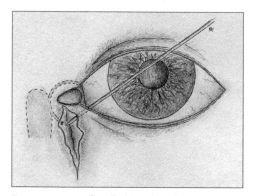

FIGURE 9.2.7 ✦ *Canalicular probing:* Several methods exist for identifying the cut canalicular ends. The simplest entails inserting a punctal probe. As it is advanced, the probe should exit the proximal cut end, and point to the distal cut end. The canaliculus is 1 to 1.5 mm in diameter and the distal end may be hard to identify in the setting of significant tissue edema.

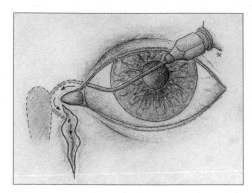

FIGURE 9.2.8 ✦ *Canalicular irrigation:* In difficult cases with significant tissue swelling, dilute fluorescein or another distinctive liquid can be injected into the opposite canaliculus to facilitate identification of the distal cut end.

- *Stenting:* After the proximal and distal cut ends are identified, a silicone stent with metal probes attached to both ends is threaded through the canaliculi and passed down the nasolacrimal duct into the ipsilateral nare. The probes are then removed, and the free ends of the stent are tied.
- *Suture Repair:* After stenting, end-to-end anastomosis of the cut canaliculus is performed with fine sutures. Alternatively, the ends can be indirectly approximated by placing horizontal

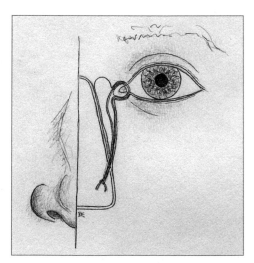

FIGURE 9.2.9 ✦ *Canalicular intubation:* After the proximal and distal cut ends have been identified, a silicone stent with attached metal probes is threaded through the canaliculi and passed down the nasolacrimal duct into the ipsilateral nare. The probes are then removed, and the free ends of the stent are tied.

mattress sutures in the adjacent lid tissue. The cut ends will then heal together over the stent.

COMPLICATIONS

1. Corneal erosion may be caused by the initial injury, aggressive cleaning, abrasion from suture tails or knots, or postoperative lid retraction.
2. Ptosis can become apparent with the resolution of tissue edema if levator aponeurosis injuries were not initially identified and repaired.
3. Infection of the lids is rare because they are highly vascular, but it may occur with inadequate cleaning, debridement, or antibiotic prophylaxis.

POSTOPERATIVE CARE

- Apply ice compresses and elevate the head of bed for 48 hours to decrease postoperative swelling, then switch to warm compresses.
- Apply antibiotic ointment to the wound for 2 to 3 days.
- Prescribe nonsteroidal anti-inflammatory drugs (NSAIDs) or mild narcotic medications for pain management.
- Alert the patient to signs of wound infection, including escalating pain, erythema, edema, or purulent discharge. Caution to avoid heavy lifting or Valsalva to prevent additional bleeding or dehiscence.

- Remove the skin sutures at 5 to 7 days for optimal cosmetic results (lengthier placement will result in more prominent scarring). The lid margin sutures should remain in place for 10 to 14 days to ensure a stable repair.
- During the cicatricial phase of wound healing (3 to 4 weeks), the patient can reduce contraction by massaging the scar.
- Leave canalicular stents in place for at least 3 months. Earlier removal may result in stricture formation and chronic epiphora.

Further Reading

Text

Green JP, Cheronis GC, Goldberg RA. Eyelid trauma and reconstructive techniques. In: Yanoff M, Duker J, eds. *Ophthalmology.* 3rd ed. Philadelphia, PA: Mosby; 2009:1443–1449.

Nelson CC. Management of eyelid trauma. *Aust N Z J Ophthalmol.* 1991;19(4):357–363.

Reifler DM. Management of canalicular laceration. *Surv Ophthalmol.* 1991;36(2):113–132.

Wagner P, Lang GK. The eyelids. In: *Ophthalmology: A Pocket Textbook Atlas.* 2nd ed. New York, NY: Georg Thieme Verlag; 2007:17–49.

Primary Sources

Jordan DR, Ziai S, Gilberg SM, Mawn LA. Pathogenesis of canalicular lacerations. *Ophthal Plast Reconstr Surg.* 2008;24(5):394–398.

Slonim CB. Dog bite-induced canalicular lacerations: a review of 17 cases. *Ophthal Plast Reconstr Surg.* 1996;12(3): 218–222.

9.3 ORBITAL FLOOR FRACTURE REPAIR

- Repair of orbital floor fracture and placement of implant to prevent entrapment of orbital tissue and prevent or reverse enophthalmos after traumatic injury

of the area of the orbital floor, or extraocular muscle entrapment:

- Inferior rectus: most commonly entrapped muscle

INDICATIONS

- Most commonly done for floor fractures significant enough to cause diplopia within 30 degrees of primary gaze, enophthalmos greater than 2 mm, fracture greater than 50%

ALTERNATIVES

Medical Therapy (for minor floor fractures)
- Prophylactic oral antibiotics
- Short course of oral prednisone (expedites resolution of orbital and muscle edema)

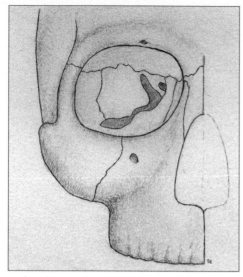

FIGURE 9.3.1 ◆ *Orbital anatomy:* The orbit is a conical structure with contributions from the frontal, lacrimal, ethmoid, zygomatic, maxillary, palatine, and sphenoid bones.

- Nasal decongestants (*Note:* Blowing the nose can lead to worsening orbital emphysema if medial wall is also fractured, due to communication with ethmoid sinus.)

RELEVANT PHYSIOLOGY/ANATOMY

Orbital Anatomy (FIG. 9.3.1)

- Orbital floor bones: maxilla, zygomatic bone (laterally), and palatine bone (posteriorly)
- Medial wall bones (from anterior to posterior): frontal process of maxilla (strongest bone), lacrimal bone, ethmoid bone (lamina papyracea: largest contribution), and lesser wing of sphenoid bone (optic nerve traverses through adjacent canal).
- Orbital foramina/opening (See table below)

Floor Fracture Theories

- Hydraulic or "Blowout" Theory: A blunt object hits globe leading to a sudden increase in intraocular pressure (IOP). This rapid pressure increase leads to compression of the orbit with fracturing of the orbital bones at their weakest points (most commonly the floor, posteriorly and medially to the infraorbital canal).
- Buckling Theory: A blunt object hits inferior orbital rim, compressing it, and causing buckling of the orbital floor, which fractures at the weakest point.

PREOPERATIVE SCREENING

- Involves complete H&P (history and physical), VA (visual acuity) measurement and pupillary function, visual fields measurement, and ocular motility exam
- Specifically, assess for:
  - Proptosis: concern for retrobulbar or peribulbar hemorrhage
  - Enophthalmos: outward fracturing of orbit increasing orbital volume
  - Diplopia: particularly vertical as inferior rectus is most commonly entrapped
  - Extraocular motility exam: forced ductions help determine entrapment of muscle or fascia
  - Bony step-offs and point tenderness of orbital rim: assess for palpable fractures
  - Ipsilateral hypesthesia of cheek and upper gum: infraorbital nerve contusion or damage
- Seidel test: application of fluorescein to assess for leakage and rule out globe rupture
- High-resolution orbital CT (computed tomography; axial and coronal views) without contrast to visualize bony defects

Foramen/Canals	Nerves Passing Through	Vessels Passing Through
Optic canal	Optic nerve	Ophthalmic artery
Superior orbital fissure	CN III (superior and inferior divisions); CN IV; CN V_1 (lacrimal, frontal, and nasociliary branches); CN VI; and sympathetic fibers from cavernous sinus	Ophthalmic vein (superior and inferior divisions)
Inferior orbital fissure	CN V_2 (maxillary nerve)	Infraorbital artery and vein
Infraorbital foramen	Infraorbital nerve	Infraorbital artery and vein
Supraorbital foramen	Supraorbital nerve	Supraorbital artery and vein

CN, cranial nerve.

TABLE 9.3.1 Rapid Review of Steps

(1) Prep and drape.
(2) Inject local anesthetic in lower lid extending to lateral orbital rim.
(3) Place lower lid traction suture.
(4) Perform lateral canthotomy and cantholysis (optional; provides greater floor exposure for larger fractures).
(5) Incise transconjunction.
(6) Place conjunctival traction suture.
(7) Dissect periosteum plus elevation.
(8) Remove prolapsed or entrapped tissue (case-specific).
(9) Implant placement.
(10) Close periosteum.
(11) Close conjunctiva.
(12) Close lateral canthotomy incision.

- Timing of surgical repair is controversial. For typical adult floor fractures, the general consensus is to perform the surgery within 2 weeks of the initial trauma in order to prevent fibrosis and/or tissue contracture.

ANESTHESIA

- General anesthesia is required. Local lidocaine is injected into lower lid margin prior to first incision.

PROCEDURE

See Tables 9.3.1 Rapid Review of Steps and 9.3.2 Surgical Pearls, and Web Tables 9.3.1 to 9.3.4 for equipment and medication lists.

The following narrative describes a transconjunctival incision (vs. transcutaneous) with lateral canthotomy and cantholysis. The lateral canthotomy and cantholysis permits broader exposure for significant floor fractures but is not always necessary for simpler cases. This summary is intended to illustrate basic principles of an orbital floor fracture repair, which can be abstracted to other cases.

1. *Placement of traction suture:* 1% to 2% lidocaine with epinephrine is first injected into the lower lid margin extending temporally to the lateral canthus and to the depth of the lateral orbital rim. A traction suture is placed centrally through the lower lid margin to the depth of the tarsus (through the meibomian orifices). With inferior traction, the lid is adequately everted allowing for exposure of the palpebral conjunctiva.

2. *Lateral canthotomy and cantholysis:* After adequate lidocaine/epinephrine is given, a 1 to 1.5 cm incision is then placed at the lateral canthus extending temporally toward the orbital rim. Using scissors, this incision is completed (full-thickness). The lower lid is elevated with forceps to visualize the lateral canthus tendon. Using sharp scissors with the tips pointing toward the nose,

TABLE 9.3.2 Surgical Pearls

Preoperative:
- Reviewing preoperative imaging (CT scan of orbits with axial and coronal cuts) is essential.
- Exophthalmometry (Hertel) is important to determine amount of enophthalmos present.
- Motility examination helps determine limitation of gaze, which correlates with the fracture pattern.
- Forced ductions is helpful to determine if soft tissue or muscle is entrapped in the fracture. The presence of entrapment may necessitate more urgent surgical intervention.

Intraoperative:
- Leave the unoperated eye in the surgical field to allow for comparison. Palpation of the unoperated and operated eye as well as direct observation allow for evaluation of correction of enophthalmos.
- Forced ductions prior to incision; after releasing entrapped tissue, placement of implant, and wound closure is key. This ensures that entrapment is improved, and that placement of the implant or wound closure does not induce entrapment.
- Wound closure should NOT include the orbital septum. This will cause lower eyelid retraction.

Postoperative:
- No nose blowing for the first 2 weeks after surgery. Consider nasal decongestants during the postoperative period.
- Perioperative and postoperative steroids may help decrease anticipated postoperative edema which may limit evaluation of motility.

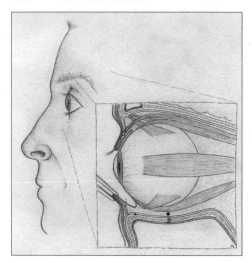

FIGURE 9.3.2 ✦ *Surgical approach to floor fractures:* A parasaggital section of the orbit demonstrating anatomical relationships; the dashed arrow represents the surgical plane for the transconjunctival incision, which is anterior to the orbital septum. The depicted orbital floor fracture (solid arrow) is accessed by elevating the periosteum of the orbital floor.

the tendon is cut allowing adequate exposure of the lower lid conjunctiva.

3. *Transconjunctival approach* (FIGS. 9.3.2 & 9.3.3): The lower lid is held taut by the traction suture. Using sharp scissors, an incision is placed at the inferior border of the tarsus. This surgical plane is extended posterior to the orbicularis oculi muscle and anterior to the orbital septum. Con-

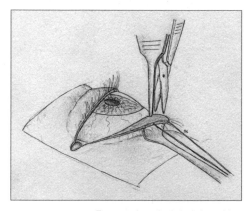

FIGURE 9.3.3 ✦ *Transconjunctival incision:* After passing a traction suture through the lower lid margin, the lid is everted over a Desmarres retractor. This exposes the surgical incision site inferior to the tarsal plate.

tinuing deeper in the surgical plane, the orbital rim is identified. *Note:* This approach to the orbital rim is entirely preseptal.

4. *Conjunctival traction suture:* Once the orbital rim has been identified, a traction suture is placed through the conjunctiva and clipped superiorly (toward the head of the patient) in order to provide adequate exposure of the orbital rim while covering and protecting the globe.

5. *Periosteal elevation* (FIGS. 9.3.3 & 9.3.4): Using a scalpel or Bovie electrocautery, an incision is placed through the periosteum just inferior to the orbital rim (FIG. 9.3.4). Using a sharp periosteal elevator, the periosteum is lifted off of the bone, starting medially and extending laterally and posteriorly into the orbit (FIG. 9.3.5). Once the fracture site is identified, the periosteal dissection must be continued to the most posterior extent of the fracture line. Prolapsed or entrapped orbital tissue is carefully dissected away from the fracture site. For significant floor fractures, care must be taken during this step to avoid the infraorbital groove so as to not damage the neurovascular bundle located there.

6. *Implant placement* (FIG. 9.3.5): Once all entrapped orbital tissue is free, an implant fitted to

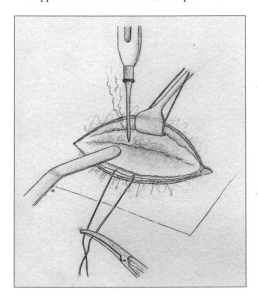

FIGURE 9.3.4 ✦ *Periosteal incision:* After the surgical field has been exposed with placement of a conjunctival traction suture, blunt dissection is carried down to the periosteum overlying the orbital rim. While pressure is applied to the orbital septum with a maleable retractor, the periosteum is incised with a scalpel or electrocautery.

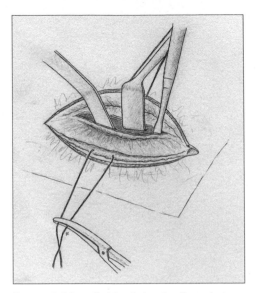

FIGURE 9.3.5 ✦ *Periosteal elevation:* The periosteum is then raised from the underlying orbital floor using a periosteal elevator. Retractors facilitate floor exposure and permit identification of the fracture site.

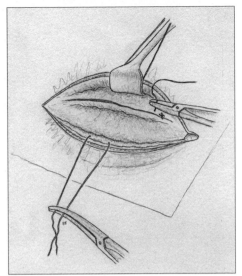

FIGURE 9.3.7 ✦ *Periosteal closure:* The orbital rim periosteum is then reapproximated with sutures. In some instances, this closure is suffcient to stabilize the orbital floor implant. In others, additional stability can be achieved by suturing or screw fixation of the implant.

the site of the fracture can be placed to prevent subsequent prolapse and entrapment. A forced duction test of the inferior rectus can be performed to ensure adequate release of the entrapped muscle (FIG. 9.3.6). Various implant materials can be used based on the clinical scenario. These include polyethylene, metallic mesh, metallic plates, resorbable materials, or silicone plates. These implants can be sutured to the

orbital rim, nailed to the orbital floor, or held in place by periosteal closure.

7. *Closing of periorbita:* The periosteum that was initially incised over the orbital rim is closed over the implant using interrupted sutures with a 5-0 polyglactin (Vicryl, Ethicon, Somerville, NJ). This prevents anterior displacement of the implant (FIG. 9.3.7).

8. *Closing of conjunctiva* (FIGS. 9.3.8 & 9.3.9)*:* Both traction sutures are removed and the conjunctiva is closed with a fine running suture.

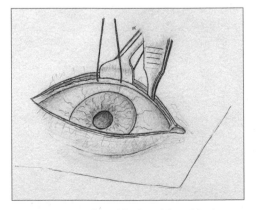

FIGURE 9.3.6 ✦ *Forced ductions:* A forced duction test is performed wih forceps to ensure that inferior rectus entrapment has been alleviated with blunt dissection and implant placement.

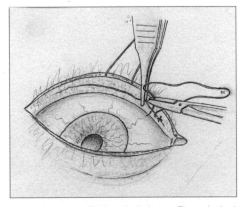

FIGURE 9.3.8 ✦ *Conjunctival closure:* The palpebral conjunctiva is then reapproximated with sutures.

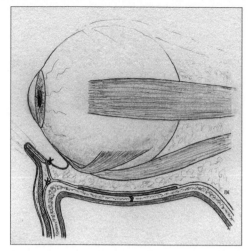

FIGURE 9.3.9 ◆ *Implant in situ:* Parasagittal section of the orbit demonstrating implant placement between the orbital floor periosteum and orbital floor fracture. This prevents subsequent soft tissue entrapment or enophthalmos. Suture closure of the orbital rim periosteum and palpebral conjunctiva is also demonstrated.

9. *Closing of lateral canthotomy incision:* After adequate hemostasis, the lateral commissure is reformed with an interrupted resorbable suture (with careful attention to realign the gray line). The skin is closed with a simple running suture.

COMPLICATIONS

Intraoperative

- Optic nerve injury from retractors, pupillary reaction, or looking for an afferent pupillary defect (APD) would all indicate injury
- Excessive globe pressure from retractors leading to decreased visual acuity due to optic nerve injury

Postoperative

- Orbital hemorrhage: inadequate cauterization, vessel tear on bony edge (Patient presents with proptosis, orbital pain, and decreased visual acuity.)
- Persistent or new-onset diplopia: may resolve spontaneously or require subsequent strabismus

surgery. (*Note:* Forced duction test intraoperatively ensures adequate inferior rectus mobility.)

- Dysesthesias: burning, tingling, or numbness in infraorbital nerve distribution
- Implant extrusion
- Late enophthalmos due to orbital fat atrophy

POSTOPERATIVE CARE

- Assess VA and pupillary reflexes frequently in first 2 hours postoperatively.
- Follow up in clinic within 24 hours to screen for complications.
- Elevate patient's head to at least 30 degrees to improve drainage and minimize inflammation.
- Systemic antibiotics (i.e., first generation cephalosporin) and nasal decongestants should be given for 1 week.
- Apply topical antibiotic ointment on incision for 1 week plus mild analgesia.
- Oral steroids should be given to reduce swelling (but is not always given).
- Skin sutures should be removed around 1 week.

Further Reading

Text

Dutton JJ. Atlas of clinical and surgical anatomy. Philadelphia, PA: WB Saunders; 1994.

Dutton JJ. Orbital surgery. In: Yanoff M, Duker J, eds. *Ophthalmology*. 3rd ed. Philadelphia, PA: Mosby; 2009:1466–1473.

Whitcher J, Riordan-Eva P. *Vaughan and Asbury's General Ophthalmology*. New York, NY: Lange Medical Books/ McGraw-Hill; 2004.

Primary Sources

Greenwald HS, Keeney AR, Shannon GM. A review of 128 patients with orbital fractures. *Am J Ophthalmol.* 1974;78:655–664.

Putterman AM, Stevens T, Urist MJ. Nonsurgical management of blow-out fractures of the orbital floor. *Am J Ophthalmol.* 1974;77:232–239.

Smith B, Regan WFJ. Blow-out fracture of the orbit. Mechanism and correction of internal orbital fracture. *Am J Ophthalmol.* 1957;44:733–738.

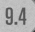

9.4

OPEN GLOBE REPAIR

- Suture closure of a globe that has been damaged by penetrating, perforating, or blunt trauma

INDICATIONS

- With an open globe, prompt evaluation and closure is essential to prevent endophthalmitis and other vision-threatening complications.
- Treatment of life-threatening injuries, however, always takes precedence.
- Types of open globe injuries include:
  - Penetrating or perforating trauma: full-thickness penetration of the cornea or of the conjunctiva and sclera. A projectile may enter and exit the eye, or be retained as an intraocular foreign body (IOFB). If the foreign body is not inert, it may cause infection or inflammation and must be removed prior to closure.
  - Blunt trauma: significant blunt trauma can cause ocular rupture. This is particularly likely upon contact with objects smaller in diameter than the orbital rim. In eyes without prior surgery, rupture most often occurs under the rectus muscle insertions, where the sclera is thinnest. Other anatomical locations at risk from rupture include the corneal limbus and optic nerve insertion. Rupture is more common, however, at prior surgical incision sites, which do not regain full strength, even after normal wound healing. Large incisions, such as those made for penetrating keratoplasty (see Chapter 3.1 Keratoplasty), confer the highest risk of traumatic rupture.

ALTERNATIVES

Medical Therapy
- Antibiotic prophylaxis may be adequate if the penetrating injury forms a small, self-sealing flap with no retained IOFB.

Surgery
Alternative and Adjunctive Techniques
- Pars plana vitrectomy (PPV): Superficial closure alone may be adequate in many cases, but adjunctive PPV is necessary in the presence of endophthalmitis, significant intraocular trauma, or noninert posterior segment IOFBs.
- Cyanoacrylate glue: If the edges of a corneal wound are small and linear with no prolapse of intraocular contents, cyanoacrylate glue or other tissue adhesives can be used to seal the wound in conjunction with a bandage contact lens. The duration of efficacy, however, is more variable than suture closure.

OCULAR TRAUMA OVERVIEW

Classification
- Open vs. closed globe injury: It is very important to make this distinction on the initial exam, because these injuries have very different treatment algorithms and risk profiles.
- Mechanism of injury (MOI): Details of the injury should be elicited with a careful history. This can provide important clues as to whether the trauma was blunt or penetrating, as well as to the likelihood that an IOFB is present.
- IOFBs:
  - May cause aqueous leakage with loss of anterior chamber depth, but often create self-sealing flaps that can disguise the injury.
  - Can rupture the lens capsule, permitting aqueous penetration that leads to edema and traumatic cataract development.
  - May be left in place if they do not pose a risk of additional damage to intraocular structures and are small, inert, and cannot be easily retrieved during primary repair.
  - Special cases necessitating removal include:
    1. Copper IOFBs, which can cause chalcosis, resulting in significant intraocular inflammation
    2. Iron IOFBs, which can cause siderosis that damages photoreceptors
    3. Organic or contaminated IOFBs, which pose a high risk of endophthalmitis

PREOPERATIVE ASSESSMENT

- History: Investigate mechanism of injury, history of ocular surgery, and use of protective eyewear.

A story that involves metal striking on metal or use of cutting or grinding tools should raise suspicion for IOFBs.

- Signs/symptoms: Signs commonly include pain, tearing (epiphora), photophobia, blepharospasm, and variable loss of visual acuity. It may be necessary to use topical anesthetic drops to obtain an adequate exam.

- Document visual function: Poor visual acuity at the time of presentation is predictive of poor long-term visual outcomes. Good vision at presentation is reassuring, but does not rule out the development of vision-threatening complications, such as endophthalmitis. It is also very important to check for an afferent pupillary defect (APD), which suggests significant retinal or optic nerve damage.

- General exam principles: Obtain as complete an exam as possible while protecting the eye from further injury. If the globe is clearly open, a protective shield should be placed and the patient should be taken directly to the operating room (OR) if stable.

- Gross exam: Evaluate for loss of anterior chamber depth, pupil displacement, intraocular tissue prolapse, and hemorrhagic chemosis.

- Slit lamp/external exam: Check the cornea and conjunctiva for lacerations. If lacerations are discovered, the surrounding conjunctiva should be mobilized with an anesthetic-wetted cotton swab to determine whether there is underlying scleral damage. Surgical incision sites should also be examined with particular care.

- Seidel test: Apply fluorescein dye to the ocular surface to see if it is diluted or washed away by leaking aqueous.

- Anterior segment exam: Check for hyphema, hypopyon, cell and flare (signs of inflammation or early infection), pupillary irregularity, iris retroillumination defects (the red reflex of the fundus will be visible through lacerations), and traumatic cataract.

- Posterior segment exam: Check for retinal detachments or tears, IOFBs, and vitreous, retinal or choroidal hemorrhage.

- Ancillary tests: A computed tomography (CT) scan may demonstrate orbital fractures or metallic IOFBs. An ultrasound is useful for detecting nonmetallic IOFBs, posterior scleral rupture, retinal detachment, and subretinal or choroidal hemorrhage.

ANESTHESIA

- General anesthesia (GA) has traditionally been used for open globe repair out of concern that patient movement may increase the risk of intraocular content extrusion. It can, however, result in coughing and vomiting, which can elevate the risk of extrusion and suprachoroidal hemorrhage.

- Succinylcholine is avoided as a GA depolarizing agent because it can induce extraocular muscle contraction, which may increase the risk of extrusion.

- A retrospective study was conducted, suggesting that local anesthesia with intravenous (IV) sedation may be an acceptable alternative for open globe repair in appropriately selected patients.[1] It may be particularly beneficial in the elderly, who are at greater risk of significant complications from general anesthesia.

PROCEDURE

 SEE TABLES 9.4.1 Rapid Review of Steps and 9.4.2 Surgical Pearls, and WEB TABLES 9.4.1 to 9.4.4 for equipment and medication lists.
Open globe repair is highly individualized. Some guiding principles are outlined as follows.

1. *Medications:* Broad-spectrum systemic antibiotics are initially administered to all open globe patients. If there is strong clinical suspicion for endophthalmitis, aqueous and vitreous specimens should be taken for culture and sensitivity. Intraocular antibiotics can be toxic to the tissues they contact and are not routinely used in

TABLE 9.4.1 Rapid Review of Steps
(1) Apply general anesthesia.
(2) Carefully insert eyelid speculum.
(3) Carefully explore the cornea or scleral wound with gentle dissection of the conjunctiva.
(4) Reapproximate corneal and scleral wounds.
(5) Close limbal wound first.
(6) Close corneal wound with 10-0 nylon.
(7) Close scleral wound with 9-0 nylon.
(8) Reform anterior chamber with BSS.
(9) Close Tenon's plus conjunctive with 7-0 Vicryl.
(10) Evaluate the wound closure for leaks.

BSS, balanced salt solution.

TABLE 9.4.2	Surgical Pearls

Preoperative:
- Communicate with the patient that the postoperative course is variable and that it may take a few weeks for recovery.
- Communicate that additional surgeries may be needed. In cases of severe trauma, the eye may need to be eviscerated or enucleated.
- Include in the consent the increased possibility for repeat surgery and the risk of sympathetic ophthalmia.

Intraoperative:
- Perform a thorough evaluation of the open globe to assess the full extent of the wound before starting wound closure. Necrotic iris should be removed before closure. Vitreous in the wound should be removed with a vitrector (if available). Viable intraocular tissue should be replaced into the eye.
- Ensure proper orientation of the corneal and scleral wound to minimize astigmatism.
- The rectus muscle may need to be isolated and removed in cases where the rupture extends under the muscle. After scleral closure, the rectus muscle is reattached with Vicryl suture.
- Avoid unnecessary or excessive manipulation and pressure on the open globe during exploration and suturing. Meticulous closure and evaluation for wound leaks during the surgery can reduce the risk of infection and sympathetic ophthalmia. In addition, gentle wound closure can help with more rapid healing facilitating any additional surgery.
- The corneal wound is closed with interrupted 10-0 nylon sutures. The scleral wound is closed with interrupted 9-0 nylon sutures. All surgical knots should be buried for patient comfort. The conjunctiva is closed with a 7-0 Vicryl suture. The wound should be thoroughly examined for wound leaks after reforming the globe and anterior chamber with BSS. Carefully check for wound leaks with a fluorescein strip. Small corneal wound leaks will often close with the aid of a bandage contact lens.
- If the wound is contaminated or there is an intraocular foreign body present, administer an intravitreal injection of antibiotics.

Postoperative:
- In patients with a large wound, intraocular foreign body, or long duration prior to repair, suspect endophthalmitis if there is significant postoperative inflammation.
- Communicate with the patient that they should not bend, strain, or lift heavy objects until cleared by the primary surgeon.
- Monitor for excessive postoperative inflammation. Consider oral or periocular depot steroids to control excessive inflammation.
- Carefully assess the presence of inflammation in the uninjured eye. Presence of panuveitis in both eyes indicates sympathetic ophthalmia, necessitating aggressive prednisone therapy.

BSS, balanced salt solution.

uncomplicated cases. If the case involves organic contamination, foreign bodies, or significant rupture, an intravitreal antibiotic injection may be warranted at the time of closure due to the increased risk of endophthalmitis. The need for tetanus prophylaxis should also be evaluated based on the patient's vaccination record and the nature of his or her exposure.

2. *Anterior chamber reconstruction:* If intraocular tissue has been extruded from the globe, it may be replaced if clearly viable. Extruded tissue should be excised, however, after prolonged exposure or heavy contamination. Corneal wounds are closed with interrupted nylon sutures to restore anterior chamber integrity. Injecting viscoelastic into a flattened anterior chamber (AC) may help to recreate the original corneal curvature. It must be aspirated following repair to avoid trabecular meshwork congestion and subsequent intraocular pressure (IOP) elevation. Scleral wounds should also be closed with sutures. If scleral rupture occurs beneath a rectus muscle insertion, significant dissection may first be necessary prior to repair.

3. *IOFB removal:* Superficial foreign bodies should be removed at the time of closure if they are readily accessible. If noninert IOFBs are deeply embedded, pars plana vitrectomy must be performed to permit removal with magnetic or grasping tools.

4. *Repair of intraocular damage:* There are two fundamental approaches:
    a. Delayed repair: The surface wound is closed immediately but vitrectomy and intraocular repairs are delayed for 4 to 10 days. Significant hemorrhagic choroidal detachments may necessitate this approach, because immediate vitrectomy would eliminate intraocular tamponade and result in rapid expansion.

       Advantages: It is easier to view the posterior segment through the repaired cornea. There is also a decreased risk of intraocular bleeding.
    b. Primary repair: Vitrectomy and intraocular repairs are performed with or shortly after primary closure. Endophthalmitis, traumatic retinal detachment, and deep IOFBs may necessitate immediate action.

       Advantages: Prompt removal of intraocular blood, lens fragments, and other debris may reduce scarring and proliferative vitreoretinopathy (PVR), which can lead to complicated retinal detachment.

5. *Pars plana lensectomy:* If vitrectomy is performed, a shattered or dislocated lens can be removed through the sclerostomy incisions. Intraocular lens placement is generally delayed until after inflammation has subsided.

COMPLICATIONS

1. *Endophthalmitis:* The risk increases with delayed repair, inadequate antibiotic prophylaxis, involvement of organic material, or failure to remove a contaminated IOFB.

2. *Retinal detachment:* A traumatic injury that involves the posterior segment, which can result in retinal detachment. Pigment in the vitreous, vitreous hemorrhage, or traumatic vitreous detachment are possible indicators of significant posterior segment trauma. Delayed detachment may also occur due to vitreo-retinal traction from PVR or scar tissue.

3. *Glaucoma:* Secondary angle closure glaucoma can result from the formation of inflammatory adhesions in the anterior chamber or from traumatic damage to the trabecular meshwork or angle structure.

4. *Sympathetic ophthalmia:* A rare but severe granulomatous inflammatory response that affects both eyes after unilateral penetrating trauma. It is believed that this immune response arises due to sensitization of the immune system to specific uveal antigens. If the injured eye has limited visual potential, it is prophylactically enucleated to protect the undamaged eye.

POSTOPERATIVE CARE

- Frequent examinations are essential to evaluate wound leakage and healing, as well as to rule out the development of inflammation or infection.

- IOP checks and gonioscopy should be performed to assess the possibility of traumatic glaucoma.

- Posterior segment examination or B-scan ultrasonography is performed to assess the possibility of retinal detachment.

- Visual acuity is documented at regular intervals.

- Protective eyewear or polycarbonate lens glasses should be used to safeguard the uninjured eye.

Further Reading

Text

Bhatia SS. Ocular surface sealants and adhesives. *Ocul Surf.* 2006;4(3):146–154.

Colby K. Management of open globe injuries. *Int Ophthalmol Clin.* 1999;39(1):59–69.

Kubal WS. Imaging of orbital trauma. *Radiographics.* 2008;28(6):1729–1739.

Lang GK. Ocular trauma. In: *Ophthalmology: A Pocket Textbook Atlas.* 2nd ed. New York, NY: Georg Thieme Verlag; 2007:507–536.

Mittra RA, Mieler WF. Controversies in the management of open-globe injuries involving the posterior segment. *Surv Ophthalmol.* 1999;44(3):215–225.

Rubsamen PE. Posterior segment ocular trauma. In: Yanoff M, Duker J, eds. *Ophthalmology.* 3rd ed. Philadelphia, PA: Mosby; 2009:744–749.

Primary Sources

1. Scott IU, Mccabe CM, Flynn HW, et al. Local anesthesia with intravenous sedation for surgical repair of selected open globe injuries. *Am J Ophthalmol.* 2002;134(5):707–711.

De Souza S, Howcroft MJ. Management of posterior segment intraocular foreign bodies: 14 years' experience. *Can J Ophthalmol.* 1999;34(1):23–29.

Ophthalmology Acronyms

5-FU:	5-fluorouracil	LASEK:	laser subepithelial keratomileusis
AC:	anterior chamber	LASER:	light amplification by stimulated emission of radiation
ACIOL:	anterior chamber intraocular lens	LASIK:	laser-assisted in situ keratomileusis
AION:	arteritic ischemic optic neuropathy	LMN:	lower motor neuron
ALK:	anterior lamellar keratoplasty	LPS:	levator palpebrae superioris
AMD:	age-related macular degeneration	MAC:	monitored anesthesia care
APD:	afferent pupillary defect	MLF:	medial longitudinal fasciculus
BPH:	benign prostatic hyperplasia	MMC:	mitomycin C
BRVO:	branch retinal vein occlusion	MRD:	marginal reflex distance
BSS:	balanced salt solution	NAION:	nonarteritic anterior ischemic optic neuropathy
CME:	cystoid macular edema	Nd:YAG:	neodymium-doped yttrium aluminum garnet
CN:	cranial nerve		
CPC:	cyclophotocoagulation	NLP:	no light perception
CRAO:	central retinal artery occlusion	NSAID:	nonsteroidal anti-inflammatory drug
CRP:	C-reactive protein	NVD:	neovascularization of the disc
CRVO:	central retinal vein occlusion	NVE:	neovascularization elsewhere
CSCR:	central serous chorioretinopathy	OCP:	ocular cicatricial pemphigoid
DALK:	deep anterior lamellar keratoplasty	OCT:	optical coherence tomography
DCR:	dacryocystorhinostomy	PAS:	peripheral anterior synechiae
DLEK:	deep lamellar endothelial keratoplasty	PCIOL:	posterior chamber intraocular lens
DLK:	diffuse lamellar keratitis	PCO:	posterior capsular opacity
DMEK:	Descemet's membrane endothelial keratoplasty	PDR:	proliferative diabetic retinopathy
		PDT:	photodynamic therapy
DSAEK:	Descemet's stripping automated endothelial keratoplasty	PKP:	penetrating keratoplasty
		PO:	per os ("by mouth")
DSEK:	Descemet's stripping endothelial keratoplasty	PPRF:	pontine paramedian reticular formation
		PPV:	pars plana vitrectomy
ECCE:	extracapsular cataract extraction	PRP:	panretinal photocoagulation
ESR:	erythrocyte sedimentation rate	PVD:	posterior vitreous detachment
GA:	general anesthesia	PVR:	proliferative vitreoretinopathy
GAG:	glycosaminoglycan	R/O:	rule out
HSV:	herpes simplex virus	RPE:	retinal pigment epithelium
ICCE:	intracapsular cataract extraction	SPK:	superficial punctate keratitis
IFIS:	intraoperative floppy iris syndrome	UMN:	upper motor neuron
ILM:	internal limiting membrane	VA:	visual acuity
IOFB:	intraocular foreign body	VEGF:	vascular endothelial growth factor
IOL:	intraocular lens		
IOP:	intraocular pressure		

Glossary

5-Fluorouracil: An antimetabolite/antiproliferative agent commonly used during filtration surgery (e.g., trabeculectomy). It inhibits fibroblast proliferation at the filtration site, thus decreasing the risk of episcleral fibrosis (one of the leading causes of filtration surgery failure).

Accommodation: Increase in the refractive power of the lens to bring near objects into focus. The ciliary muscle contracts, leading to an increased lens curvature (likely via relaxation of the zonules/lens capsule), resulting in additional positive diopters.

Age-related macular degeneration (AMD): Progressive deterioration of the macula results in central vision loss. It occurs in two forms. Nonexudative ("dry"): subacute degeneration of the macula characterized by atrophy and subretinal deposits (drusen) that can distort the central vision. Frequently progresses to "wet" (neovascular) AMD: development of choroidal neovascularization (CNV) leads to acute fluid extravasation and serous detachment of the retinal pigment epithelium. This can produce varying degrees of vision loss from mild metamorphopsia to severe loss of central vision. Macular degeneration is the leading cause of irreversible vision loss in the elderly.

Akinesia: Inability to initiate movement. After a retrobulbar block, the patient is no longer able to move the extraocular muscles (leading to globe akinesia).

Amblyopia: Decreased visual acuity in an eye that is otherwise physically normal. The most common etiology is early deprivation of visual stimuli (e.g., congenital cataracts or the nondominant eye of a child with strabismus). Defects cannot be corrected with lenses, as they represent altered function of the visual cortex.

Ametropia: Presence of refractive error.

Amniotic membrane graft: Placement of a vascularized graft (banked human amniotic membrane) on the ocular surface during the acute phase of an inflammatory condition (e.g., Stevens-Johnson, corneal ulcer) may reduce corneal damage by providing a substrate for epithelialization. This has also been shown to inhibit inflammation, neovascularization, and fibrosis. The graft may also be used for selective pterygium repair or for bleb leaks.

Aniseikonia: A significant difference in the perceived size or shape of images, usually arising because of asymmetric refractive error (anisometropia).

Anisometropia: A difference in refractive error between the two eyes. In children, this can lead to monocular amblyopia if the image from the more blurry eye is ignored.

Anterior levator aponeurosis advancement: Used for moderate to severe ptosis with some degree of preserved levator function. The upper lid margin is elevated by shortening the levator aponeurosis.

Aphakia: Absence of the lens due to surgery, trauma, or congenital abnormality. These patients are hyperopic and are unable to accommodate.

Applanation tonometry: Measures intraocular pressure (IOP) using a calibrated probe. The force required to flatten a fixed corneal surface area corresponds to the IOP in millimeters of Mercury (mm Hg). The Goldmann tonometer, which necessitates use of fluorescein dye, is considered the gold standard, but the Pascal Dynamic Contour tonometer is an alternative growing in popularity. Since the probe makes contact with the corneal surface, a topical anesthetic must be administered before IOP measurement.

Argon laser trabeculoplasty (ALT): Laser procedure intended to lower intraocular pressure (IOP); uses thermal energy to create small burns in the trabecular meshwork. The burns are thought to increase flow via mechanical effects and trabecular meshwork endothelial cell proliferation.

Astigmatism: Irregular, cylindrical corneal, or lens shape that leads to different degrees of refraction and multiple focal points, resulting in image distortion.

Astigmatism, "against the rule": A regular astigmatism in which the horizontal meridian is the steepest. The principle meridians must be at right angles, with the steeper axis within 20 degrees of the horizontal plane. Against the rule astigmatism is more common in adults.

Astigmatism, irregular: Produced by an irregularly shaped cornea in which the principle meridians are not perpendicular and have variable power.

Astigmatism, oblique: The principle meridians are more than 20 degrees from the horizontal or vertical meridian.

Astigmatism, regular: The cornea or lens is shaped like a football, with two regular but different radii (one shorter than the other) that are 90 degrees apart. This produces two different focal points in two different planes (meridians).

Astigmatism, "with the rule": A regular astigmatism in which the vertical meridian is the steepest. The principle meridians must be at right angles with the steeper axis within 20 degrees of the vertical plane. This is more commonly seen in children.

Blepharochalasis: A familial angioneurotic edema syndrome that causes periodic lid inflammation, leading to thinning and wrinkling of periorbital skin in younger females.

Blepharophimosis syndrome: A rare autosomal dominant genetic syndrome characterized by abnormal narrowing of the palpebral fissures, upper lid ptosis, inner canthal folds, and laterally displaced inner canthi.

Blepharoplasty: Surgical excision of redundant upper lid skin (dermatochalasis) and prolapsed orbital fat (steatoblepharon) to improve cosmetic appearance and/or visual function (if lid tissue redundancy is severe enough to partially obstruct the visual axis).

Blepharospasm: An abnormal tic or spasm of the eyelid. Although some patients may have a history of dry eyes or light sensitivity, the etiology remains unknown. Localized botulinum toxin injection is the most common therapy.

Browplasty: Correction of significant sagging of the forehead and brow (brow ptosis), which can lead to sagging of upper lid skin. Accordingly, this procedure is often combined with lid ptosis repair.

Bruch's membrane: The innermost layer of the choroid. It is composed of five layers (from inside to out): basement membrane of the RPE, inner collagenous zone, central elastic fiber band, outer collagenous zone, and the basement membrane of the choriocapillaris. It separates the retina from the choroid; breaks in this membrane have been implicated in the development of choroidal neovascularization (CNV).

Bullous keratopathy: Small vesicles or bullae that form on the cornea due to endothelial cell dysfunction. This is generally preceded by stromal edema and corneal opacification. Precipitating factors include inflammation, trauma, endothelial dystrophies, and anterior segment surgery.

Capsulopalpebral fascia: A fibrous extension of inferior rectus sheath that inserts on the inferior tarsus. It stabilizes the tarsus and depresses the lower eyelid with downgaze. As a lid retractor, its function is analogous to the levator aponeurosis of the upper lid.

Capsulorrhexis: Prior to cataract phacoemulsification, a cystotome or pair of forceps is used to produce a controlled circular tear in the anterior capsule, permitting access to the underlying lens cortex and nucleus.

"Cell and flare": Clinical finding requiring the use of a slit-lamp biomicroscope. Signs of anterior segment inflammation can be seen within an off-centered, 1×1 mm beam of light directed through the pupillary aperture. Discrete inflammatory cells can be seen and counted within this beam, while presence of a diffuse haze (flare) indicates the presence of proteinaceous material suspended within the aqueous.

Central serous chorioretinopathy: Leakage of choroidal fluid into the subretinal space overlying the macula, distorting and blurring vision. Although the etiology remains unknown, it is believed to be a disorder of the retinal pigmented epithelium, and stress appears to be involved. The vision loss is usually temporary and unilateral, affecting males (ages 20 to 50) more commonly than females.

Chemosis: Fluid collection between the conjunctiva and sclera. May be serous or hemorrhagic.

Choroidal neovascularization (CNV): Vessel growth originating from the choroid and entering the subretinal space through breaks in Bruch's membrane. This is commonly seen in "wet" age-related macular degeneration (AMD) but may also arise in high myopes, after trauma, or as a complication of retinal laser photocoagulation.

Conjunctiva: Nonkeratinized epithelium that lines the anterior sclera (bulbar conjunctiva) and the posterior aspect of the eyelids (palpebral conjunctiva). The conjunctiva is a continuous mucous membrane that inserts at the limbus, where the cornea meets the scleral, reflects back on itself in the fornix, and terminates at the lid margin. The conjunctiva contains numerous mucous producing goblet cells that are critical for stabilizing the tear film.

Corneal endothelium: The innermost portion of the cornea is a single, cell layer in direct contact with the aqueous that regulates stromal hydration with an

ATP driven pump-leak system (critical to maintaining corneal transparency). The cells are unable to regenerate, and cell density normally decreases with age. Trauma, toxicity, inflammation, degenerative diseases, and anterior segment surgery hasten endothelial cell loss. A normal adult cell count is 2,500 cells/mm^2. Corneal edema typically develops when cell density drops below 300 cells/mm^2 due to inadequate pumping of fluid out of the cornea. Elevated intraocular pressure (IOP) can overwhelm corneal endothelial cell function, driving fluid into the cornea.

Cryopexy: Use of a liquid nitrogen-cooled probe to produce chorioretinal adhesions around a retinal tear or hole. Along with physical reapposition of the retina (e.g., with a scleral buckle), these adhesions prevent subretinal extravasation of vitreous fluid and redetachment. Laser photocoagulation is a commonly employed alternative.

Cycloplegic: A drug (e.g., atropine, tropicamide) that paralyzes accommodation by relaxing the ciliary muscle.

Cystoid macular edema: Accumulation of fluid in the outer plexiform layer of the macula, which consists of the synapses connecting cones and bipolar cells. The edema distorts central vision and produces cystic spaces visible on optical coherence tomography (OCT). This is commonly seen in conditions such as diabetic retinopathy, central retinal vein occlusion (CRVO), and branch retinal vein occlusion (BRVO). It can also arise after cataract or other intraocular surgery.

Dacryocystitis: Inflammation or infection of the nasolacrimal sac. The patient commonly presents with pain, erythema, and edema over the medial portion of the lower lid. The most common etiology is nasolacrimal obstruction, so epiphora is commonly seen as well.

Dacryocystorhinostomy (DCR): A surgical procedure intended to bypass an occluded nasolacrimal duct by creating an alternative drainage route (epithelium-lined tract) between the lacrimal sac and nasal mucosa.

Dehiscence: A surgical term indicating separation of sutured tissues.

Dermatochalasis: Upper lid skin redundancy and loss of tissue elasticity. This is a common age-related change that may be addressed with blepharoplasty.

Descemet's membrane: The thick corneal basement membrane generated by underlying endothelial cells. Lying between the corneal stroma and the en-

dothelium, it is the strongest layer of the cornea and helps to define the shape of the anterior chamber.

Diffuse lamellar keratitis (DLK): A complication of laser-assisted in situ keratomileusis (LASIK) surgery characterized by an inflammatory response at the flap/stromal bed interface. Diffuse, white granular deposits are seen on slit-lamp exam. The patient often presents with tearing, pain, foreign body sensation, and photophobia 1 week postoperatively. Etiology remains unknown but is thought to be related to debris at the flap interface.

Diopter: A measurement of refractive power that is the reciprocal of the focal length (D = 1/f).

Diplopia: The perception of two images while fixating on one object ("double vision"). Diplopia may be binocular (e.g., cranial nerve palsy) or monocular (e.g., refractive error). Monocular diplopia generally presents with split images while binocular diplopia may produce images displaced horizontally, vertically, or obliquely, depending on ocular misalignment.

Distichiasis: A rare acquired or congenital condition in which eyelashes arise from the orifices of the meibomian glands on the posterior lamella. These aberrant lashes are directed toward the globe and can cause irritation.

Duction test, forced: Under anesthesia, the eye is moved with forceps to determine whether there are external impingements on ocular motility (e.g., scar tissue or entrapment of a muscle in a blow-out floor fracture).

Ectropion: The lower lid margin and punctum are everted from the globe, which can lead to tearing, lagophthalmos, and corneal exposure. Causal factors include horizontal lower lid laxity, dehiscence or attenuation of the capsulopalpebral fascia, mid-face droop, and scarring causing vertical shortening of the anterior lamella or maxillary skin.

Electroretinography (ERG): Retinal function is assessed by measuring the electrical responses from various cell types (e.g., photoreceptors, amacrine cells, ganglion cells). After exposure to a standardized stimulus, the cells cumulatively produce a characteristic waveform. Deviations from this waveform may aid in the diagnosis of retinal pathology.

Emmetropia: Absence of refractive error.

Endophthalmitis: Inflammation within the eye that affects the aqueous and/or vitreous humor, commonly due to an infection. Symptoms include ocular pain, decreased visual acuity, conjunctival injection, chemosis, hypopyon, and presence of anterior chamber cell and flare on slit lamp examination. This is most often a complication of intraocular surgery, but may also result from penetrating ocular trauma. Less common causes include hematogenous spread from a distant site of infection, known as metastatic or endogenous endophthalmitis (e.g., endocarditis with septic emboli or intravenous drug use with a contaminated needle).

Enophthalmos: Recession of the globe within the orbit; most commonly seen after trauma (e.g., orbital floor fracture). In the elderly population, senile atrophy or orbital fat may produce physiologic enophthalmos (bilateral).

Entropion: The lid margin is inverted with the eyelashes directed toward the globe. This may result in keratitis, conjunctivitis, and/or epiphora. Causal factors include horizontal lower lid laxity, dehiscence or attenuation of the capsulopalpebral fascia, spasticity or override of the preseptal orbicularis muscle, and scarring causing vertical shortening of the posterior lamella.

Enucleation: Removal of the entire globe and a portion of the optic nerve with preservation of the extraocular muscles and orbital contents. Indications include irreparable ocular trauma with no light perception (due to concern for sympathetic ophthalmoplegia), presence of malignant ocular tumors (e.g., choroidal melanoma, retinoblastoma), and pain relief in blind eyes.

Epiblepharon: A developmental abnormality in which a redundant fold of pretarsal skin and orbicularis extends beyond the lid margin, pressing the eyelashes inward toward the globe.

Epicanthal fold: A congenital skin fold of the upper eyelid that covers the medial canthus. This is commonly seen in patients of Asian descent but may also be seen in patients with various genetic syndromes (e.g., Down syndrome, Cri du chat).

Epiphora: Overflow of tears onto the face rather than through the nasolacrimal system. Etiologies include obstruction of the drainage system (e.g., canalicular or nasolacrimal duct blockage), punctal malposition (e.g., entropion, ectropion), and reflex tearing due to ocular irritation (e.g., trichiasis, dacryocystitis).

Epiretinal membranes: Membranes composed of glial cells, fibroblasts, RPE cells, and inflammatory cells that tightly adhere to the retina (e.g., cellophane maculopathy, macular pucker, surface-wrinkling retinopathy). These membranes are often vascular in proliferative diabetic retinopathy (PDR) and avascular when associated with proliferative vitreoretinopathy. Both types may result in traction on the retina, which may cause no visual changes, mild metamorphopsia, a macular hole, or a tractional retinal detachment.

Evisceration: Removal of all intraocular contents (lens, uvea, retina, and vitreous) with preservation of the sclera and optic nerve. In some cases, the cornea is also preserved. This procedure is most often used to manage endophthalmitis or for blind, painful eyes, but may also be indicated following significant ocular trauma. *Note*: Unlike enucleation, the risk of sympathetic ophthalmoplegia remains postevisceration if globe rupture and exposure of intraocular contents to the systemic immune system occurred during or after the trauma.

Excimer laser: The "excited dimer" laser is a 193-nm laser (ultraviolet spectrum) that ablates finite amounts of tissue without damaging adjacent structures. The laser is produced by a combination of an inert gas (argon, krypton, or xenon) with a reactive gas (fluorine or chlorine). Common clinical uses include ablations for refractive surgery (e.g., photorefractive keratectomy [PRK] and laser-assisted in situ keratomileusis [LASIK]) and removal of superficial corneal scars.

Exenteration: Removal of the globe and all adjacent orbital soft tissues. This procedure is most often performed to treat life-threatening malignancies or infections such as with mucormycosis. The extent of exenteration depends on the pathology. Subtotal exenteration involves removal of the globe and adjacent tissues with preservation of the periorbita and some or all of the eyelids. Total exenteration includes removal of the globe, soft tissues, and periorbita. Radical exenteration involves removal of the globe, soft tissues, periorbita, bone, sinuses, muscle, and skin (depending on the extent of the pathology).

Eyelid crease: This crease in the upper lid delineates the inferior extent of the orbital septum and fat pads as well as the insertion point of the levator aponeurosis on the lid skin. It is generally located 8 to 10 mm above the lid margin in the midpupillary axis, but may be significantly lower in Asians.

Floppy eyelids syndrome: Extreme bilateral laxity of lid tissues with tarsal thickening and low-grade chronic inflammation; leads to ectropion. This is most commonly seen in overweight males and is associated with obstructive sleep apnea.

Fluorescein angiography: A diagnostic procedure used to evaluate the retinal and choroidal vasculature. After intravenous injection of sodium fluorescein, an angiogram of the fundus (specialized photograph measuring fluorescence at 490 nm) is taken to directly visualize the dye within the vasculature. Under normal circumstances, the fluorescein dye remains intravascularly. Under pathologic conditions associated with increased vascular permeability (e.g., diabetes or inflammation), the dye extravasates and collects within the retinal layers. Fluorescein may also help highlight abnormal vascular structures such as neovascularization associated with a central retinal vein occlusion (CRVO).

Frontalis muscle: The major muscle of the forehead, which raises the eyebrows; supplied by temporal branch of cranial nerve (CN) VII.

Frontalis suspension: A form of ptosis repair for patients with severe ptosis and poor levator function (but an intact frontalis muscle). The tarsal plate is anchored to the frontalis muscle with a strip of fascia or silicone sling. The patient must then learn to use the frontalis muscle to elevate and depress the lid.

Fuchs endothelial dystrophy: A slowly progressive endothelial dystrophy characterized by corneal guttata (discrete, granular deposits) and stromal edema. Patients often present with increased sensation of glare or blurred vision after the development of corneal edema. With corneal decompensation, this may result in severe pain. Definitive treatment involves penetrating keratoplasty (PKP) or posterior lamellar keratoplasty (Descemet stripping endothelial keratoplasty [DSEK], Descemet membrane endothelial keratoplasty [DMEK]).

Fusional vergence: Corresponding eye movements that enable fusion of monocular images to produce binocular or stereoscopic vision. Noncorresponding eye movements are referred to as disjunctive vergences. Convergence: eyes move inward. Divergence: eyes move outward.

Glaucoma drainage implant: An intraocular pressure (IOP) lowering device that bypasses the trabecular meshwork with an anterior chamber silicone tube that drains aqueous to a plate ("bleb spreading device") implanted beneath the conjunctiva. This is commonly preferred for conditions where trabeculectomy is likely to fail, such as for neovascular or uveitic glaucoma. Implants are available as valveless (Molteno and Baerveldt) or valved (Ahmed). Examples include glaucoma drainage device, aqueous drainage device, tube shunt, and seton implant.

Glaucoma, neovascular: Neovascularization of the iris (rubeosis iridis) and anterior chamber angle typically caused by ischemic retinal disorders (e.g., diabetic retinopathy, central retinal vein occlusion). Neovascularization causes fibrovascular membranes that initially cause secondary open angle glaucoma due to obstruction, then secondary angle closure due to the progressive formation of synechial scar tissue that closes off access of aqueous to the trabecular meshwork.

Glaucoma, uveitic: Anterior chamber inflammation that can lead to trabecular meshwork dysfunction and secondary open angle glaucoma and/or synechiae formation, resulting in secondary angle closure glaucoma.

Gonioscopy: Because of an optical phenomenon related to the different refractive indices of the tear film and air, and the curvature of a normal cornea, it is necessary to use special lenses to overcome the critical angle of light. Gonio lenses (e.g., three-mirror Goldmann lens or four-mirror Sussman lens) are used in conjunction with a slit lamp, which allows visualization of the ocular structures between the iris and the cornea, the anterior chamber angle. This technique permits the evaluation of conditions that predispose to angle closure glaucoma, trabecular meshwork obstruction, or some occult pathology such as tumors.

Grave's ophthalmopathy: A presumed autoimmune process that leads to extraocular myositis with lymphocytic infiltration along with proptosis from glycosaminoglycan deposition in the retrobulbar space. Severe cases can result in poor cosmesis, persistent diplopia, exposure keratitis, and compressive optic neuropathy.

Hering's law: Corresponding extraocular muscles (yoke muscles) are equally innervated. Thus, movement of one eye or lid triggers the corresponding contralateral muscle to fire equally. This principle becomes relevant after surgical repair of unilateral ptosis; due to bilateral innervation of the levator muscle from a single nucleus, significant elevation of one lid during ptosis repair may unmask ptosis in the other lid.

Hertel's exophthalmometer: Device that measures the position of the globe in relation to the lateral orbital rims. The average distance between the lateral orbital rim and apex of the ipsilateral cornea is 12 to 20 mm. While there is considerable individual and racial variation, shorter measurements may indicate enophthalmos, whereas longer measurements may suggest exophthalmos. A difference in measurements greater than 2 mm should raise suspicion for unilateral or asymmetric disease.

Hyperopia: *"Farsightedness"*; images converge posterior to the retina in an unaccommodated eye. Without accommodation, the retinal image is out of focus and requires a plus lens for adequate correction.

Hyperopia, latent: The degree of hyperopia corrected by accommodation (prepresbyopic patients can overcome a few diopters of hyperopia by accommodation). The extent of latent hyperopia is revealed by cycloplegic refraction (eliminates accommodation). As a patient ages and loses the ability to accommodate his or her hyperopia will become apparent.

Hyperopia, manifest: Hyperopia that cannot be corrected by accommodation. If congenital, this may be a cause of deprivation amblyopia.

Hyphema: Blood in the anterior chamber of the eye, most commonly due to blunt trauma. The blood generally layers inferiorly due to gravity.

Hypopyon: Leukocytic exudates in the anterior chamber of the eye. This is a sign of anterior chamber infection or uveitis. Hypopyon is often accompanied by conjunctival injection. The leukocytes generally layer inferiorly due to gravity.

Hypotony: An intraocular pressure (IOP) of 5 mm Hg or less. This is a relatively common complication of filtration surgery (overfiltration) and can result in maculopathy, corneal decompensation, and accelerated cataract development.

Intraocular lens (IOL): Usually after cataract removal, an artificial lens is placed in the eye to restore its refractive power. The optic, or refracting portion of the lens, is typically centered and anchored in the capsular bag via attached haptics, but can be placed in various alternative locations. Special IOLs are available to correct high refractive errors in patients with clear crystalline lenses (phakic IOLs).

Intraocular lens (IOL), monofocal: An IOL that corrects vision at one set distance. Although generally selected for distance vision, near or intermediate distances can be chosen based on patient preference.

Intraocular lens (IOL), multifocal: An IOL that focuses light at multiple planes, correcting vision for near and far vision simultaneously.

Intraocular lens (IOL), pseudoaccomodative: An IOL that is designed to be pliable, moving anteriorly with accommodative effort, mimicking the presurgical accommodative process.

Intraocular lens (IOL), toric: An IOL that corrects astigmatism. Correct orientation of the lens and haptics during surgery is very important because even slight rotations in the IOL can drastically reduce the refractive power of the lens or even exacerbate the existing astigmatic error.

Iridocorneal endothelial (ICE) syndrome: A group of disorders (progressive iris atrophy, Chandler's syndrome, and Cogan-Reese syndrome) characterized by abnormal corneal endothelium that behaves more like epithelium. The abnormal corneal endothelium can cause corneal edema, iris atrophy, and/or secondary angle closure glaucoma from peripheral anterior synechiae (PAS) formation.

Iridoplasty: A laser procedure performed to deepen a narrowed iridocorneal angle. Circumferential application of nonpenetrating laser burns contracts the peripheral iris, widening the angle. This is sometimes done prior to trabeculoplasty to provide better visualization of the trabecular meshwork.

Keratectomy, phototherapeutic: Removal of superficial corneal scars by ablating up to 20% of the stromal thickness with an excimer laser ablation.

Keratitis: Inflammation of the cornea.

Keratitis, exposure: Inflammation of the cornea due to the inability to fully close the eyelids. This may progress to ulceration and even perforation if left untreated.

Keratitis, neurotrophic: A degenerative corneal disease caused by impaired corneal sensation (CN V_1). The patient does not receive appropriate sensory stimuli prompting eye closure and may develop epithelial defects and ulcers.

Keratoconjunctivitis sicca: Commonly called "dry eye," this condition can be caused by decreased tear production or increased tear evaporation. Patients often present with intermittent or persistent blurred vision, and burning and persistent foreign body sensation. Cases may be idiopathic, associated with systemic autoimmune diseases such as Sjögren's, or a side effect of systemic medical therapy.

Keratoconus: Progressive thinning of cornea causes conical protrusion with severe, irregular astigmatism. Acute decompensation with corneal edema and opacification may result from tears in Descemet's membrane. Initial treatment involves placement of a hard contact lens or placement of intrastromal corneal implants. New research suggests that riboflavin cross-linking can prevent the formation or progression of keratoconus, and may improve the corneal steepness. Keratoconus can progress at variable rates. The definitive treatment of keratoconus is a penetrating keratoplasty.

Keratometer: An ophthalmic instrument that measures corneal shape (e.g., extent of astigmatism) and power/refractive error of the central cornea (e.g., myopia/hyperopia). More advanced techniques such as videokeratography are now available to provide a precise, automated map of corneal topography.

Keratoplasty, anterior (ALK): Partial-thickness removal of diseased anterior corneal tissue, followed by replacement with donor tissue. This is performed if the defect is limited to the superficial stroma; the remaining Descemet's membrane and endothelium should be healthy.

Keratoplasty, deep anterior (DALK): Partial-thickness removal of diseased anterior corneal tissue, followed by replacement with donor tissue. Performed for defects deeper in the stroma; Descemet's membrane and endothelium must be healthy. DALK permits a more even dissection of the recipient cornea compared to ALK, theoretically benefitting postoperative visual acuity (VA).

Keratoplasty, penetrating (PKP): Full-thickness removal of diseased corneal tissue followed by replacement with equivalent donor tissue; performed if defect is full thickness, involves the endothelium, or if other techniques are not likely to achieve desired results.

Keratoplasty, posterior lamellar: Partial-thickness removal of pathologic posterior corneal tissue, followed by replacement with healthy donor tissue. This is the preferred treatment for endothelial defects without stromal damage (e.g., Fuchs endothelial dystrophy or pseudophakic bullous keratopathy). Many techniques have been developed, including deep lamellar endothelial keratoplasty (DLEK), Descemet stripping endothelial keratoplasty (DSEK), and Descemet membrane endothelial keratoplasty (DMEK).

Keratoprosthesis: A clear synthetic prosthesis, secured to a ring of donor tissue, used to replace a pathologic host cornea for cases where traditional penetrating keratoplasty (PKP) is unlikely to succeed, such as after repeated graft rejection, or severe ocular adnexal disease. The Boston Type 1 is the most commonly used prosthesis. The prosthetic, button-like implant is secured to a donor cornea, which is then sutured to the host corneal rim. Visual improvement can be rapid, but complications are fairly common including glaucoma, formation of inflammatory membranes, extrusion of the implant, and infection.

Lagophthalmos: Inability to close the eyelids completely, commonly due to facial nerve palsy (paralyzed orbicularis oculi) or excessive tissue removal during blepharoplasty. If prolonged, keratitis and corneal ulcers may develop.

Lamella, anterior: Includes skin, underlying connective tissue, and orbicularis oculi muscle.

Lamella, posterior: Includes palpebral conjunctiva, tarsus, and lid retractors.

Laser-assisted in situ keratomileusis (LASIK): A surgical procedure that corrects refractive error by modifying the radius of curvature of the anterior cornea. A hinged lamellar flap is created using an automated microkeratome or laser (flap thickness = 100 to 180 microns). The underlying corneal stroma is then reshaped with excimer laser ablation, followed by sutureless flap replacement.

Laser iridotomy: A laser procedure commonly done to treat or prevent acute or chronic angle closure glaucoma associated with pupillary block. Creation of a peripheral iris defect equalizes anterior and posterior chamber pressures, eliminating pupillary block and opening the anterior chamber angle.

Laser photocoagulation: Use of a thermal argon laser to burn small portions of the retina. Therapeutic goals include sealing leaky, abnormal blood vessels and forming chorioretinal adhesions to reappose detached sensory retina with the underlying retinal pigment epithelium (RPE).

Laser retinopexy: In this technique, laser spots are applied to the region surrounding an area of retinal attachment. This creates focal adhesions between the retina and underlying choroid, which act as "spot welds" preventing extension of the detachment.

Laser subepithelial keratomileusis (LASEK): A surgical procedure that corrects refractive error by modifying the radius of curvature of the anterior cornea. A 50-micron hinged, lamellar flap is created using an automated microkeratome. Excimer laser ablation at the level of Bowman's membrane is followed by sutureless flap replacement.

Latent hyperopia: Please see *Hyperopia, Latent.*

Lateral canthotomy and cantholysis: Canthotomy entails dividing the lateral canthus with a horizontal incision that extends temporally toward the orbital rim. This is often combined with the cantholysis, or transection of the inferior arm of the lateral canthus tendon. This is done emergently to relieve pressure on the globe (e.g., in cases of retrobulbar hemorrhage), or electively to provide surgical access to the lateral orbital rim and orbital floor.

Levator excursion: Levator function/power is estimated by measuring elevation of the upper lid from full downgaze to full upgaze (normally 16 to 20 mm).

Levator palpebrae superioris: The main upper lid retractor, innervated by cranial nerve (CN) III. It originates on the lesser wing of the sphenoid bone, and inserts on the tarsal plate and upper lid skin after interdigitating with orbicularis fibers.

Limbal stem cell transplant: Stem cells located at the limbus are responsible for regenerating the corneal epithelium; successful transplant from the contralateral or cadaverous eye may restore a healthy ocular surface if pathology does not involve the full corneal thickness. In select cases, this may be used in place of a corneal transplant or prior to a corneal transplant depending on the ocular pathology. The patient will require chronic, systemic immunosuppression.

Limbus: The junction of the peripheral cornea and adjacent sclera. It is the site of insertion of the conjunctiva and is populated by stem cells critical to regeneration of the corneal epithelium.

Macular hole: A small retinal break overlying the macula. Although the precise etiology remains unknown, posterior vitreous detachment (PVD) and epiretinal membrane formation have been implicated. Holes are also related to high myopia as well as trauma. They are staged using a 1 to 4 scale, where 1 = decreased/absent foveal depression with a yellow ring, 2 = a full-thickness hole less than 400 microns in diameter, 3 = a full-thickness hole greater than 400 microns in diameter, and 4 = a full-thickness hole greater than 400 microns with vitreous detachment and a Weiss ring.

Macular pucker: Wrinkling of the retinal surface overlying the macula due to tractional forces exerted by epiretinal membranes. This may lead to significant visual distortion (metamorphopsia) and decreased visual acuity (VA).

Manifest hyperopia: Please see *Hyperopia, Manifest.*

Marginal reflex distance (MRD): The distance from the pupillary light reflex to the upper lid margin in primary gaze (normally ~4 mm).

Metamorphopsia: A perceived distortion of images typically due to macular pathology. This is often assessed by the use of an Amsler grid. The straight lines will appear distorted or bent in a positive test.

Microkeratome: An ophthalmic instrument with an oscillating blade, used to make corneal flaps with thicknesses ranging from 50 to 180 microns. This device is commonly used in laser-assisted in situ keratomileusis (LASIK) and laser subepithelial keratomileusis (LASEK) surgery, although femtosecond lasers are gaining popularity as an alternative.

Mitomycin C (MMC): An antimetabolite/antiproliferative agent commonly used during filtration surgery (e.g., trabeculectomy). MMC inhibits fibroblast proliferation at the filtration site, thus decreasing the risk of episcleral fibrosis (one of the leading causes of filtration surgery failure).

Muller's muscle: An accessory upper lid retractor innervated by sympathetic fibers. It originates on the underside of the levator palpebrae superioris and inserts on the superior tarsal margin.

Muller's muscle resection (Fasanella-servat): A technique used to repair mild ptosis via posterior excision of a segment of tarsus, Muller's muscle and palpebral conjunctiva.

Mydriatic: A pharmacologic agent that dilates the pupil by sympathomimetic stimulation of the iris dilator muscle (e.g., phenylephrine) or anticholinergic inhibition of the sphincter muscle (e.g., atropine, tropicamide). Of note, anticholinergics also achieve cycloplegia (render the patient unable to accommodate).

Myopia ("nearsighted"): Distant images converge anterior to the retina in an unaccommodated eye. Distance vision is out of focus and requires a minus lens for adequate correction.

Nasolacrimal duct: A conduit permitting drainage from the tear meniscus to the nasal mucosa. This may be congenitally obstructed, leading to epiphora, but this generally resolves with conservative management.

Nd:YAG capsulotomy: Pulses from a neodymium-doped yttrium aluminum garnet (Nd:YAG) laser induce the formation of plasma to create a shock wave that can mechanically breakdown intraocular tissues. Nd:YAG lasers are commonly used to remove an opacified posterior lens capsule ("secondary cataract") from the pupillary axis after cataract phacoemulsification or to create a laser peripheral iridotomy.

Ocular cicatricial pemphigoid (OCP): An autoimmune disease affecting the skin and mucous membranes. Primary ocular manifestations include fibrosis and scarring of the conjunctiva; secondary manifestations include dry eyes and trichiasis, which can lead to corneal scarring and vascularization.

Optical coherence tomography (OCT): Use of a special near-infrared laser to produce high-resolution cross-sectional images of the retina (wavelength = 810 nm) or anterior segment (wavelength = 1,310 nm). The laser is exceptionally precise, permitting differentiation of tissues only 10 microns apart. This technology is now routinely used to aid in the diagnosis of most macular and disc pathologies (e.g., macular edema and glaucoma, respectively), while anterior segment applications are being explored.

Orbicularis oculi: This muscle forcefully closes the eye, and consists of orbital, preseptal, and pretarsal components. It is supplied by the zygomatic branch of cranial nerve (CN) VII.

Orbital decompression: Controlled removal of one or more orbital walls to permit partial prolapse of orbital contents and decompression of the orbital space.

Pachymetry: A device used to measure central corneal thickness to assess or monitor corneal edema or contribute to the management of glaucoma. Typically, an ultrasound is used to measure corneal thickness, although other modalities are available.

Palpebral fissure: The space between the upper and lower lid margins. The normal height is 6 to 10 mm, while the normal width is approximately 28 to 30 mm.

Panretinal photocoagulation (PRP): In proliferative diabetic retinopathy, retinal ischemia from microangiopathic changes stimulates the production of vascular endothelial growth factor (VEGF). This in turn promotes the growth of fragile new blood vessels, which are easily disrupted, resulting in vitreous and retinal hemorrhage. PRP entails applying upwards of 1,000 small laser burns to the outer retina. This destroys tissue that is not critical to central vision, thus decreasing the oxidative demand of the retina and the stimulus for VEGF production.

Pars plana: A 4 mm section of the posterior ciliary body, bordered anteriorly by the highly vascular ciliary processes (pars plicata) and posteriorly by the ora serrata and peripheral retina. This region is used for posterior segment surgery and intravitreal injections because it provides access to the vitreous cavity without high risk of hemorrhage or retinal damage.

Pars plana vitrectomy (PPV): A surgical procedure that involves the cutting and removing of the vitreous. This provides access to drain subretinal fluid, relieve retinal traction, perform endolaser, etc., and allows for safe maneuvering within the vitreous cavity without causing vitreoretinal traction.

Pellucid marginal degeneration: A rare degenerative corneal condition characterized by bilateral, peripheral corneal thinning (ectasia). Patients present with increasing astigmatism. This condition is commonly confused with keratoconus. It is an absolute contraindication for refractive surgery.

Periorbita: The periosteum lining the orbit; it is loosely adherent to the orbital bones. It converges with external periosteum at the arcus marginalis to form the orbital septum.

Phacodonesis: Movement of the lens.

Phacoemulsification: Use of an ultrasonic transducer, which converts electrical energy to mechanical vibratory energy, to fragment the lens for removal.

Photodynamic therapy: Use of a special laser-activated dye (verteporfin) to selectively target areas of pathologic neovascularization while minimizing retinal tissue damage. The photosensitizing dye has an affinity for low-density lipoprotein (LDL) receptors, which are abundant in neovascular tissue. A special laser (wavelength = 689 nm) is applied to the neovascular areas, activating the verteporfin dye and causing coagulation of the vessels.

Photophobia: A nonspecific symptom of excessive sensitivity to light, which causes pain or discomfort. Nonocular causes include migraine and meningitis. Ocular causes include conjunctivitis, episcleritis, keratitis, iritis, angle-closure glaucoma, and pupillary dilation.

Photopsia: The perception of flashes of light. This is commonly associated with posterior vitreous detachment (PVD), retinal detachment or breaks, and migraines.

Photorefractive keratectomy (PRK): A surgical procedure that corrects refractive error by modifying the radius of curvature of the anterior cornea. After removing the epithelium with alcohol, an excimer laser is used to ablate Bowman's membrane tissue. This reshapes the cornea and provides the necessary refractive correction.

Phototherapeutic keratectomy (PRK): A surgical procedure that can correct corneal surface anomalies. After removing the epithelium with alcohol, an excimer laser is used to ablate Bowman's membrane tissue. This reshapes the cornea, can diminish anterior opacities and can provide improved surface adherence for the corneal epithelium (in cases of recurrent corneal erosions).

Phthisis bulbi (Globe phthisis): A shrunken, atrophic, nonfunctional eye that is the result of severe trauma or inflammation. Characteristic ocular findings include blood or exudate between the ciliary body and the sclera, a cyclitic membrane extending from one part of the ciliary body to the next, retinal detachments, and optic nerve atrophy.

Pinguecula: Thickening and discoloration of exposed bulbar conjunctiva. It is histologically identical to a pterygium, but does not extend across the cornea.

Pneumatic retinopexy: Injection of an expandable gas bubble into the vitreous to treat small retinal breaks. The bubble tamponades break against the retinal pigment epithelium (RPE) and prevents fluid from tracking underneath the retina, permitting reattachment. As head position is critical to keeping the bubble over the detachment, this procedure is mostly used for superior retinal breaks. It is commonly done in conjunction with cryopexy or laser photocoagulation.

Posterior capsule opacity (PCO): Opacification of the posterior capsule after cataract extraction from the capsular bag. This is a very common complication, occurring in 50% of patients within 5 years of surgery. Residual lens epithelial cells that are adherent to the capsule proliferate and differentiate, obstructing the visual axis. PCO can be treated with neodymium-doped yttrium aluminum garnet (Nd:YAG) capsulotomy, an office-based procedure.

Presbyopia: Loss of accommodation with aging.

Prism diopter: The distance in centimeters that light is bent by a prism at 1 meter.

Proliferative vitreoretinopathy (PVR): Formation of cellular membranes (scar tissue) on the retina following a retinal break. This scar tissue may contract, leading to retinal traction and possibly to further detachment. This is the most common complication after retinal detachment.

Proptosis (Exophthalmos): Anterior protrusion of the globe from the orbit. The condition may be bilateral (e.g., thyroid eye disease in greater than 80% of presentations) or unilateral (e.g., tumor). The extent of protrusion may be measured with an exophthalmometer (see *Hertel's exophthalmometer*).

Pseudophakia: Presence of an artificial intraocular lens within the eye, typically placed during cataract extraction surgery or clear lens exchange (in refractive surgery).

Pseudopterygium: A fibrovascular extension of the bulbar conjunctiva onto the cornea at a site of prior damage (e.g., inflammation, ulceration, chemical injury). It is differentiated from true pterygium by its atypical location (may originate from conjunctiva not exposed to the elements within the palpebral fissure) and lack of adhesion to the limbus.

Pseudoptosis: The illusion of unilateral ptosis due to ipsilateral globe recession (enophthalmos).

Pterygium: Benign, fibrovascular proliferation and elastotic degeneration of collagen of the bulbar conjunctiva, which has been exposed to the elements within the palpebral fissure. Pterygia grow across the cornea, damaging Bowman's membrane. Originates nasally in 90% of cases. They may be small and benign, cosmetically significant, or visually significant if they induce corneal astigmatism or obstruct the visual axis.

Punctum: A small orifice located on the medial portion of the lid margin in each eyelid, which drains tears into the nasolacrimal sac via its corresponding canaliculus.

Pupillary block: Posterior chamber pressure becomes higher than anterior chamber pressure due to blockage of aqueous flow through the pupil. This pressure differential causes the iris to bow forward (iris bombé), narrowing the angle and preventing outflow through the trabecular meshwork (resulting in closed angle glaucoma). Laser iridotomy or surgical iridectomy equalizes the pressure across the anterior and posterior chambers, relieving the block, and deepening the anterior chamber angle.

Quickert-Rathbun sutures: A temporizing treatment for entropion. Placement of several full-thickness sutures originating at the deepest extent of the inferior fornix and exiting 1 to 2 mm from the eyelid margin helps to evert the lid. Subsequent fibrosis around the sutures reinforces the everted lid position.

Recession, surgical: A strabismus surgery technique performed to correct extraocular muscle misalignment. One of the muscles is detached from its scleral insertion and reinserted more posteriorly to improve alignment. This is commonly done in conjunction with a resection (shortening) of its antagonist.

Resection: A strabismus surgery technique performed to correct extraocular muscle misalignment. One of the muscles is transected, shortened, and sutured to its original scleral insertion. This is commonly done in conjunction with a recession of its antagonist.

Retinal detachment, rhegmatogenous: A full-thickness break or tear in the retina that allows fluid from the vitreous to extravasate between the sensory retina and underlying retinal pigment epithelium (RPE; subretinal space).

Retinal detachment, serous/exudative: Fluid accumulates in the subretinal space due to inflammation, injury, or vascular abnormalities. The sensory retina is elevated from the underlying retinal pigment epithelium (RPE), but no break is present.

Retinal detachment, traction: Traction on the retina from abnormal fibrovascular tissue exceeds the adhesion between the retina and retinal pigment epithelium (RPE), causing detachment.

Retinoschisis: Abnormal, but frequently benign, intraretinal splitting that must be differentiated from true retinal detachment on funduscopic exam. Subgroups include degenerative, hereditary, tractional, and exudative. Degenerative retinoschisis is the most common, affecting 7% of the population, but does not require any treatment. It generally occurs in the outer plexiform layer.

Rose bengal: This stain is used to identify areas of dead or devitalized epithelium that has not sloughed off of the corneal surface. By contrast, fluorescein stain binds to basement membrane, identifying full epithelial defects (areas where the cells have already sloughed off).

Scanning laser ophthalmoscopy (SLO): A narrow laser beam is used to image ocular structures, producing high-resolution, real-time images of the cornea or retina.

Schirmer test: A test frequently used in the evaluation of dry eyes. Filter paper is placed between the globe and outer third of the lower eyelid, and the eyes are closed for 5 minutes. The distance of tear migration along the filter paper can then be quantitatively assessed. Less than 10 mm of wetting in nonanesthetized eyes is considered abnormal.

Schwalbe's line: The outer limit of Descemet's membrane, which marks the anterior border of the trabecular meshwork on gonioscopy.

Scleral buckle: A surgically placed silicone insert that treats rhegmatogenous retinal detachment with scleral indentation. The primary goal is to reappose the sensory retina to the retinal pigment epithelium (RPE). This surgery is often done in conjunction with cryopexy or laser photocoagulation to produce stabilizing chorioretinal adhesions.

Scleral spur: A circumferential scleral prominence that anchors the trabecular meshwork and serves as the insertion site of the longitudinal ciliary muscle fibers.

Seidel Test: Fluorescein dye is applied to the ocular surface. A positive Seidel test indicates globe rupture or wound leak, and occurs when the fluorescein is diluted or washed away by draining aqueous.

Selective laser trabeculoplasty (SLT): A laser procedure intended to lower intraocular pressure (IOP) that uses neodymium-doped yttrium aluminum garnet (Nd:YAG; "YAG") laser technology to treat pigmented cells in the trabecular meshwork without damage to surrounding structures. Treatment may increase flow via expulsion of pigment and debris from the meshwork and/or via the stimulation of trabecular meshwork endothelial cell function.

Serpiginous corneal ulcer: A rapidly progressing infectious ulcer, most often bacterial, that may result in corneal perforation and loss of the eye.

Staphyloma: An abnormal protrusion of uveal tissue through a thinned outer layer of the eye (e.g., sclera). This is most commonly the result of an inflammatory or degenerative condition.

Steatoblepharon: Bulging of orbital fat through a weakened orbital septum. This is a common age-related change and may be addressed via blepharoplasty.

Stevens-Johnson syndrome: A hypersensitivity reaction affecting the skin and mucous membranes, which can be triggered by exposure to various drugs or pathogens. Primary ocular manifestations include fibrosis and scarring of the conjunctiva; secondary manifestations include dry eyes and trichiasis, leading to eventual corneal scarring and vascularization.

Strabismus: Due to ocular misalignment, object images are projected to noncorresponding points on the retina. This can result in diplopia in adults and amblyopia in young children.

Strabismus, concomitant: The deviating eye follows the lead eye such that the angle remains constant in all directions of gaze. This is more common in children.

Strabismus, incomitant (Paralytic): Paralysis of one or more extraocular muscles results in an angle of deviation that varies depending on gaze position. This is more common in adults.

Subretinal space: The potential space between the sensory retina and retinal pigment epithelium (RPE).

Superficial punctate keratitis: Nonspecific corneal inflammation, which is characterized by small, scattered areas of epithelial loss or damage. Patients may present with conjunctival injection, tearing, photophobia, and decreased visual acuity (VA). Common causes include conjunctivitis, blepharitis, and contact lens overuse.

Sympathetic ophthalmoplegia: A very rare but severe granulomatous inflammatory response seen in the uninjured (contralateral) eye after penetrating trauma. This is thought to arise from immunologic sensitization to uveal antigens. Systemic findings include vitiligo (patches of skin depigmentation) and poliosis (whitening) of the eyelashes. This may be prevented by enucleating eyes with ocular damage severe enough to preclude visual potential.

Synechia: Adhesions between the iris and cornea (anterior synechia) or between the iris and lens (posterior synechia). Causes include trauma, inflammatory conditions, and iatrogenic damage (e.g., from ALT [argon laser trabeculoplasty]/SLT [selective laser trabeculoplasty]). If significant, anterior or posterior synechia may precipitate acute angle closure glaucoma or cause chronic angle closure glaucoma.

Tarsoligamentous sling: An important lid structure formed by the tarsal plates as well as the medial and lateral canthal tendons. It provides mechanical support to the lid and keeps the lid margin apposed to the globe. Any or all parts may develop laxity, resulting in ectropion or entropion.

Tarsorrhaphy: A surgical procedure used to prevent corneal decompensation. Temporary tarsorrhaphy is often complete and promotes corneal healing. Long-term tarsorrhaphy entails partial lateral eyelid closure. This reduces corneal exposure often at the expense of partial visual axis obstruction. Prolonged use is cosmetically undesirable and may result in lid-margin scarring and trichiasis. Accordingly, lid reanimation techniques may be preferred in such cases.

Tarsus: A dense connective tissue plate found in the posterior lamella of each eyelid, which contributes important structural support. It extends to the lid margin and is an important point of insertion for the lid retractors.

Tear film breakup time test: A test commonly used to evaluate dry eye conditions. After fluorescein application, the time required for dry patches to appear on the cornea after the patient blinks is measured using the slit lamp. This occurs when the tear film loses its cohesive force. Normal breakup time is 10 to 12 seconds; if the breakup time is shorter than the average blink rate, the corneal surface is unprotected, resulting in the symptoms of dry eye.

Tenon's capsule: A dense fascial layer that surrounds the globe from the optic nerve to the limbus. It merges with the fascial sheaths of the extraocular muscles and separates the globe from the orbital fat posteriorly.

Trabecular meshwork: Spongy tissue in the anterior chamber angle that is lined by trabeculocytes and permits aqueous drainage into Schlemm's Canal.

Trabeculectomy: A glaucoma filtration procedure that decreases intraocular pressure (IOP) by creating a limbal fistula that allows aqueous to drain across a conjunctival bleb and wash away in the tear film. Usually used in conjunction with antiscarring agents such as mitomycin C (MMC) or 5-fluorouracil (5-FU).

Trephine: A cutting instrument with a cylindrical blade that is used to make partial thickness corneal incisions in keratoplasty and keratoprosthesis cases. The incision depth depends on the several trephine revolutions (one-fourth turn equals approximately 60 microns).

Trichiasis: An acquired condition in which the eyelashes originate from the normal position in the anterior lamella, but are directed posteriorly toward the globe as a result of inflammation and scarring. This is commonly seen in the developing world as a result of *Chlamydia trachomatis* infection (trachoma).

Upper lid reanimation: Use of a lid weight, palpebral spring, or temporalis muscle transfer to increase upper lid excursion with blinking. This permits adequate lid closure, preventing exposure keratitis and corneal breakdown.

Viscoelastics: Various polymers used during anterior segment intraocular surgery (e.g., cataract phacoemulsification) to stabilize the anterior chamber and manipulate intraocular tissue, while protecting the corneal endothelium from damage.

Visual function index: A survey that assesses visual impairment due to cataract symptoms. This provides a subjective measure of cataract related disability.

Weiss ring: Glial tissue that remains attached to the posterior vitreous cortex after posterior vitreous detachment over the optic nerve head. Funduscopic exam reveals a gray to brown partial or complete ring, which may be apparent to the patient as a large floater.

Zonules: A ring of fibrous strands that connect the ciliary body with the equator of the lens capsule, holding the lens in place.

Appendix

A.1 INTRAOCULAR LENS CALCULATION

- There are many variables that must be taken into account to determine the correct power of the implanted intraocular lens (IOL). These variables are typically measured and calculated before cataract extraction or clear lens exchange (in refractive surgery).

- The first formula to determine appropriate IOL power was developed by S. Federov in 1967. It incorporated the following variables: axial length (L), net corneal power or average keratometry (K), effective lens position (ELP), desired postoperative refraction (Post Rx), and vertex distance (V).

- A common initial formula is the SRK (Sanders, Retzlaff, and Kraft) formula: $P = A - 0.9\,K - 2.5\,L$, where
  - P is the power of the IOL
  - A is a constant determined by the manufacturer of the lens based on its refractive index and refractive power
  - K is the average keratometry
  - L is the axial length

- From the SRK formula, one can determine that the axial length is relatively more important to measure accurately than keratometry since errors in axial length will be magnified by a power of 2.5. The postoperative refraction will be 1 D off target for every 0.4 mm the axial length is miscalculated.

- More complex modern formulas now exist, including the SRK/T, Holladay, Holladay II, Haigis, and Hoffer Q, but they are all variants of the original formula. In practice, the dependent variables are frequently plugged into a computer program that calculates IOL power.
  - Most modern formulas are appropriate for eyes with Ls ranging between 22.0 and 26.0 mm and Ks between 41.00 and 46.00 D.
  - Haigis, Hoffer Q, or Holiday 2 formulas are best for very short eyes.

- Haigis, Hoffer Q, and Holiday 1 or 2 formulas are best for very long eyes.

Dependent Variables to Determine IOL Power Include

- Axial length (L): distance from the anterior cornea to the retinal surface; normal length ~23 mm; original formula must be modified for very short (<20 mm) or long eyes (>26 mm)
  - Axial length is most commonly measured by ultrasound (applanation or immersion) or optical coherence biometry (IOL Master).
  - Compressing the eye during applanation biometry can artificially shorten the eye, making applanation biometry the least reproducible.

- Average keratometry (K): Corneal power measured in diopters. Generally, multiple modalities, such as manual keratometry and videokeratography, are performed to confirm this measurement.

- Effective lens position (ELP): Position of the lens with respect to axial length. This measurement is indirectly calculated by combining keratometry and axial length data. It is the most difficult variable to determine since lens location significantly affects ELP. In most uncomplicated cataract extractions, a posterior chamber IOL is placed in the capsular bag but alternative placements are occasionally necessary. Other potential positions include the ciliary sulcus, pars plana, and anterior chamber. Accordingly, due to the potential variability in ELP, the surgeon should know the appropriate IOL power calculation (P) for various IOL placements in advance. This prevents the need for intraoperative IOL power calculations if complications arise.

- Desired postoperative refraction (Post Rx): This is a relatively patient-driven variable. The patient might opt for low myopia if he or she wants to be independent of reading glasses and has a history of low myopia. Alternatively, the patient may choose emmetropia in order to achieve optimal distance vision. One rule (with caveats) is that the Post Rx should not be more than 3 D different from the nonoperative eye in order to prevent anisometropia. If the patient is having cataract extraction on the contralateral eye in the near future, and may tolerate anisometropia in the short term, or if the patient is willing to wear a contact lens to overcome the anisometropia, then this principle does not apply.

- Vertex distance (V): If preoperative refraction is determined with glasses on, the V must be calculated. V is the distance between the back of the spectacle lens and the front of the cornea. Generally, this distance is 14 mm.

Factors to Consider

- When undergoing bilateral cataract extraction, patients may opt for monovision in which the dominant eye is corrected for distance vision and the nondominant eye is corrected for near vision. Patients should undergo a trial with contact lenses or spectacles (with the desired correction) before proceeding with this surgery as the different refractive powers may be initially disorienting. Some studies have indicated that women are more likely to tolerate monovision than men.

- Multifocal lenses and accommodative lenses exist that allow for both near and distance correction and can reduce spectacle dependence. These premium lenses are generally considered if bilateral cataract extraction is anticipated.

- Previous keratorefractive surgery changes the net corneal power because it alters the contour and thickness of the cornea. In general, traditional keratometry readings on a patient with a history of laser correction of myopia will result in an overestimation of the refractive power of the cornea (artificially high K readings), resulting in an undesirable hyperopic refractive outcome (known as a "hyperopic surprise"). There are further mathematical formulas and/or procedures beyond the scope of this appendix that can be used to adjust for the change in net corneal power after corneal refractive surgery.

Federov's Original Formula (for the Mathematically Inclined)

$$IOL\ Power = (1336/[L - ELP]) - (1336/[1336/\{1000/PostRx\} - V) + K\} - ELP])$$

Further Reading

Text

Rosen ES. Refractive aspects of cataract surgery. In: Yanoff M, Duker J, eds. *Ophthalmology*. 3rd ed. Philadelphia, PA: Mosby; 2009:451–458.

Primary Sources

Federov SN, Galin MA, Linskz A. A calculation of the optical power of the intraocular lens. *Vestn Ophthalmol.* 1967;80(4): 27–31.

Gimbel H, Sun R, Kaye GB. Refractive error after previous refractive surgery. *J Cataract Refract Surg.* 2000;26(1): 142–144.

Retzlaff JA, Sanders DR, Kraff MC. Development of the SRK/T intraocular lens implant power calculation formula. *J Cataract Refract Surg.* 1990;16(3): 333–40.

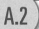

A.2   LASERS IN OPHTHALMOLOGY

- **LASER:** **L**ight **A**mplification by **S**timulated **E**mission of **R**adiation
- Special properties that make it apt for therapeutic/clinical use include:
  - Coherency (does not spread; emitted light or photons are all of equal frequency and phase)
  - Monochromacy (single wavelength)
  - High energy
- Ophthalmic lasers are almost exclusively gas lasers (discussion follows).

GENERAL PRINCIPLES

- There are three types of interactions between photons and atoms:
  - Absorption: A low-energy electron absorbs a photon and jumps to a higher energy orbit. The photon's energy must equal the energy difference between the two electron orbits in order for absorption to occur.

- Spontaneous emission: A high-energy electron spontaneously drops into a lower energy orbit, emitting a photon of energy equal to the difference between the two electron orbits. This is a random process.
- Stimulated emission: A high-energy electron encounters a passing photon (the stimulating photon) and is stimulated to drop into a lower-energy orbit, while releasing a second photon (emitted photon). In order to cause emission, the stimulating photon's energy must equal or exceed the energy difference between the two electron orbits. This nonrandom process yields a lower-energy electron and two photons of equal frequency and phase (coherent).

PRINCIPLES OF GAS LASERS

- A gas (e.g., argon, krypton) is enclosed in a transparent tube with two mirrors (a fully reflecting mirror and a partially reflecting mirror at opposite ends). Surrounding the tube, there is an electrical power source.

- At baseline, there are more electrons in low-energy orbits. A few electrons, however, are in high-energy orbits. These electrons undergo spontaneous emission, producing photons. If these photons encounter low-energy electrons, absorption occurs. If, however, they encounter high-energy electrons, stimulated emission occurs.

- Population inversion is a condition in which several stimulated emissions occur. When engaged, the power source activates electrons to enter higher energy states. This increases the probability that photons will interact with high-energy electrons, resulting in stimulated emission. These photons continue to encounter high-energy electrons setting off a chain reaction production of all coherent photons.

- Photons bounce off the fully reflective mirror and perpetuate the chain reaction by interacting with more high-energy electrons. Some are able to escape through the partially reflective mirror, thus transmitting a coherent stream of photons (the actual laser beam).

LASER WAVELENGTHS

Lasers come in various wavelengths (from the ultraviolet to the infrared spectrum), which can significantly alter their function (discussion follows). Listed are some of the commonly used lasers in clinical ophthalmology and their associated wavelengths.

Ultraviolet Lasers
- Acute renal failure (ArF) excimer ("excited dimer") laser: 193 nm

Visible Light Lasers
- Argon-blue laser: 488 nm
- Argon-green laser: 514 nm
- Tunable dye laser: 570 to 630 nm
- Krypton-red laser: 647 nm

Near-Infrared Laser
- Solid-state diode laser: 488 nm

Infrared Laser
- Neodymium-doped yttrium aluminum garnet (Nd:YAG) laser: 1064 nm

MECHANISM OF ACTION AND CLINICAL USES

Photocoagulation
- Thermal lasers with wavelengths between 488 (argon-blue laser) and 1064 (Nd:YAG laser) nm.
- When light energy is absorbed, it is converted to thermal energy, coagulating and denaturing the exposed tissue.

Applications
- Treatment of retinal tears or holes: Photocoagulation results in adhesions between the choroid and retina. These adhesions or scars function like thumb tacks, attaching the retina to the underlying retinal pigment epithelium. In the context of a retinal tear or hole, such adhesions prevent fluid in the vitreous cavity from entering the subretinal space and dissecting the retina.
- Treatment of neovascularization via peripheral retinal destruction: Panretinal photocoagulation is performed when there is neovascularization in the setting of retinal hypoxia (e.g., proliferative diabetic retinopathy, after central retinal vein occlusion [CRVO]). Neovascularization is promoted by diffusible vasoproliferative

substances (e.g., vascular endothelial growth factor [VEGF]) produced largely by the retina. Photocoagulation destroys much of the retina (the loss of nonessential peripheral retina is well tolerated) and results in decreased levels of these substances, hence less neovascularization.

- Treatment of macular edema: Application of laser to the macula (focal grid laser) is believed to reduce the production of vasoproliferative substances (these substances are not well defined, although VEGF appears to be one them) that promote edema of the macula. This scenario is commonly seen in the setting of diabetic retinopathy (diabetic macular edema). Visual loss as a result of direct photocoagulation of the macula is remarkably minor, since the percentage of nerve tissue destroyed is small and the macula has some redundancy of nerve function.

- Treatment of choroidal neovascularization: Direct destruction of proliferating blood vessels is desirable when blood vessels are growing from the choroid into the subretinal space, as occurs in exudative or "wet" macular degeneration. This procedure has largely been supplanted by injectable anti-VEGF agents into the vitreous.

- Argon laser trabeculoplasty (ALT): Scarring of the trabecular meshwork (where aqueous humor drains out of the anterior chamber) appears to facilitate aqueous drainage.

- Peripheral iridotomy (PI): Application of laser to the iris produces a small hole, enabling aqueous humor to move from the posterior to the anterior chamber in situations where its normal pathway (through the pupil) is blocked.

- Cyclophotocoagulation: Laser is applied to the ciliary body through the sclera in attempts to destroy the ciliary body and reduce aqueous humor production. This procedure is sometimes useful in the treatment of advanced glaucoma after medical and surgical therapies have failed.

Photodisruption

- Infrared (Nd:YAG) laser emits a high-energy pulse over a few nanoseconds.
- This extremely high-power pulse can physically strip electrons from their nuclei (optical breakdown) producing the physical matter state of plasma (approximately 10,000° C).
- The plasma momentarily expands during optical breakdown and immediately collapses afterward, producing an acoustic shock wave that disrupts the tissue targeted. This disruption essentially cuts the tissue focused on, but due to the small plasma size, there is little effect adjacent to the laser impact.

Applications

- YAG capsulotomy: After placement of an intraocular lens, the Nd:YAG laser may be used to treat visually significant posterior capsular opacification. The laser produces many small holes in the capsule, which connect to result in an entire section of posterior capsule falling back into the vitreous, effectively clearing the visual pathway.

- Selective laser trabeculoplasty (SLT): application of laser to pigmented trabecular meshwork appears to facilitate aqueous drainage (see Chapter 5.3 Laser Trabeculoplasty for more details)

- Peripheral iridotomy (PI): use of the Nd:YAG laser to produce a hole in the peripheral iris (see previous)

Photoablation

- The ultraviolet laser breaks the chemical bonds of biologic materials (due to the short wavelength of the laser), converting larger polymers into smaller molecules that essentially vaporize or diffuse away.

- The ArF excimer laser can remove approximately 25 microns of tissue (per pulse) without damaging surrounding tissue.

Applications

- Keratorefractive surgery: The excimer laser is used to reshape the cornea in order to correct refractive error. Laser in-situ keratomileusis (LASIK) and photorefractive keratectomy (PRK) are the most commonly performed keratorefractive procedures.

- Removal of superficial corneal scars: The laser may be used to remove scars no greater than 20% of the corneal thickness. This procedure, however, is infrequently performed largely due to inaccessibility of the laser.

OTHER LASER USES

Photodynamic Therapy

- Therapy includes the use of a special laser-activated dye (verteporfin) to selectively target areas of pathologic neovascularization while minimizing retinal tissue damage.
- The photosensitizing dye has an affinity for low-density lipoprotein (LDL) receptors, which are abundant in neovascular tissue.
- A special laser (wavelength = 689 nm) is applied to the neovascular areas, activating the verteporfin dye and causing coagulation of the vessels.
- *Note:* The laser itself does not cause any damage; its only function is to activate the dye, which in turn destroys whatever tissue it is bound to.
- It is used to treat choroidal neovascularization and several tumors (e.g., choroidal melanomas).

Diagnostic Lasers

- Optical coherence tomography (OCT): Use of special near-infrared laser (wavelength = 810 nm) to produce high-resolution cross-sectional images of the retina. The laser is exceptionally precise, being able to differentiate tissue only 10 microns apart. This technology is now used to aid in the diagnosis of most macular and disc pathologies (i.e., macular edema and glaucoma, respectively).
- Scanning laser ophthalmoscopy (SLO): Use of a narrow laser beam to illuminate the fundus, producing high-resolution, real-time retinal images.

Further Reading

Text

Atebara NH, Thall EH. Principles of lasers. In: Yanoff M, Duker J, eds. *Ophthalmology*. 3rd ed. Philadelphia, PA: Mosby; 2009:41–48.

Whitcher, J, Riordan-Eva P. *Vaughan and Asbury's General Ophthalmology*. New York: Lange Medical Books/McGraw-Hill; 2004.

Primary Sources

The Glaucoma Laser Trial Research Group. The glaucoma laser trial (GLT) and glaucoma laser trial follow-up study: results. The Glaucoma Laser Trial Report number 7. *Am J Ophthalmol.* 1995; 120:718.

LOCAL ANESTHESIA IN OPHTHALMOLOGY

A.3

- Most commonly achieved using topical medication or injections, including sub-Tenon's, peribulbar, and retrobulbar blocks.
- Typically combined with monitored anesthesia care (MAC), in which a sedative and systemic analgesic (e.g., midazolam and fentanyl) are given to achieve amnesia and minimize anxiety.
- May require general anesthesia for patients who are unable to comfortably remain still throughout surgery or in whom topical or periocular medication is contraindicated (e.g., open globes).

GENERAL PRINCIPLES

- Topical anesthesia:
  - Topical ocular medication, either drops or gels, provide corneal and a small degree of conjunctival anesthesia by blocking the lacrimal, nasociliary, and short and long ciliary nerves.
  - Globe movement is not altered because the anesthetic does not penetrate deeply enough to affect the nerves supplying the extraocular muscles.
  - Commonly used agents include 2% or 4% lidocaine, 0.5% to 0.75% bupivacaine, 0.4% benoxinate, 0.5% tetracaine, 0.5% amethocaine, and 0.5% proparacaine.
  - Anesthesia may be combined with intracameral preservative-free lidocaine to reduce sensitivity of intraocular structures such as the iris.
- Regional anesthesia (retrobulbar, peribulbar, and sub-Tenon's):
  - Like topical anesthetics, these injections block the ciliary nerves, providing corneal and conjunctival anesthesia.

- Successful regional anesthesia should also provide akinesia (globe immobility) by blocking the cranial nerves that supply the rectus and oblique muscles (CN III, IV, and VI). The sub-Tenon's block is the exception; it does not afford true akinesia and requires use of a traction suture to ensure globe immobility.
- Commonly used agents include a 50:50 mixture of 2% lidocaine with or without epinephrine and 0.5% to 0.75% bupivacaine. Hyaluronidase, which breaks down connective tissue facilitating diffusion of the periocular medication, may be added to the block to facilitate the diffusion of anesthetic.
- The addition of epinephrine to the anesthetic constricts blood vessels, prolonging anesthesia by reducing clearance of the anesthetic agent, and reducing local bleeding.
  - *Note:* Some surgeons avoid epinephrine in periocular injections out of a concern that epinephrine's constriction of blood flow could cause an ischemic optic neuropathy.

TECHNIQUES OF ORBITAL BLOCKS

Retrobulbar Block

A 25- to 27-gauge 1.5 inch blunt tipped needle is used to inject anesthetic into the posterior intraconal space (the soft tissue within the "cone" formed by the extraocular muscles).

Typically, the anesthesiologist will administer a larger dose of systemic anesthetic (e.g., Propofol) prior to the placement of a retrobulbar block. The surgeon should communicate with the anesthesiologist regarding the appropriate level of sedation for a patient prior to initiating the block.

An operating room (OR) assistant or anesthesiologist can help to stabilize the patient's head during administration of the block.

- Insertion site: With the globe in primary gaze, the surgeon's finger palpates and verifies the space between the globe and the inferior orbital rim. The needle with bevel toward the eye penetrates the skin of the inferolateral orbit just above the inferior orbital rim and halfway between the lateral canthus and lateral limbus.
- Needle advancement: The needle is directed parallel to the orbital floor until the tip reaches the equator of the globe (~15 mm of needle advancement based on normal axial length), typically a "first pop" is felt as the needle passes through the anterior orbital septum. The needle is then aimed medially and superiorly, toward the orbit apex, in order to penetrate the intraconal space, where typically a "second pop" is felt as the muscle cone is penetrated. The needle should not be permitted to cross the midsagittal plane of the eye as this increases the risk of optic nerve penetration. Total needle advancement is ~25 to 35 mm based on the size of the orbit. In most patients, the needle is too short to reach and penetrate the optic nerve.
- Injection: Aspiration is first performed to confirm that the needle tip is not intravascular or subdural. Anesthetic (3 to 7 ml) is then slowly injected.

Peribulbar Block

A 25- to 27-gauge three-fourths to 1-inch needle is used to inject anesthetic into the orbital soft tissue surrounding the extraocular muscle cone. Anesthesia is obtained after diffusion of the anesthetic agent throughout the orbital soft tissue. This reduces the risk of optic nerve damage, but requires a greater volume of anesthetic.

- Insertion site: Generally, two injections are performed. This is because a single extraconal injection may not satisfactorily paralyze the superior oblique in addition to the other extraocular muscles. The first (inferotemporal) needle insertion site is identical to that used for a retrobulbar injection. The second (medial) insertion site is between the medial canthus and the caruncle.
- Needle advancement: The first needle is advanced posteriorly, parallel to the orbital floor for a distance of ~25 mm (corresponding to the distal point of an average globe). The second needle is advanced posteriorly, parallel to the medial orbital wall, to a depth of ~15 mm.
- Injection: For both injections, aspiration is first performed to confirm that the needle tip is not intravascular or subdural. Anesthetic (3 to 7 ml) is slowly injected inferolaterally and another 5 ml of the same anesthetic is placed medially.

- Pressure lowering: A Honan balloon or alternate pressure-lowering device is placed for approximately 10 to 20 minutes prior to initiating the surgical procedure. In addition to lowering intraocular pressure (IOP) by vitreous compression and dehydration, a compression device can facilitate appropriate diffusion of the anesthetic.

Sub-Tenon's Block

A special curved needle or cannula is used to inject anesthetic just deep to Tenon's capsule. Unlike other blocks, a sub-Tenon's block requires conjunctival dissection and pretreatment with a topical anesthetic.

- Approach to Tenon's capsule: After adequate topical anesthesia is given, a traction suture may be placed in order to immobilize the globe. The conjunctiva and underlying Tenon's capsule are then dissected with fine scissors in the infranasal quadrant, approximately 3 to 5 mm from the limbus. The site of dissection may be in any quadrant, but the infranasal location is commonly used to avoid damage to the vortex veins.
- Cannula advancement: The cannula (or curved needle) is then placed through the incision site into sub-Tenon's space. The curvature of the cannula (flat profile with curvature resembling the letter "D") allows appropriate advancement just posterior to Tenon's capsule. Resistance through sub-Tenon's space is overcome with infusion of anesthetic, allowing for blunt dissection in the potential space. Full cannula insertion is achieved when the tip is just past the equator of the globe. Note: This is an approximate distance assuming normal axial length.
- Injection: Once again, slow injection of anesthetic while the cannula is advanced provides adequate dissection through the potential space. A total volume of 3 to 5 ml is injected.
- Local subconjunctival/sub-Tenon's may be utilized with a blunt cannula or small gauge needle to augment topical anesthesia for conjunctival surgery (trabeculectomy/glaucoma drainage tubes).

Partial Facial Nerve Block (Van Lindt Block/ Modified Van Lindt Block)

A subcutaneous anesthetic injection may be given around the lateral orbit rim, just temporal to the lateral canthal angle. The purpose of the injection is to temporarily weaken or paralyze the orbicularis oris muscle to reduce lid squeezing or closure during surgery.

ADVANTAGES/DISADVANTAGES

Topical Anesthesia
Advantages
- It is easy to administer and has rapid onset.
- It achieves adequate corneal and moderate conjunctival anesthesia for anterior segment surgery with virtually no risk of extraocular damage from the anesthetic administration such as retrobulbar hemorrhage, ruptured globe, diplopia, or ptosis.
- Patients maintain a normal ability to blink and more rapid, same-day visual recovery. Patients can be discharged without a patch.

Disadvantages
- Patients are more aware of some surgical sensations such as pressure changes or shifts of the lens–iris diaphragm.
- Significant conjunctival and intraocular manipulation can be painful.
- No akinesia is achieved.
- It does not eliminate photophobia.
- Some patients require more systemic anesthesia to offset ocular motion or to improve overall comfort.
- It alters tear film properties. It also may be toxic to the epithelium (delays wound healing if epithelial defect is present) or endothelium.

Retrobulbar Block
Advantages
- It achieves relatively rapid onset anesthesia and akinesia (~4 to 5 minutes).
- It is a more complete anesthesia for manipulation of ocular structures such as conjunctiva, sclera, and iris.
- It decreases or eliminates sensitivity to bright light of operating microscope.
- It produces less chemosis compared to peribulbar blocks, because less anesthetic is injected and it is confined to the intraconal space.

Disadvantages
- Most patients require more significant systemic anesthesia during the administration of

the block. If the primary surgeon is administering the block, the additional effort and time to instill a block may slow down turnover between cases.

- It has higher levels of pain and anxiety upon administration of periocular anesthesia compared with topical anesthesia (when penetrating the skin, orbital septum, and/or contact with the periosteum).

- It may create a temporary increase in IOP due to increase of orbital volume, but no adjunctive treatment is generally required. A Honan balloon or alternative pressure-lowering device may be necessary to decrease intraocular pressure.

- It typically requires postoperative patching due to decreased blink reflex. Many patients temporarily lose light perception if the anesthetic agent(s) affects the optic nerve.

- Rare but severe complications (1% to 3% risk for each) include retrobulbar hemorrhage, optic nerve injury, retinal artery/vein occlusion, globe perforation, oculocardiac reflex, ocular muscle injury, prolonged ptosis, and central nervous system depression.

Peribulbar Block

Advantages

- It achieves adequate anesthesia and akinesia with a theoretically lower risk of complications compared to retrobulbar block (most comparative series do not show a difference between complication rates).

- It is similar to retrobulbar block for more complete anesthesia compared to topical anesthesia for manipulation of ocular structures such as conjunctiva, sclera, and iris.

- It decreases or eliminates sensitivity to the bright light of the operating microscope.

Disadvantages

- It often requires more significant systemic anesthesia during the administration of the block. If the primary surgeon is administering the block, the additional effort to instill a block may slow down turnover between cases.

- It may include higher levels of pain and anxiety upon administration of anesthesia (when penetrating the skin, orbital septum, and/or nicking the periosteum).

- There is a longer period of time before adequate akinesia is achieved (~30 minutes).

- It requires a higher volume of anesthesia compared to retrobulbar block. This may result in an increase in IOP and typically requires a Honan balloon application or ocular compression before proceeding with anterior segment surgery.

- Chemosis commonly occurs and may complicate the surgical approach.

- Possible complications are the same as retrobulbar block and includes retrobulbar hemorrhage, optic nerve injury, retinal artery/vein occlusion, globe perforation, oculocardiac reflex, ocular muscle injury, prolonged ptosis, and central nervous system depression.

Sub-Tenon's Block

Advantages

- It achieves adequate anesthesia with a lower risk of the serious complications seen in retrobulbar/peribulbar blocks.

- The block only lasts 60 minutes (good for short procedures).

- It involves a small volume of fluid with no increase in IOP.

- Patient can voluntarily move eyes. Alternatively, if akinesia is desired, a traction suture may be placed to prevent globe movement.

- Use of epinephrine with anesthetic agent can improve hemostasis.

Disadvantages

- Conjunctival dissection may be necessary; if the conjunctiva is perforated while advancing the needle, the anesthetic will leak, decreasing the efficacy of the block. Furthermore, if the cannula does not form a seal around the incision site, the anesthetic may not adequately dissect through sub-Tenon's space (due to retrograde leakage through the incision site).

- It may result in local chemosis.

- There is a possible increased risk of infection due to dissection of tissue surrounding the insertion site of the needle.

Further Reading

Text

Greenhalgh, DL. Anesthesia for cataract surgery. In: Yanoff M, Duker J, eds. *Ophthalmology. 3rd* ed. Philadelphia, PA: Mosby; 2009:441–446.

McGoldrick KE. *Anesthesia for Ophthalmic and Otolaryngologic Surgery*. Philadelphia, PA: WB Saunders; 1992.

Mostafa SM. *Anaesthesia for Ophthalmic Surgery*. Oxford, United Kingdom: Oxford University Press; 1991.

Whitcher, J, Riordan Eva P. *Vaughan and Asbury's General Ophthalmology*. New York: Lange Medical Books/McGraw-Hill; 2004.

Primary Sources

Katsev DA, Drews RC, Rose BT. An anatomic study of retrobulbar needle path length. *Ophthalmology*. 1989; 96:1221.

Sullivan KL, Brown GC, Forman AR, et al. Retrobulbar anesthesia and retinal vascular obstruction. *Ophthalmology*. 1983;90:373.

A.4 PHACOEMULSIFICATION PRINCIPLES AND TECHNIQUES

- A phacoemulsification handpiece consists of a surgical probe containing a transducer (converts electrical energy to mechanical vibratory energy) to disassemble the lens, an irrigation component to maintain anterior chamber stability and regulate thermodynamics, and an aspiration component to remove the lens fragments.

- When combined with foldable intraocular lenses, phacoemulsification permits cataract extraction through an incision as small as 1.8 mm for Food and Drug Administration (FDA) approved lenses in the United States.

GENERAL PRINCIPLES

- Phaco handpiece: A combination of mechanisms is thought to contribute to breakup of the cataract nucleus.
  - Mechanical vibratory energy: The phaco tip vibrates at approximately 44 kHz (44,000 times/second). These vibrations are transmitted to a titanium tip, producing a jack-hammer effect, effectively fragmenting the nucleus.
  - Sound waves: The tip vibrations also produce acoustic shock waves, which are sufficiently strong to emulsify the nucleus.

- Irrigation/aspiration: Balanced saline solution (BSS) flows from the phaco tip to maintain an expanded anterior chamber. Stable chamber depth maximizes the room for surgical maneuvers, reducing the likelihood of complications (e.g., capsular tear). In order to prevent anterior chamber collapse, irrigation must at least equal aspiration plus incisional outflow (leakage through the incision site).

- Vacuum: When the aspiration port is blocked, a vacuum is created that holds the nucleus against the phaco tip, permitting direct mechanical fragmentation. After the nucleus has been broken into sufficiently small pieces, it is aspirated into a collection reservoir. The more completely the aspiration port is occluded, the larger the vacuum that is created. This has important implications for various methods for nuclear disassembly (described under Basic Phacoemulsification Principles).

- Irrigation, aspiration, and phaco power are all controlled by the surgeon via a foot pedal. There are three levels of engagement based on depth of pedal depression (1 = minimal foot depression, 3 = pedal fully depressed):
  - Foot placement 1: Irrigation
  - Foot placement 2: Irrigation and aspiration
  - Foot placement 3: Irrigation, aspiration, and phaco power

PHACODYNAMICS AND PHACOEMULSIFICATION SETTINGS

- Phacodynamics refers to the complex relationship between variables that affect intraocular pressure, fluid flow, phacoemulsification power, aspiration, and vacuum. Modification of various parameters can result in different intraoperative experiences and facilitate (or complicate) each surgical step and various intraoperative techniques.

- Bottle height refers to the height in centimeters of the irrigation bottle above the eye, and affects the hydrostatic pressure inside the eye. Elevating bottle height can increase anterior chamber depth and stability, but may stress zonules or push fluid into a posterior capsule tear.

TABLE A.4.1				
Step	**Bottle Height**	**Power**	**Aspiration**	**Vacuum**
Sculpting	90 cm	70%	25 ml/min	80 mm Hg
Quadrant removal	110 cm	70%	35 ml/min	350 mm Hg
Chopping	*120 cm*	*70%*	*40 ml/min*	*400 mm Hg*
Cortex removal	110 cm	0%	35 ml/min	400 mm Hg
Viscoelastic removal	120 cm	0%	40 ml/min	500 mm Hg

- Phacoemulsification power is titrated to achieve safe and efficient clearance of lenticular material at the phaco probe without causing damage to intraocular structure such as the corneal endothelium or lens capsule. Soft cataracts need little, if any, ultrasonic power to clear the phaco tip; dense cataracts may require a few minutes of 100% ultrasonic power. Phacoemulsification was traditionally performed with continuous linear movements of the phacoemulsification tip. Also, as the foot pedal was depressed in position 3, higher levels of power were achieved. Some strategies have been developed to reduce overall phacoemulsification power, including:
  - Torsional phaco: Side-to-side motion of the phaco tip decreases repulsion of lenticular material improving followability of the material and efficiency of lens removal.
  - Burst mode: Fixed levels of phaco power are dispersed in small increments in a pattern (e.g., on-off-on-off). As the foot pedal is depressed through position 3, the time in the "off" position decreases.
  - Pulse mode: As with burst mode, there is cycling between phaco energy delivered in an on-off-on-off pattern, but the time between each cycle is fixed. As the foot pedal is depressed through position 3, the amount of power in the "on" phase is increased.
- Aspiration refers to the rate of flow of BSS within the eye. Higher rates of aspiration allow for faster clearance of material from the eye, but increase the speed at which materials (wanted: lens, and unwanted: capsule or iris) move to the phaco tip.
- A vacuum occurs only when the phaco tip is occluded. Increasing a vacuum improves the ability of the phaco tip to purchase and hold lenticular material. A vacuum is particularly important during maneuvers that involve holding lenticular material, such as during chopping. When a piece of the lens, held at the phaco tip

under high vacuum, is rapidly cleared, a post-occlusion surge can drive fluid out of the eye and result in a momentary loss of anterior chamber pressure. During this surge and chamber collapse, intraocular structures such as the corneal endothelium or lens capsule can be damaged.

- For common phacoemulsification settings for a 2+ NS cataract, SEE TABLE A.4.1

NOTE: *In the setting of floppy iris syndrome or zonular weakness, it is useful to reduce some parameters, such as decreasing bottle height, aspiration, and vacuum.*

BASIC PHACOEMULSIFICATION PRINCIPLES

- Sculpting: The phaco tip is used to shave the nucleus with moderate flow and low vacuum (the tip is generally not completely occluded).
  - This allows for nuclear disassembly within the capsular bag with minimal risk of sucking the capsule into the tip and damaging it.
- Nucleus consumption: The phaco tip is used to disassemble and aspirate the nucleus under high-flow/high-vacuum conditions. The tip is angled so that it is almost completely occluded during this technique.
  - Allows for rapid emulsification and removal of the nucleus.
  - Must be performed away from the capsule to prevent inadvertent aspiration and tearing of the capsule.

REPRESENTATIVE TECHNIQUES

Multiple techniques have been devised to fragment and remove the lens based on the principles of sculpting and nucleus consumption. Most techniques, however, involve a combination of these principles in order to completely fragment the lens. Two representative techniques are described.

- Divide and conquer:
  - After hydrodissection, a horizontal groove is shaved in the anterior lens surface. The groove is extended away from the limbal incision and under the capsulorrhexis margin. During this process, the phaco tip is generally angled to avoid complete occlusion. This permits peripheral phacoemulsification near the capsule.
  - The nucleus is then rotated and the central groove is extended on the opposite end. This groove is deepened until the red reflex becomes more visible. A second groove is typically created 90° from the first, resulting in a "Maltese Cross." A thin rim of nucleus remains between the quadrants of the nucleus at the floor of the grooves. The nucleus can be cracked using the phaco probe and a second instrument moving away from each other against the walls of the groove. Alternatively, a single nucleus-cracking instrument may be used. This instrument has opposing, scissor-like arms that result in similar forces acting against the groove walls.
  - The quadrants of the lens are purchased under high vacuum, lifted anteriorly out of the capsular bag, emulsified, and aspirated from the eye. Each section is typically brought centrally, away from the capsule, before emulsification and aspiration.
- Horizontal phaco chop:
  - After hydrodissection and hydrodelineation, the phaco tip is embedded into the center of the nucleus. In this orientation, the quadrant will occlude the tip, creating high-vacuum conditions. A fine curved hook called a "nucleus chopper" is then placed at the equator of the nucleus. The chopper is pushed toward the stationary phaco tip, which cleaves the intervening nuclear material. This step is repeated several times to segment the nucleus into small fragments.
  - Each nuclear segment is brought centrally, away from the capsule, and subsequently emulsified and aspirated from the eye.

OTHER PHACOEMULSIFICATION TECHNIQUES

- These techniques are beyond the scope of this text but are briefly described to provide a further

understanding of lens phacoemulsification methods:

- Chip and flip: similar to phaco chop requiring separation of the endonucleus from the epinucleus via hydrodelineation. The procedure involves sculpting a central crater in the middle of the nucleus followed by removal of the rim under high vacuum. The final "chip" (thinned nuclear plate with no rim) is "flipped" into the anterior chamber and can then be emulsified and aspirated after bringing it centrally away from the capsule. The epinucleus is removed last.
- Vertical phaco chop: The phaco tip is buried into the nucleus and a sharp, hook-like second instrument is driven down into the nucleus while the phaco tip and nucleus is held anteriorly. The opposing movements create a cleavage line between the two pieces. This step is repeated several times to separate the nucleus into multiple fragments.
- Stop and chop: The nucleus is divided into two halves via the divide-and-conquer sculpting and separating method. The remaining halves are then horizontally chopped.
- Bimanual phacoemulsification: Irrigation is separated from the aspirating/ultrasonic handpiece, resulting in two instruments that can each fit through a 1.2-mm incision. The nucleus can then be disassembled by various techniques.

Further Reading

Text

Allen D. Phacoemulsification. In: Yanoff M, Duker J, eds. *Ophthalmology*. 3rd ed. Philadelphia, PA: Mosby; 2009: 447–450.

Maloney WF, Grindle L. *Textbook of Phacoemulsification*. Fallbrook, CA: Lasendra Publishers; 1988.

Seibel, BS. *Phacodynamics: Mastering the Tools and Techniques of Phacoemulsification Surgery*. 4th ed. Thorafore, NJ: Slack Inc.; 2005.

Primary Sources

Anis A. Understanding hydrodelineation: The term and related procedures. *Ocular Surgical News*. 1991;9: 134–137.

Fine IH. The chip and flip phacoemulsification technique. *J Cataract Refract Surg*. 1991;17(3):366–371.

Gimbel HV. Divide and conquer nucleofractis phacoemulsification: Development and variations. *J Cataract Refract Surg*. 1991;17(3):281–291.

Index

Page numbers followed by *t* or *f* indicate tables or figures, respectively.